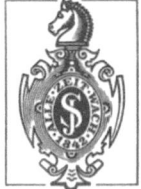

Neurosecretion — The Final Neuroendocrine Pathway

VI International Symposium on Neurosecretion,
London 1973

Edited by
Francis Knowles and Lutz Vollrath

With 92 Figures

Springer-Verlag Berlin Heidelberg GmbH 1974

Sir Francis Knowles F.R.S.†, Professor of Anatomy, King's College, Strand, London WC2R 2LS, Great Britain

Lutz Vollrath, Professor of Anatomy, King's College, Strand, London WC2R 2LS, Great Britain. Present address: Anatomisches Institut der Johannes-Gutenberg-Universität, D-6500 Mainz, Saarstr. 19—21/Federal Republic of Germany

Library of Congress Cataloging in Publication Data

Neurosecretion — the final neuroendocrine pathway.
International Symposium on Neurosecretion, 6th, London, 1973.

1. Neurosecretion-Congresses. 2. Neuroendocrinology-Congresses. I. Knowles, Sir Francis Gerald William, bart., 1915—   ed. II. Vollrath, Lutz, 1936—   . III. Title. [DNLM: 1. Neurosecretion-Congresses. W3IN92Q 1973n/WL312 I61 1973n]   QP356.4.I59   1973   591.1'88   74-13218

ISBN 978-3-662-12589-2   ISBN 978-3-662-12587-8 (eBook)
DOI 10.1007/978-3-662-12587-8

Preface

This volume marks the end of twenty years of neurosecretion during which there were five symposia, namely Naples (1953), Lund (1957), Bristol (1961), Strasbourg (1966), and Kiel (1970). In comparison with these symposia an exceptionally large number of papers were read at this the sixth symposium, in London, and for economic reasons it has not been possible to publish all the papers *in extenso*. The editors have therefore been obliged to undertake the unenviable work of selection, a task made all the more difficult by the excellence and importance of contributions of the symposium. We felt that it was of the utmost importance at this moment in the history of neurosecretion to present as complete a picture as possible of the present state of the subject in relation to the past and opportunities for the future. We have therefore given some preference to papers with a strong review element, research papers in areas of current importance and contributions which deal with recently developed techniques with promise for the future. We have moreover attempted to strike some balance between the different areas of research on neurosecretion so that the volume as a whole may be of interest to the general reader, and that he will find in it a reasonably coherent pattern of thought which demonstrates neurosecretion as the final neuroendocrine pathway.

We have attempted a certain degree of uniformity of spelling, symbols, etc. but in cases where there is some difference of opinion, as in spelling which differs on both sides of the Atlantic or in a word such as "neuron/neurone" which seems to have no geographical boundaries we have not attempted any value judgements but have left the spelling as it was intended by the authors.

Finally we should like to acknowledge our gratitude to the authors who met our demands in the preparation of manuscripts and especially to those who responded so splendidly to the request that they should not write in their mother tongue but, instead, in English so that the volume could have complete uniformity of language. A special mention should also be made of those who presented results of great importance in the symposium yet are represented in this volume by abstracts only. They knew, and we knew, that their work should be presented in a longer form yet they accepted without complaint the need for selection so that the many areas of research in neurosecretion could each be adequately represented.

Acknowledgements: The members of the VI International Symposium on Neurosecretion are all indebted to the following for financial support of our symposium: Ciba-Geigy (U. K.) Ltd; Hoechst Pharmaceuticals; Imperial Chemical Industries Ltd; Organon International B. V. Some members of the symposium were given financial aid by British Council.

The success of the symposium was in no small measure due to the enthusiasm and efforts of Miss Wendy Charnell and Miss Jeannie Paterson, who did the essential secretarial and art work. The organisers of the symposium are deeply indebted to these and the many other helpers for their assistance.

London, Summer 1974

FRANCIS KNOWLES
LUTZ VOLLRATH

It is with deep regret that owing to his sudden and unexpected death on July 13th, 1974, Sir Francis Knowles is unable to see the completion and publication of this present volume. Especially so because he found great pleasure and satisfaction in both the organising of the VI International Symposium on Neurosecretion, into which he put so much effort, and in editing the present Proceedings of this conference. Sir Francis' review, published as the Introduction to the present volume, of twenty years of neurosecretion in which he played such an important role reflects very clearly that neurosecretion has lost both a great pioneer and an aristocratic ambassador. He was one of the few who attended all six Symposia on Neurosecretion held so far and he will be greatly missed by all.

LUTZ VOLLRATH

Contents

c) Electrophysiology

B. Hypophysiotropic Neurosecretion

III. Aminergic Mechanisms in Neuroendocrine Control

IV. Summaries

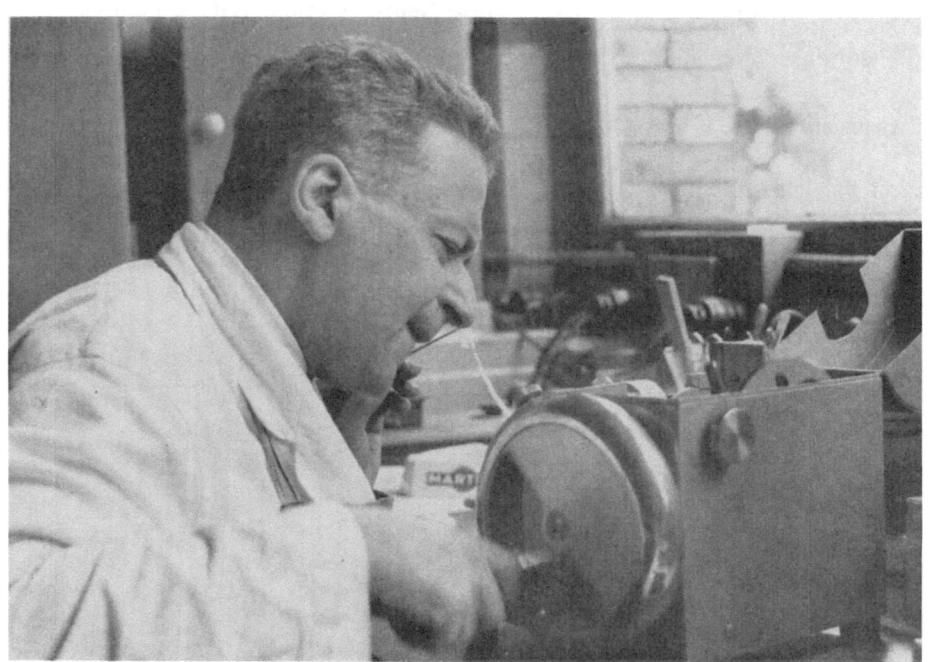

Dr. Manfred Gabe 1916—1973

The sad news of the death of Dr. Manfred Gabe came during the Symposium and his friends thought that it would be appropriate that this volume should be dedicated to his memory, in recognition of his place among the pioneers of neuro-secretion.

Dr. M. Gabe, of Rumanian origin, was born in Vienna, Austria on the 28th January 1916. After early studies in Rumania he came to Paris and there studied simultaneously Natural Sciences at the Sorbonne and at the Institute Pasteur and the Faculty of Medicine. After he qualified he became Médecin-externe at The Hôpital de la Pitié until, in November 1942, he was arrested and in February 1943 he was deported to the concentration camp of Golleschau, an annexe of Auschwitz. There for 32 months he cared for the prisoners working in the quarries.

After the war he returned to France and resumed his scientific studies as a director of research at the C.R.N.S.

Dr. Gabe was a man of prodigious energy and skill whose 356 publications included many substantial works, such as the following: —

Histochimie des polysaccharides chez les Invertébrés. Gustav Fischer Verlag, Stuttgart. *Hdb. der Histochemie*, 1962, *2* (1), 95–393, 133 fig.

Neurosecretion. Pergamon, Oxford, 1966, pp. 872, 586 fig.

Neurosécrétion. Gauthier-Villars, Paris, 1967, pp. 1091, 586 fig.

Techniques histologiques. Masson, Paris, 1968, pp. 1113.

Polysaccharides in lower Vertebrates. Hdb. der Histochemie, Gustav Fischer, Stuttgart, 1971, *2* (3), 1–543, 203 fig.

In the field of neurosecretion he will probably be best remembered for his detailed studies on the sinus gland and other invertebrate neurohaemal organs, his histochemical studies on vertebrate neurosecretion and for his discovery of the moulting-gland of crustaceans (named by him the Y organ), as also for his massive reviews of neurosecretion illustrated by his superb histological preparations. In his book Neurosecretion (1966) he wrote, "The charitable silence which one may be tempted to observe when writing an original work would be entirely misplaced in critical surveys, when the aim is to arrive at a true picture". This remark was characteristic of the man, a dedicated pursuer of truth and perfection, who could be merciless in scientific combat yet exquisitely polite and helpful in personal contacts with other research workers. Currently eighty of Dr. Gabe's colleagues and friends are preparing a memorial volume to be entitled "Recherches bio-logiques contemporaines" to be published in the near future.

In reply to a letter begging him to attend our symposium he wrote, "I have a horror of voyages — I have travelled too much in my youth — but the principal reason for my refusal is that I feel too old and much too tired". We must all feel a sadness that he was not able to make one more voyage to attend our meetings so that we could all have met hime once more and he could have seen the development of the concept he did so much to pioneer. His death was untimely and he will be sadly missed.

SIR FRANCIS KNOWLES

I. Introduction

Twenty Years of Neurosecretion

FRANCIS KNOWLES

Department of Anatomy, King's College, London (Great Britain)

"We have just heard some very interesting things, — and also a great deal of nonsense"!

Those were words that were addressed to Ernst Scharrer, in this city, twenty years ago, when he presented the concept of neurosecretion at a meeting at the Ciba Foundation. They epitomised a not uncommon reaction to the revolutionary idea that a part of the nervous system might have an endocrine function.

Today the words neurosecretion and neurohaemal organs are commonplace in our scientific vocabulary and it is quite difficult to communicate to you the atmosphere — the excitement — of that first conference at Naples in 1953 when this distinct new function of the nervous system crystallized before us. Those have been called the heroic days of neurosecretion and I think it is an appropriate phrase for the founders then encountered a wide spectrum of opposition, ranging from polite doubt to disbelief. Some of us have been privileged to attend the birth of the concept, and then watch its gradual progression — an unfolding of the design.

Before we look at the first symposium at Naples it may be well first to glance at some of the events that led to it. This audience will be familiar with the first report by Speidel in 1919 of what seemed to be glandular cells in the spinal cord of fishes and the startling proposal by Ernst Scharrer in 1928 that the hormones of the posterior pituitary might be made in certain hypothalamic nuclei, a theme pursued by Ernst Scharrer in the 30's in the face of strong opposition. Less generally known is the importance of studies on the invertebrates in those early days. As early as 1917 Kopêc had demonstrated that in Lepidoptera the brain was the source of a secretion necessary to induce pupation. During the 30's and 40's the precise and painstaking experiments of Wigglesworth, Williams, the Thomsens and others combined with the morphological studies by Hanström laid firm foundations for the concept of neurosecretion among the invertebrates.

In the early 30's Frank Brown suggested that in crustaceans the nerve cord might be, in addition to the eyestalk, a source of hormones controlling the chromatophores and my good friend Kleinholz suggested to me a critical experiment to disprove this heretical idea. I carried out this experiment — but obtained evidence strongly supporting Brown. That was my first publication and I must say that I have been a convert to neurosecretion ever since!

I have spoken of early workers on invertebrate neurosecretion but I have reserved at the end a very special place for Berta Scharrer and the great contributions she made to insect physiology and the neurosecretion concept. It must be very rare, if not unique in the history of science, to find such a husband and wife team with interests so perfectly complementary for the formulation of a new concept. Ernst on the vertebrates — Berta on the invertebrates — how excited they must have been as they found new correlations in their studies and saw correlations in the work of others substantiating the universality of their neurosecretion concept. The late 1940's were significant for neurosecretion for then the Scharrers published an important review, Harris and Green enunciated their releasing factor theory and in 1947 a conference on arthropod endocrinology was held in Paris, at which many papers dealt with neurosecretion.

From Hanström and Cazal we heard the confirmation and extension of the discovery by Berta Scharrer a few years before that nerves from the pars intercerebralis of the insect brain contained secretory material. From Carrol Williams we heard that experiments had shown that the pars intercerebralis cells of the insect brain produce a substance which triggers the release of a prothoracic gland hormone essential for development. Clearly neurosecretion could be a vital link between the nervous and the endocrine systems. It was not long before Berta Scharrer showed by lesion experiments in insects that neurosecretory material passed from the brain along the pericardial nerves, thus demonstrating in an invertebrate a passage of neurosecretory material along a nerve, as had been postulated by Ernst Scharrer but not yet demonstrated in vertebrates.

The situation was soon to be transformed by the publication in 1949 of Bargmann's inspired discovery that the Gomori Chrome-alum-haematoxylin stain clearly differentiated the hypothalamic neurosecretory system in the mammalian brain and made possible the detection of neurosecretory material along the course of axons. Soon this method was to be used by many investigators and particularly in Bargmann's school where the names of Hild, Eichner, Kratzsch, Ortmann, Rodeck, Zetler, Schiebler, Knoop and Thiel will be remembered for their contributions. Soon the evidence for vertebrate neurosecretion became overwhelming and in the spring of 1951 Bargmann suggested to Ernst and Berta Scharrer that the time had come to bring together investigators in the field and lay firm foundations for the concept of neurosecretion. Accordingly we met in Naples.

Naples 1953. At the Naples conference the concept of neurosecretion in vertebrates was dominated by the "classical" neurosecretory pathway, namely the hypothalamo-neurohypophysial system. Yet coming events are said to cast their shadows before them and it is interesting to see how some further developments in neurosecretion were adumbrated at that first symposium. Benoit and Assenmacher for example described fine droplets of gomori staining material in the external zone of the median eminence of birds. Hanström drew attention to a probable neurosecretory activity of the nuclei tuberis, the nerve fibres of which constitute the external layer of the median eminence and do not form part of the classical neurosecretory pathway.

There was therefore already then some morphological support for the Harris-Green postulate. On the other hand the experimental evidence for neurosecretory control of the pituitary was confusing. From Birmingham Sir Solly Zuckerman brought news of ferrets which succeeded in maintaining normal sexual cycles though it was claimed that the portal vessels from the hypothalamus to the pituitary had been effectively interrupted but Benoit and Assenmacher reported contradictory results in comparable experiments on ducks, and there was therefore at that time an aura of uncertainty over the status of neurosecretion in pituitary pars distalis control.

The evidence for a neurosecretory control of endocrine function in insects was far more convincing. The results which had been reported in Paris some years previously were greatly extended by the Thomsens, De Lerma, Bounhiol, Arvy,

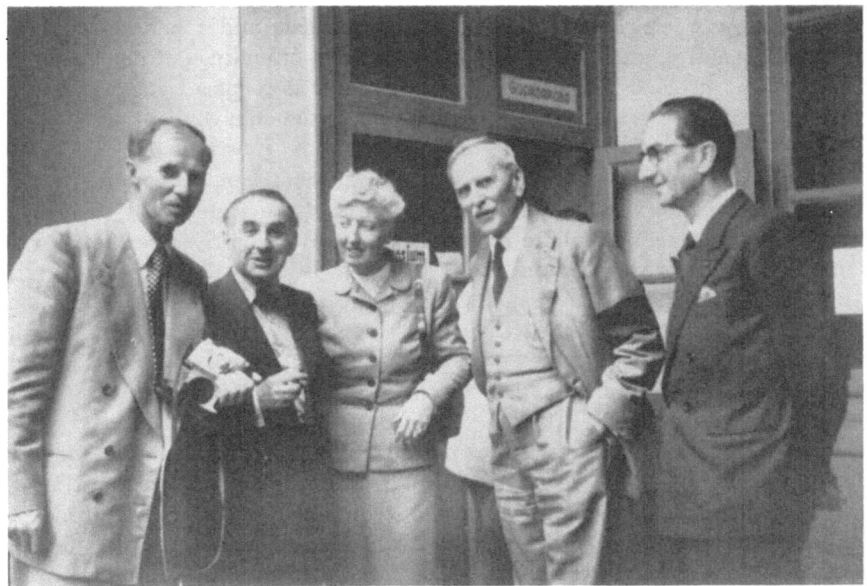

Fig. 1. Naples, 1953; at the Stazione Zoologica [Left to Right: E. Scharrer, W. Bargmann, B. Scharrer, R. Dohrn (Director of the Stazione Zoologica), J. Benoit]

Gabe, Possompès, Grandori and others, all of whom demonstrated clearly the morphology of that neurosecretory system which passes from the pars inter-cerebralis to the corpora cardiaca-allata complex. Neurosecretory systems in crustaceans also were described in detail by Enami, Passano and others.

It is noteworthy that approximately 60% of the papers at that first neuro-secretion symposium dealt with invertebrates. Also that the emphasis was on the morphological characteristics of the neurosecretory cell. One carried away a conviction that early in evolution a special kind of nerve cell had appeared which showed features characteristic of gland cells such as the elaboration and discharge of colloid droplets in addition to the general features of neurones. These special cells were organized into distinct groups and furthermore the apparent uni-versality of the Gomori stain to pick out neurosecretory systems in vertebrates and invertebrates further supported the view that neurosecretion could be recognised as a clearly definable sub-function of the nervous system.

At the same time Ernst Scharrer emphasised that neither the Gomori nor the equally effective aldehyde fuchsin stains were cytochemical in value and pointed out that the terms Gomori substance, Gomori positive and Gomori negative, were not to be recommended. These very wise remarks were unfortunately not heeded by later workers, many of whom used these staining methods alone as criteria for neurosecretory activity.

To some of us at Naples it seemed that not only the morphological features of neurosecretory cells were significant criteria for identification but also that the relation of neurosecretory neurons to the body fluids might distinguish them from other elements of the nervous system. Stutinsky drew attention to the fact that in the eel neurosecretory perikarya projected into the c.s.f. of the third ventricle. A few weeks before the symposium Carlisle and I had proposed the name neurohaemal organ to describe the collections of endings of neurosecretory fibres abutting on blood-vessels in crustaceans, and at Naples I suggested that a definition of neurosecretion might include the neurohaemal concept.

Lund 1957. Four years later we met at Lund, as guests of our much-loved Bertil Hanström. From the start the neurohaemal concept became a matter of controversy. The intervening years had shown that the stainability of neurones by itself was not a reliable guide to their endocrine properties. Perhaps for this reason Ernst Scharrer was anxious that we should officially define neurosecretion (at the Lund Symposium) and that the discharge of hormones at neurohaemal organs would be a fundamental feature distinguishing neurosecretory neurones from what our French colleagues charmingly call "neurones banales". Wigglesworth opposed this for he felt that to make a formal definition at that stage would be premature.

Eventually no formal definition was passed by the Symposium but we all agreed in our own minds that at least a working definition of neurosecretion was clear. Cytologically neurosecretory neurones combined features of neurones and gland cells and their axon terminals did not appear to make synaptic junctions with effector organs but instead discharged secretory products into the circulation at a neurohaemal organ.

The Lund Symposium confirmed and extended many of the observations at Naples. By now the electron microscope had revealed small vesicles, some $1000 \text{ Å} - 3000 \text{ Å}$ in diameter in neurosecretory perikarya and axons, as was demonstrated by Bargmann.

A new precision was introduced by Sloper who demonstrated a histochemical test for neurosecretory material and a radioisotope method for studying the dynamics of the process, both dependent on the presence of cysteine. He was able to show that neurosecretory material moves down the axon in fine particulate form.

The discovery of elementary neurosecretory vesicles presented opportunities but also problems. Did these vesicles contain the hormones or had they some other function? Where were they produced? Were these vesicles perhaps a feature which would distinguish neurosecretory neurones from other elements of the nervous system? These were themes which dominated the next symposium at Bristol in 1961.

Bristol 1961. The problem of the identification of vesicles with hormones was very elegantly resolved by Heller and Lederis who combined methods of centrifugation, bioassay and electron microscopy to show that the oxytocin and vasopressin were indeed contained in elementary neurosecretory vesicles. Bern and co-workers indicated that these were formed in the Golgi apparatus.

The other question — whether the presence of elementary vesicles might be a criterion for neurosecretion — raised fundamental issues. Certainly the E.M. studies of Palay and others had shown that elementary vesicles *were* a feature of neurosecretory systems but it was *also* becoming clear that membrane-bound electron-dense granules were fairly ubiquitous in the c.n.s. especially in the lower animals. Once more the special nature of neurosecretion was questioned, this time by De Robertis in unequivocal terms. He said, "We shall maintain here that there are no essential differences between synaptic processes and those secretory processes from which the active product acts by way of the circulation upon distant receptors". This unitary concept of the neurosecretory activity of all neurones reflected earlier ideas of Welsh and Koelle.

The fact that secretion is a feature of neurones could not be contested and as Bern put it, "the presence of elementary neurosecretory granules cannot in itself be diagnostic of the phenomenon of neurosecretion". On the other hand, as Ernst Scharrer summed up, "the proposition to expand the concept of neuro-secretion to include all nerve cells was not received with enthusiasm by the members of this conference. Nothing would be gained by such an indiscriminate use of the term. The definition of the neurosecretory cell has been quite clear since the Naples Symposium. It is not solely based on the presence of neuro-secretory granules but also on the fact that neurosecretory cells do not form synapses with other neurones or effector organs. Their axons end at blood spaces into which they release the neurosecretory material".

Once again the neurohaemal concept proved to be a useful criterion to which the neurosecretologists could point when pressed by the neurologists, but it was clear that the pressure was increasing and that amine-containing neurones might present some problems. I was myself very conscious of this for I had recently found two kinds of neurosecretory fibre with different elementary vesicles in the pericardial organs of a crustacean, both apparently discharging into the blood-stream. It was known that two active principles, one an amine and the other a peptide, were present in this neurohaemal organ, and there was a possibility therefore that these two fibres which I termed A and B, were respec-tively peptide and amine containing.

From other directions also came evidence of the likelihood of more than one kind of neurosecretion. At Bristol Stahl and Leray presented clear evidence of two fibre systems in the pituitary of teleosts, one which stained with Gomori and aldehyde fuchsin (AF) while the other did not. This latter system of the tuberal nucleus showed secretory activity correlated to sexual maturity.

In birds Oksche and Farner gave a very clear demonstration of two kinds of neurosecretory systems in the median eminence, and very tentatively suggested that a gonadotropin-releasing principle may be related to neurosecretory material of the zona externa of the median eminence. Certainly the changes in AF + ve material after photostimulation were remarkable. It is interesting to note that in the discussions Farner put forward what he called wild speculation suggesting that the tuberal nucleus AF − ve fibres might in some way modulate the activity of the AF positive system.

At Bristol, like previous symposia, papers on the invertebrates dominated and in addition to the arthropods annelids were shown to have important neurosecretory systems. Looking back on that symposium though it was the studies in ultrastructure and cytophysiology that are most memorable. The E.M. demonstrations showed that although some modification of neurosecretory material might take place in the axon it was the perikaryon where the bulk of synthesis occurred. The beautiful histochemistry of Arvy and Gabe which supported the view that many neurosecretory stains coloured the so-called carrier substances rather than the hormones. These are some impressions that remain.

Between the Bristol Symposium in 1961 and the Strasbourg Symposium in 1966 a number of significant events occurred. First in place I shall put the discovery by Falck, Hillarp and their colleagues of a method which demonstrated catecholamines histochemically. Thereby, for example, certain tracts from the tuberal nuclei to the median eminence were clearly delineated and identified.

A second development was the discovery of a direct neurosecretory innervation of cells of the pituitary pars intermedia of the dogfish by at least two fibre types — a Type A or peptidergic fibre at the synthetic pole and a Type B or aminergic fibre at the release pole. Here for the first time was proof of a direct synaptoid contact between a peptidergic neurosecretory fibre and an epithelial cell. Here was a hypothalamo-hypophysial system in which no neurohaemal organ was concerned. In presenting these results at a meeting of endocrinologists in Paris in 1964 I suggested that the neurohaemal concept was no longer universally valid, and thereby questioned my own definition of ten years before. At this same meeting, in the same session, Ernst Scharrer developed a theme which he and Berta had been postulating for some years, namely that the real significance of neurosecretion was that it provided a final common pathway — linking the nervous and endocrine systems. Like many other brilliant ideas this was essentially simple, but it made many of our problems fall into place and changed the direction and emphasis of the neurosecretion concept. For instance in the case of the dogfish pituitary it was not of fundamental importance that here a peptidergic neurosecretory axon was not ending on a neurohaemal organ — what was important was that it was providing a final pathway from the c.n.s. to an endocrine gland. This was the conclusion reached after a very lively and prolonged discussion which took place at that session in Paris and in which Howard Bern took a very energetic part.

Strasbourg 1966. Sadly Ernst Scharrer did not live long enough to crystallize this concept of the final common pathway in an overall review of the nature of neurosecretion. I have no doubt he would have done so and I hope that his direction of thought would have lain along the lines which Howard Bern and I proposed at the symposium at Strasbourg. A few months prior to this symposium we, in consultation with Berta Scharrer, had suggested that neurosecretory systems consist of "neuronal elements which are engaged directly or indirectly in endocrine control and form all or part of an endocrine organ; as such they provide the final common pathway for neuroendocrine regulation". According to this concept the classical peptidergic neurosecretory systems were unquestionably neurosecretory while the precise neurosecretory status of aminergic systems and ependymal systems remained to be determined (I shall return to this point later).

At the Strasbourg Symposium for the first time the number of vertebrate papers greatly exceeded those on invertebrates and we begin to see the growing importance of studies on the catecholamines in relation to neuroendocrine control. In particular the clear demonstration by Fuxe and Hökfelt of changes in the catecholamine density in the median eminence in relation to changes in pituitary activity. This was but one of a number of papers dealing with pituitary regulation.

Kiel 1969. Three years after at Kiel we find the trends which appeared at Strasbourg continuing. Of 41 research papers presented nearly half dealt specifically with adrenergic neurones and hypothalamic control of the pituitary. In a paper by Fuxe and Hökfelt at Kiel we see outlined for the first time a postulate for the role of aminergic neurones in the median eminence as modulators of the activity of peptidergic neurones containing releasing factors. Such a concept was supported by Schneider and McCann who indicated that monoamines did not themselves act as releasing factors. Barry too emphasised the importance of aminergic systems in the regulation of releasing factor activity.

And what of the releasing factors themselves? At that time in 1969, we did not know the chemistry of these substances nor their probable location. There were however shadowy indications that they might lie in some kind of peptidergic neurone. Rinne and others had shown that after adrenalectomy of a rat an AF + ve material appeared in the external zone of the median eminence and at Kiel Rinne showed micrographs which indicated that the increase in AF + ve material was accompanied by an increase in the number of large elementary vesicles. Corresponding results were reported by Bock and Wittkowski.

Recently Dierickx has published highly significant EM studies which indicate Type A vesicles in the median eminence of an amphibian — results which accord well with those currently being obtained by my team working on fishes.

At the Kiel Symposium and in recent years interest has been focussed on those enigmatic ependymal elements in the ventrolateral walls and floor of the hypothalamus. Enigmatic because they do not seem to be indifferent to changes in activity of the pituitary gland. Indeed close correlations have been noted. But as yet we have no clear definitive evidence of the part, if any, these elements play in the regulation of pituitary function. It may however be significant that they link the c.s.f. with the tuberal nuclei and pituitary portal vessels.

And so we leave the Kiel Symposium and come to the present and face the future. This has been a general survey of trends in neurosecretion since our first symposium. It has been necessary to be selective and I am very conscious of the fact that I have been unable to record in perfectly balanced detail all the important work that has been done. It has been a *personal* account of the evolution of neurosecretion as I saw it, and I should like, if you will permit me, to conclude with a few final impressions and interpretations.

I hope that by the end of this symposium we shall be able to formulate a clearer picture of the peptidergic neurone. We shall be hearing many papers on the synthesis, transport and release in peptidergic neurones. We shall hear about their electrical properties. These data should make possible the first fairly complete description of peptidergic neurosecretion. We must not however forget that

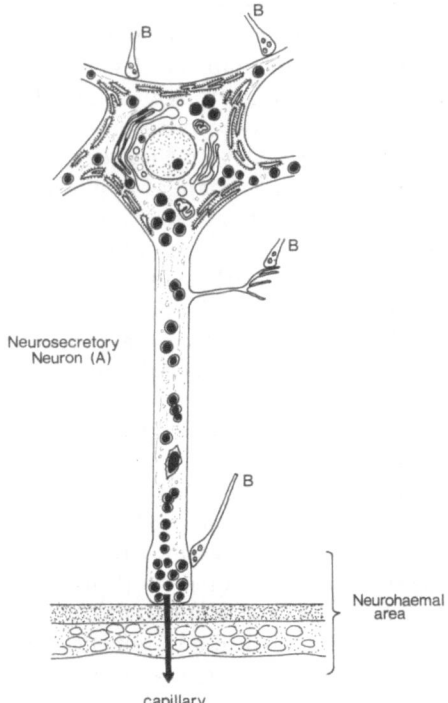

Neurosecretory
Neuron (A)

Neurohaemal
area

capillary

Fig. 2. Some features of a classical or peptidergic neurosecretory neurone (A), innervated by aminergic (B) fibres, terminating at a neurohaemal area

because we have chosen to give the name neurosecretion to those peptidergic neurones which form the final common pathways between nervous and endocrine systems, this should not blind us to the fact that it has been claimed that peptidergic neurones may be widely distributed in nervous tissue and could act as specific modulators of neuronal activity. The neurosecretion that we neuroendocrinologists study may be but one specialized form of a more widespread nervous activity.

I submit to you now that we have reached a significant moment in the history of the neurosecretion concept — a moment when we begin to see clearly a confluence of thought between the releasing factor hypothesis and peptidergic neurosecretion. The releasing factors so far identified are small peptides — unquestionably they are an essential neuroendocrine link. They are discharged at a neurohaemal area and there are various lines of evidence that they are contained within neurones. They satisfy therefore all the main historical criteria of neurosecretion and should, in my view, be embraced by the neurosecretion concept.

About the precise role of the catecholamines and their position within the neurosecretion concept I am less certain. Unquestionably they play an intimate part in the regulation of endocrine function. On the other hand is there evidence that they do this via a vascular link? In other words, can their products in any sense be described as hormones. If, as seems possible and has been suggested, the aminergic fibres in the external zone of the median eminence are modulating the activity of the peptidergic neurones, is there any clear locical distinction between these and those, say, originating in the reticular formation or limbic system ? If on the other hand some aminergic systems in the hypothalamus or elsewhere constitute final common pathways for neuroendocrine regulation it may well be appropriate to call these neurosecretory. This could well be a fruitful topic for discussion.

For a current working hypothesis I propose that it is the peptidergic neurone linking the nervous and endocrine systems which is the unquestionable neuro-secretory neurone. It may contain releasing or inhibitory factors regulating other endocrine organs, or it may produce hormones affecting other target organs. It receives synaptic efferents but itself makes no efferent synapses with other neurones[1]. Usually it releases hormones via a neurohaemal organ into the blood-stream (Fig. 2). It stands apart, by reason of these features, from the rest of the nervous system — and twenty years of neurosecretion have not fundamentally altered the original concept of Bargmann and Scharrer — they have rather enabled us to see even more clearly that twenty years ago a historic statement was made — Some nerve cells are specialized for a true endocrine function — This is neuro-secretion.

References

1. I. International Symposium on Neurosecretion: Pubbl. Staz. Zool. Napoli **24**, Suppl. 1—98 (1954).
2. II. International Symposium on Neurosecretion, Zweites Internationales Symposium über Neurosekretion (W. Bargmann, B. Hanström, B. und E. Scharrer, Eds.). Berlin-Göttingen-Heidelberg: Springer 1958.
3. III. International Symposium on Neurosecretion, Neurosecretion (H. Heller, R. B. Clark, Eds.). Mem. Soc. Endocrinol., No. 12. London-New York: Academic Press 1962.
4. IV. International Symposium on Neurosecretion, Neurosecretion (F. Stutinsky, Ed.). Berlin-Heidelberg-New York: Springer 1967.
5. V. International Symposium on Neurosecretion, Aspects of Neuroendocrinology (W. Bargmann, B. Scharrer, Eds.). Berlin-Heidelberg-New York: Springer 1970.

---

[1] This may need to be modified (see Cross this volume, p. 115).

II. Peptidergic Neurosecretion

A. Classical Neurosecretion

a) Morphology

Morphological and Physiological Reactions of the Supraoptic and Paraventricular Nuclei

F. Stutinsky

Laboratoire de Physiologie générale, Université Louis Pasteur, Strasbourg (France)

Introduction

Since the paper published by Bargmann and Scharrer (1951), in which they postulated the hypothalamic origin of the posterior lobe hormones, the experimental data have largely confirmed this hypothesis in the rat (Stutinsky, 1952; Lloyd and Pierog, 1955; Diamond, 1956; Croxatto and Zamorano, 1957), in the dog (Hild and Zetler, 1953) and in many other species. Almost at the same time a hypothesis concerning the specialisation of the SON and the PVN was put forward namely that oxytocin is primarily synthesized by the PVN (Olivecrona, 1957; Lederis, 1961; Nibbelink, 1961; Brooks et al., 1966; and others) and vasopressin by the SON (Weyl-Sokol and Valtin, 1967).

The observations leading to these conclusions were of two kinds:

— firstly, attempts were made to extract the hormones of different areas of the hypothalamus and showed that the SON contains more vasopressin than the PVN which sometimes does not contain any at all (Lederis, 1961).

— secondly, the destruction of the PVN in the rat (Olivecrona, 1957) and in the cat (Nibbelink, 1961) results in the disappearance of oxytocin in the posterior lobe, while the concentration of vasopressin remains unchanged. But such arguments can only be valid if the patterns of these nuclei are sharply delimited and this is far from being the case. The study of transverse serial sections of the rat brain shows clearly that numerous tracts of neurosecretory fibers cross the whole hypothalamus from the PVN to the SON, and that different groups of neurons scattered through this area are accessory neurosecretory nuclei. These, and the tracts are large enough to render impossible any biochemical extraction or any electric destruction of the PVN alone. Moreover, we will show, in this paper, that using all usual morphological and physiological criteria, no distinction can be drawn between these two nuclei.

Morphological Criteria

The morphology of these nuclei has been described in detail by numerous histologists, both in electron- and light-microscopy, the SON by Duncan and Alexander (1961), Sloper and Bateson (1965), Zambrano and De Robertis (1966), Cotte and Picard (1968), the PVN by Flament-Durand (1971); Klein et al. (1968), Pilgrim (1969) and Clementi and Ceccarelli (1970) have compared the two nuclei. So we can briefly summarise our description of the normal neurosecretory neuron (Stutinsky, 1970). After appropriate staining, light microscopy reveals large neurons containing Nissl bodies, a central nucleus and a large nucleolus. In electron micrographs these cells show well developed ergastoplasm and Golgi complexes which elaborate the characteristic elementary granules. The immature granules are smaller than the mature ones and possess a more opaque core which only partially fills the isolated Golgi vesicles. Their maturation occurs on the way from the Golgi complex to the periphery of the cell and the beginning of the axon. The granules originating in the SON are said to mature faster than those coming from the PVN which, after fixation at pH 8, remain dense-cored in a significantly higher proportion (Morris and Cannata, 1973). A mixture of immature and mature granules is however always seen in the normal cell. Numerous larger electron-dense bodies are present: the denser ones are lysosomes, while other more translucent bodies of similar size are multivesicular.

Under experimental conditions, morphological changes are similar in both nuclei.

(1) For instance, the incorporation of labelled cysteine follows the same pattern in the two groups of neurosecretory cells (Sloper et al., 1960; Flament-Durand, 1967).

(2) The administration of 2% saline solution as drinking water causes distinct morphological changes in the two nuclei, especially after the first week. Light microscopy shows that the cell bodies and the Golgi zone are enlarged and that the ergastoplasm is more abundant. The cell nuclei and nucleoli are also larger (Ortmann, 1951; Stutinsky, 1957). Electron micrographs show a proliferation of the rough endoplasmic reticulum. The Golgi apparatus occupies a large zone and gives rise to numerous Golgi vesicles. A great number of vesicles contain an electron dense substance, and numerous immature granules are seen in the vicinity of the Golgi zone; mature granules are rare; faster release of neurosecretory material at the axon terminal is very likely to be responsible for these observations. Similar modifications occur in the SON and in the PVN (Klein et al., 1968).

(3) Certain other experimental conditions can also modify the concentration of neurosecretory granules in the PV and SO nuclei. Following implantation into the CNS, or subcutaneous injection of oestrogen, an increased number of neurosecretory granules is observed in the entire neuron (Stutinsky, 1970); thyroidectomy, however, causes their number to decrease and also diminishes uptake of labelled cysteine or methionine (Talanti and Attila, 1972).

(4) Intraventricular injection of colchicine also increases the storage of granules in the two cell groups (Stoeckel et al., unpublished results; Flament-Durand and Dustin, see p. 304).

(5) After hypophysectomy or stalk transection, light microscopy of the SO and PV nuclei indicates an increase in neurosecretory material (Stutinsky, 1951) and degeneration of many cells, especially in the earlier stages (Klein et al., 1969, 1970). Surviving cells however show remarkable changes leading to hypertrophy and apparently normal functioning. Electron microscopy studies of hypophysectomized rats reveal the same modifications in the neurosecretory neurons

of the supraoptic and paraventricular nuclei (Klein et al., 1969; 1970). After the first 24 hours, the hypothalamic neurosecretory cells show increased secretory activity together with the appearance of multivesicular bodies and autophagy of secretory granules; after the fourth day, an enormous proliferation of ergastoplasm can be observed, as well as large quantities of glycogen, lysosomes and apparently stored granules. These observations mean that we are dealing in the same cell and at the same moment with both secretion and catabolic involution of the synthesized granules. These are the most important transformations of the early period, termed by Raisman (1973) the "obstructive" phase. In addition, between the 6th and 12th day, a second type of neuronal reaction is observed. At this stage, many cells begin to degenerate and pronounced glial reactions are observed, while once again the modifications observed are the same in the two nuclei.

Two to eight months later, the general structure of the surviving cells in the SO and PV nuclei returned progressively to almost normal ("Reconstructive" phase of Raisman). The ergastoplasm remains abundant, the Golgi complexes are very active, but there is no longer a peripheral accumulation of the granules. The large dense bodies are less numerous than in the earlier period, and it becomes very difficult to distinguish neurosecretory cells of a normal animal from those of a hypophysectomized one.

Physiological Criteria

A. Electrical Stimulation

Wistar rats of 230—280 g, anesthetized with nembutal or urethane were placed in a stereotaxic instrument, and concentric electrodes of about $600\,\mu$ in diameter were then introduced. The cells were stimulated with rectangular waves of 2—5 v, for at least 10″, at a frequency of 60 c/s, but never for longer than 1′.

The hypothalamic area explored is far from homogeneous in structure and the results will differ according to the spot stimulated (Stutinsky and Guerné, 1965). If arterial pressure is used as the peripheral test, three responses are possible:

(1) There may be no modification at all of the arterial pressure.

(2) Sometimes low hypotension, and sometimes acute hypertension are encountered.

(3) Among all the areas of the hypothalamus which can be stimulated, only the SON and the PVN present a specific response: a biphasic blood pressure variation. The first response, short and intense, is followed by a prolonged rise in pressure. The initial phase which took place without latency does not occur if a sympatholytic drug, like ergotamine tartrate, is previously injected. Previous bilateral adrenalectomy also suppresses this phase which can be simulated by the injection of a low dose of epinephrine. It seems very likely that this first modification of arterial pressure stems from liberation of epinephrine by the adrenals. The second phase has a longer latency and only begins after the first one is over. It is characterized by a slow increase of arterial pressure which reaches its maximum after 30″—60″. The maximum is maintained for several minutes and then the pressure slowly returns to its basal level some 5′—10′ later. This kind of pres-

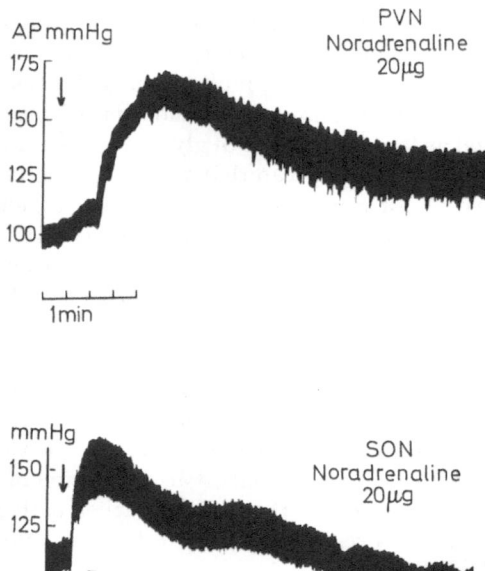

Fig. 1. Action of noradrenaline on arterial pressure in an adrenalectomized rat

sure modification can be induced by low doses of vasopressin (5—10 µU per animal). The reaction remains unchanged after the injection of a sympatholytic drug and after bilateral adrenalectomy or transection of the medulla. The phenomenon no longer occurs after hypophysectomy, posthypophysectomy or destruction of the median eminence. We can therefore conclude that the long pressure reaction is related to a secretion of vasopressin.

It must be emphasized that the electrical stimulation of the two neurosecretory nuclei produces comparable results (Stutinsky and Guerné, 1965). This also remains true if vasopressin is secreted during water diuresis. In this case, special precautions must be taken to avoid the secretion of minute quantities of endogenous vasopressin which could disturb diuresis. In order to inhibit any stress reaction resulting from the positioning of the animal in the stereotaxic instrument, we apply an observation made by Lutz et al. (1969), namely that high doses of dexamethasone prevent the secretion of both ACTH and ADH. The method used for over-hydration and anesthesia was to administer a 12% ethanol solution by stomach tube under light ether anesthesia. The total volume amounting to 7—8% of the animal's weight was given in two doses, 60' apart. Electrical stimulation under the same conditions as before and with almost the same parameters, produces—when applied to the neurosecretory nuclei — a marked antidiuresis which is directly related to the intensity of the stimulus. The only difference between this test and the pressure reaction is that the former is much more sensitive to ADH: the introduction of the electrode alone—a mechanical stimulation—is sufficient to produce an ADH release resulting in an antidiuresis lasting

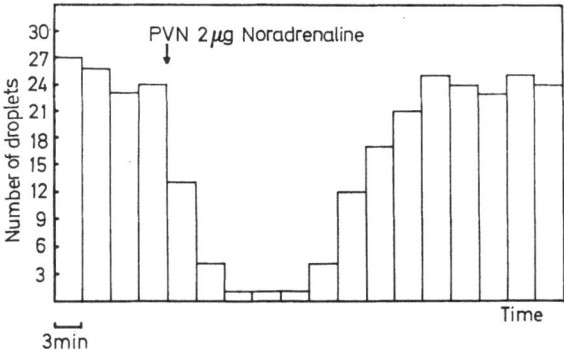

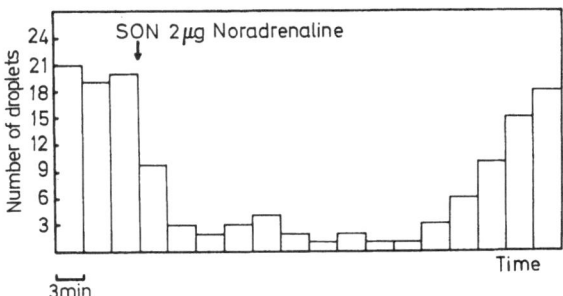

Fig. 2. Antidiuretic action of noradrenaline. Each column represents the number of urine droplets collected during 3'. The action is obviously stronger by injection of the transmitter in the SON

twenty minutes, despite the fact that the blood pressure remains unchanged. The antidiuretic reaction lasts two or three times as long as the modification of the blood pressure for an equivalent stimulation; but here again, the two neuro-secretory nuclei react similarly. The same observations can be made by recording uterine contraction or intramammary pressure.

B. Stereotaxic Drug Injections

The similarity in the functional reactions of the supraoptic and paraventricular nuclei can also be observed after the injection of some drugs, especially neuro-transmitters, acetylcholine and catecholamines.

It has long since been shown that these nuclei react to acetylcholine and that they release ADH (Pickford, 1947). It is generally accepted that acetylcholine has a stimulating effect, while the catecholamines exert an inhibitory action.

Our first observations on neurotransmitters came from the use of 6—OH dopamine. This drug destroys the nerve endings containing catecholamines

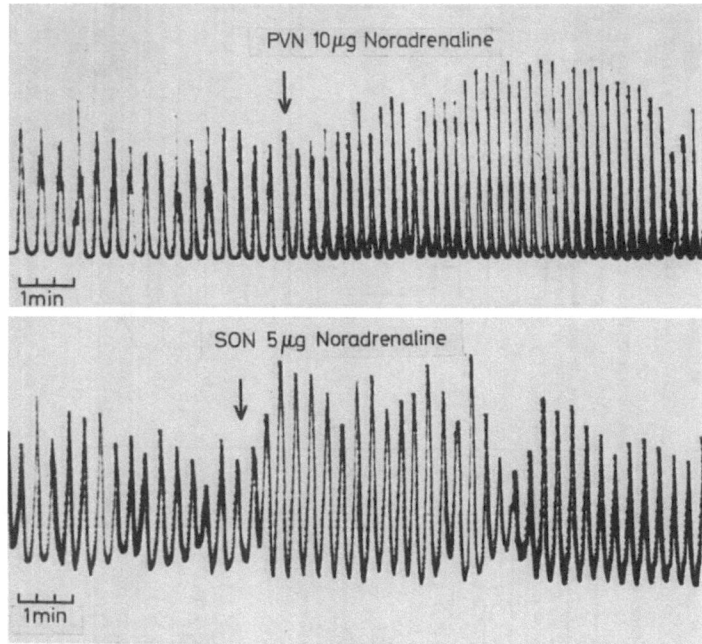

Fig. 3. Action of noradrenaline on intra-uterine pressure in an adrenalectomized rat

(Thoenen and Tranzer, 1968) and we used it to study with the electron microscope the nerve endings during their degeneration after local injection of the drug. In order to check the adequate positioning of the electrodes, the arterial pressure, water diuresis, intrauterine pressure and intramammary pressure were recorded.

The local injection into neurosecretory cells of 10—20 µg or less of 6—0H dopamine produces a rise in blood pressure and it seems very clear that during the destruction of the synapses, catecholamines were released. So we tried L-Dopa and noradrenaline, and found that both substances induce an increase in blood pressure, antidiuresis and also a rise in intrauterine pressure. No fundamental differences between the two nuclei could be detected (Stutinsky and Guerné, 1972). Atropine inhibits the reaction of acetylcholine and an α-blocker (Régitine) that of catecholamines. But the effects of the catecholamines persist after adrenalectomy or transsection of the medulla at different levels.

The following conclusions may therefore be drawn: the neurosecretory cells receive a double innervation, catecholaminergic and cholinergic. Both stimulate the release of ADH, and also of oxytocin as has been shown in other experiments (Figs. 1—3).

Discussion

The general morphological structure of the neurons of the two nuclei is very similar, and further important observations have been reported recently. It has been shown with immunofluorescent methods that vasopressin-containing cells are present not only in the SON but also in the PVN of the pig (Elde, 1973) and the rat (Elde, 1973; Burlet et al., this volume, p. 24; moreover, substitution of 2% NaCl solution for drinking water for 3 days increased electrical activity of neuro-secretroy neurons, both in the SON and in the PVN (Dyball and Morris, 1973).

The release of ADH after intraventricular injection of noradrenaline and L-Dopa has already been observed by Bhargava et al. (1972) in the dog, by Olsson (1970) in the goat and has been recently confirmed by Kuhn (1973) in the rat. Despite the generally accepted concept that catecholamines exert an inhibitory effect on the action of the posterior lobe hormones, it must be stressed that the results obtained by intracerebral injection of drugs are quite different from those obtained by systemic injection. As we know, the effect of oxytocin is inhibited by previously injected epinephrine (Cross, 1953), in which case oxytocin affects only peripheral targets (Vorherr, 1971). Our results, obtained by intracerebral injections in no wise tally with those of various investigators using microiontophoresis to apply the drugs to neurosecretory cells. This method seems to prove that most of the neurosecretory cells are stimulated by acetylcholine and inhibited by nor-adrenaline (Barker et al., 1971; Dreifuss and Kelly, 1972; Moss et al., 1971, 1972).

Exactly what this may signify needs to be explored further, but, in any case, it cannot be denied that the two nuclei are able to excrete ADH and oxytocin following either an electrical or a pharmacological stimulation. An explanation of the double innervation could be that two different kinds of afferent nerves of different origin converge on these cells, or, that in the chain of synaptic transmis-sions ending in a cholinergic synapse, a noradrenergic relay precedes the last link.

In any case, these results must be interpreted with caution, since it has been shown by electrophysiological techniques that complicated interconnections exist between these two nuclei; the electric stimulation of the SON activates or inhibits cells of the PVN and vice versa (Yamashita et al., 1970). But these observations also confirm that we must reject an oversimplified scheme for this neuronal com-plex and that its division into two completely distinct nuclei has no physiological or even morphological significance. Finally, as has already been suggested by earlier researches (Lederis, 1961; Heller, 1966) and as confirmed in some of our experiments (see for instance Fig. 2), the only distinction between these nuclei is of a quantitative nature, the SON secreting more vasopressin and the PVN probably more oxytocin.

Acknowledgments. This research was carried out by the Research Team for Comparative Neuroendocrinology n° 178 of the C.N.R.S. I am greatly indebted to Dr. A. Porte, chief of the Department of Electron Microscopy, and his co-workers Dr. M. E. Stoeckel and Miss M. L. Klein for the morphological part of this paper, and to Mrs. Y. Guerné for her active collabora-tion in the physiological experiments.

References

Bargmann, W., Scharrer, E.: The site of origin of the hormones of the posterior pituitary. Amer. Sci. **39**, 255—259 (1951).

Barker, J. L., Crayton, J. W., Nicoll, R. A.: Noradrenaline and acetylcholine responses of supraoptic neurosecretory cells. J. Physiol. (Lond.) **218**, 19—32 (1971).

Bhargava, K. P., Kulshrestha, V. K., Srivastava, Y. P.: Central cholinergic and adrenergic mechanismsin the release of antidiuretic hormones. Brit. J. Pharmacol. 44, 617—627 (1972).

Brooks, C. Mc., Ishikawa, T., Koizumi, K., Lu, H. H.: Activity of neurons in the paraventricular nucleus of the hypothalamus and its control. J. Physiol. (Lond.) 182, 217—231 (1966).

Burlet, A., Marchetti, J., Duheille, J., Boulange, M.: Immunohistochemistry of the vasopressin: study of the hypothalamohypophysial system of the normal and experimental rat. VI. Int. Symp. on Neurosecretion, London 1972.

Clementi, F., Ceccarelli, B.: Fine structure of rat hypothalamic nuclei. In: The Hypothalamus (Eds.: Martini, L., Motta, M., Fraschini, F.) p. 1—28. New York, London: Academic Press 1970.

Cotte, G., Picard, D.: Etude ultrastructurale des neurones du noyau supraoptique du rat. C. R. Ass. Anat. 141, 738 (1968).

Cross, B. A.: Sympathetico-adrenal inhibition of the neurohypophysial milk-ejection mechanism. J. Endocr. 9, 7—18 (1953).

Croxatto, H., Zamorano, B.: Effect of purified vasopressin and oxytocin on water and sodium excretion in hypophysectomized rats. Acta physiol. lat.-amer. 7, 33—38 (1957).

Diamond, M. C.: The effect of hypophysectomy, removal of the posterior pituitary, adrenal ectomy, and dehydration on the antidiuretic activity of the rat hypothalamic-neurohypophyseal system. Endocrinology 58, 461—470 (1956).

Dreifuss, J. J., Kelly, J. S.: Recurrent inhibition of antidromically identified rat supraoptic neurones. J. Physiol. (Lond.) 220, 87—103 (1972).

Duncan, D., Alexander, R.: An electron microscope study of supraoptic nucleus of the rat. Anat. Rec. 139, 223 (1961).

Dyball, R. E. J., Morris, J. F.: Ultrastructural and electrical changes in neurosecretory neurones associated with prolonged stimulation of hormone release. In: VI. Int. Symp. on Neurosecretion, London 1973.

Elde, R. P.: Methods for the localization of vasopressin-containing neurons in the hypothalamus and pars nervosa by immunoenzyme histochemistry. Anat. Rec. 175, 255—518 (1973).

Flament-Durand, J.: Contribution à l'étude de la neurosécrétion chez le rat par la méthode autoradiographique. In: Neurosécrétion (Stutinsky, F., Ed.), p. 60—76. Berlin-Heidelberg-New York: Springer 1967.

Flament-Durand, J.: Ultrastructural aspects of the paraventricular nucleus in the rat. Z. Zellforsch. 116, 61—69 (1971).

Flament-Durand, J., Dustin, P.: Further observations on the action of colchicine on the neurosecretory paraventricular neurons in the rat. In: VI. Int. Symp. on Neurosecretion, London 1973.

Heller, H.: The hormone content of the Vertebrate Hypothalamo-Neurohypophyseal system. Brit. med. Bull. 22, 227—231 (1966).

Hild, W., Zetler, G.: Experimenteller Beweis für die Entstehung der sog. Hypophysenhinterlappenwirkstoffe im Hypothalamus. Pflügers Arch. ges. Physiol. 257, 169—201 (1953).

Klein, M. J., Porte, A., Stutinsky, F.: Comparaison ultrastructurale des noyaux neurosécrétoires hypothalamiques chez le rat normal ou en état de surcharge osmotique. C. R. Ass. Anat. 142, 1066—1072 (1968).

Klein, M. J., Stoeckel, M. E., Porte, A., Stutinsky, F.: Etude ultrastructurale des noyaux neurosécréteurs hypothalamiques chez le rat hypophysectomisé. C. R. Soc. Biol. (Paris) 163, 2698—2700 (1969).

Klein, M. J., Stoeckel, M. E., Porte, A., Stutinsky, F.: Sur les modifications ultrastructurales des cellules neurosécrétoirs hypothalamiques (noyaux S.O. et P.V.) chez le rat hypophysectomisé. C. R. Acad. Sci. (Paris) 270, 386—388 (1970).

Kühn, E. R.: The release of antidiuretic hormone and electrolyte excretion after injections of cholinergic, and adrenergic agents into the third ventricle of the male rat. In: Seventh Conference of European comparative Endocrinologists, Abstracts, p. 139. Budapest 1973.

Lederis, K.: Vasopressin and oxytocin in the mammalian hypothalamus. Gen. comp. Endocr. 1, 80—89 (1961).

Lloyd, C. W., Pierog, S.: Studies of the antidiuretic activity of blood and hypothalamus of hypophysectomized rats. Endocrinology 56, 718—726 (1955).

Lutz, B., Koch, B., Mialhe, C.: Libération des hormones antidiurétique et corticotrope au cours de différents types d'agression chez le rat. Hormones et Métab. 1, 213—217 (1969).

Morris, J. F., Cannata, M. A.: Ultrastructural preservation of the dense core of posterior pituitary neurosecretory granules and its implications for hormone release. J. Endocr. 57, 517—529 (1973).

Moss, R. L., Dyball, R. E. J., Cross, B. A.: Responses of antidromically identified supraoptic and paraventricular units to acetylcholine, noradrenaline and glutamate applied iontophoretically. Brain Res. 35, 573—575 (1971).

Moss, R. L., Dyball, R. E. J., Cross, B. A.: Excitation of antidromically identified neurosecretory cells of the praventricular nucleus by oxytocin applied iontophoretically. Exp. Neurol. 34, 95—102 (1972).

Nibbelink, D. W.: Paraventricular nuclei, neurohypophysis and parturition. Amer. J. Physiol. 200, 1229—1232 (1961).

Olivecrona, H.: Paraventricular nucleus and pituitary gland. Acta physiol. scand. 40 (suppl. 136), 1—178 (1957).

Olsson, K.: Effects on water diuresis of infusions of transmitter substances into the third ventricle. Acta physiol. scand. 79, 133—135 (1970).

Ortmann, R.: Über experimentelle Veränderungen der Morphologie des Hypophysenzwischenhirnsystems und die Beziehung der sog. „Gomorisubstanz" zum Adiuretin. Z. Zellforsch. 36, 92—140 (1951).

Pickford, M.: The action of acetylcholine in the supraoptic nucleus of the chloralosed dog. J. Physiol. (Lond.) 106, 264—270 (1947).

Pilgrim, Ch.: Morphologische und funktionelle Untersuchungen zur Neurosekretbildung. Enzymhistochemische, autoradiographische und elektronenmikroskopische Beobachtungen an Ratten unter osmotischer Belastung. Ergebnisse Anat. Entwickl-Gesch. 41, 7—79 (1969).

Raisman, G.: An ultrastructural study of the effects of hypophysectomy on the supraoptic nucleus of the rat. J. comp. Neurol. 147, 181—208 (1973).

Sloper, J. C., Arnott, D. J., King, B. C.: Suphur metabolism in the pituitary and hypothalamus of the rat: a study of radioisitope-uptake after the injection of ^{35}Sdl-cysteine, methionine, and sodium sulphate. J. Endocr. 20, 9—23 (1960).

Sloper, J. C., Bateson, R. G.: Ultrastructure of neurosecretory cells in the supraoptic nucleus of the dog and rat. J. Endocr. 31, 139—150 (1965).

Stutinsky, F.: Sur l'origine de la substance Gomori-positive du complexe hypothalamo-hypophysaire. C. R. Soc. Biol. (Paris) 145, 367—370 (1951).

Stutinsky, F.: Sur l'origine diencéphalique des hormones dites "posthypophysaires". C. R. Soc. Biol. (Paris) 146, 1691—1695 (1952).

Stutinsky, F.: Recherches morphologiques sur le complexe hypothalamoneurohypophysaire. Bull. Micr. théor. appl., Mémoire h.s. 2, 8—90 (1957).

Stutinsky, F.: Hypothalamic neurosecretion. In: The Hypothalamus (L. Martini, M. Motta, F. Fraschini, Eds.), p. 45—67. New York, London: Academic Press 1970.

Stutinsky, F., Guerné, Y.: Effets des stimulations électriques hypothalamiques sur la pression artérielle du rat. C. R. Soc. Biol. (Paris) 159, 1420—1422 (1965).

Stutinsky, F., Guerné, Y.: Rôle des catécholamines dans la libération des hormones posthypophysaires. C. R. Acad. Sci. (Paris) 275, 573—576 (1972).

Talanti, S., Attila, U.: Incorporation of ^{35}S-labelled cysteine and methionine in the hypothalamic-hypophyseal neurosecretory system of the thyroidectomized rat. Life Sci. Part 1, 11, 49—54 (1972).

Thoenen, H., Tranzer, J. P.: Chemical sympathectomy by selective destruction of adrenergic nerve endings with 6-hydroxydopamine. Naunyn-Schmiedebergs-Arch. Pharmak. exp. Path. 261, 271—288 (1968).

Vorherr, H.: Catecholamine antagonism to oxytocin-induced milk-ejection. Acta endocr. (Kbh.) 67, suppl. 154 (1971).

Weyl-Sokol, H., Valtin, H.: Evidence for the synthesis of oxytocin and vasopressin in separate neurons. Nature (Lond.) 214, 314—316 (1967).

Yamashita, H., Koizumi, K., Mc C. Brokks, C.: Electrophysiological studies of neurosecretory cells in the rat hypothalamus. Brain Res. 20, 462—466 (1970).

Zambrano, D., De Robertis, E.: The secretory cycle of supraoptic neurons in the rat. A structural-functional correlation. Z. Zellforsch. 73, 414—431 (1966).

Immunohistochemistry of Vasopressin:
Study of the Hypothalamo-Neurohypophysial System of Normal, Dehydrated and Hypophysectomized Rats

A. BURLET, J. MARCHETTI, and J. DUHEILLE

Laboratory of Histology and Laboratory of Physiology, U.E.R. Sciences Médicales, Nancy-Cedex (France)

After the initial findings of Bargmann (1949), using Gomori chrome-alum-haematoxylin, several histochemical methods have been proposed for demonstrating the neurosecretory material of the mammalian hypothalamo-neurohypophysial system (HNHS)—(see References in GABE, 1966). However, most of the authors agree that none of these procedures is specific for the neurohypophysial hormones, vasopressin and oxytocin, for they stain at the same time the hormonal peptides and their carrier proteins, the neurophysins (Hild and Zetler, 1953; Rinne, 1960; Sawyer, 1961; Moses et al., 1963; Gutierrez and Sloper, 1969).

We have taken advantage of the specificity of anti-vasopressin antibodies for localizing the immunologically reactive peptide in the HNHS of the rat, in normal and experimental conditions.

Materials and Methods

a) Antisera

Anti-lysine-vasopressin antibodies (antiLVP) were produced in rabbits, using the synthetic peptide coupled to rabbit serum albumin (RSA) as antigen.

Their specificity was checked against a series of synthetic structural analogues of LVP by a quantitative radioimmunoassay. All antisera reacted with the phenylalanine residue in position 3. The hydroxyl group of the tyrosyl in position 2 of the LVP molecule is involved in the reaction. A complete cross-reaction was obtained with arginine-vasopressin (AVP), the biologically active peptide of the rat. They react neither with oxytocin, nor with RSA.

b) Immunological Procedure

Thin sections (4 μ) of fixed tissues were stained by the indirect immunofluorescence technique of Coons.

Two fixatives yielded satisfactory results:
— Zamboni and De Martino solution, pH 6.8
— Freshly prepared 4p. 100 formaldehyde solution in 0.1 M phosphate buffer containing 0.005 M $CaCl_2$; final pH 7.3.

Following fixation, the tissues were washed overnight at 4° C in phosphate buffered saline (PBS). They were then either frozen in liquid nitrogen and cut in acryostat, or rapidly embedded in paraffin and cut as usual.

The sections were mounted on glass slides and handled as follows:
— incubation with unlabelled anti-LVP suitably diluted (1 : 20), 3 hours at 6° C.
— washing in PBS, 15 minutes
— incubation with fluoresceinated goat anti-rabbit globulin serum (Institut Pasteur, Paris), 30 minutes at room temperature
— washing in PBS, 15 minutes
— mounting in buffered glycerine.

A Leitz fluorescence photo-microscope was used for immediate observation (primary filter BG 12, secondary filter K530, dark or bright-field condenser).

c) Controls

The specificity of the staining reaction was established by the absence of any fluorescent structure in sections receiving, in place of anti-LVP serum, PBS, or rabbit pre-immunization serum, or rabbit anti-angiotensin serum, or anti-LVP serum previously absorbed by LVP. Pre-incubation of anti-LVP serum with oxytocin does not alter the immunohistochemical staining.

d) Animals

We studied the HNHS of adult, normal male and female rats (Wistar WAG) and of male rats under the following conditions:
— dehydration by withdrawing water for periods of 24 hours, 3 days, a week and 12 days (n = 50)
— total hypophysectomy through the lateropharyngeal space; the results were observed after 24 hours, after 3 days and then every week for 3 months after the operation (n = 50).

All these test animals and their respective controls (isolated in the same conditions or sham operated) were killed under chloroform anesthesia by slow intraventricular infusion of the fixative. We have previously verified that this procedure, although raising the plasma vasopressin level in normal rats, did not alter, under our working conditions, the immunohistochemical staining properties of the HNHS.

Results

In normal rats, immunologically cross-reactive vasopressin is localized in the perikaryon of most of the ante- and retro-chiasmatic neurons of the supraoptic nucleus (SON) as well as in the magnocellular elements of the supero-external angles of the paraventricular nucleus (PVN). It also appears in several clusters of cells in the anterior and median hypothalamus, corresponding, according to Peterson (1966), to the anterior and posterior fornical nuclei, to the nucleus circularis, to the nucleus of the medial forebrain bundle. It appears as well in isolated neurons, some of which are closely attached to vascular walls, others which

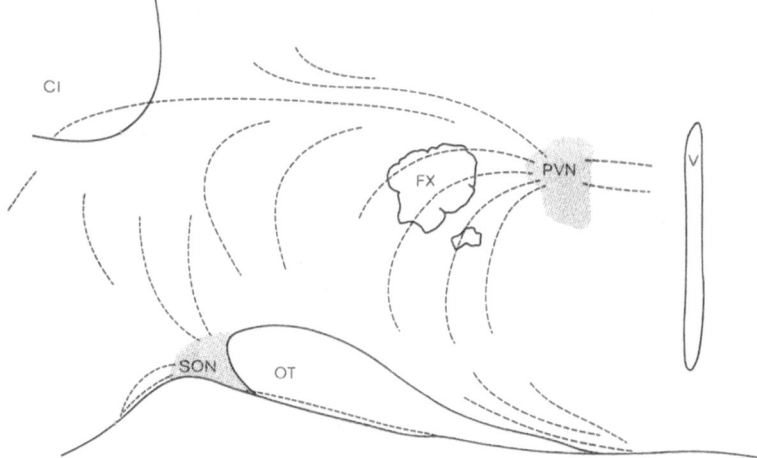

Fig. 1. Schematic drawing of the SON and PVN hypophysial fibres (frontal section). SON: Supraoptic nucleus, PVN: paraventricular nucleus, FX: fornix, OT: optic tractus, CI: internal capsule, V: third ventricle

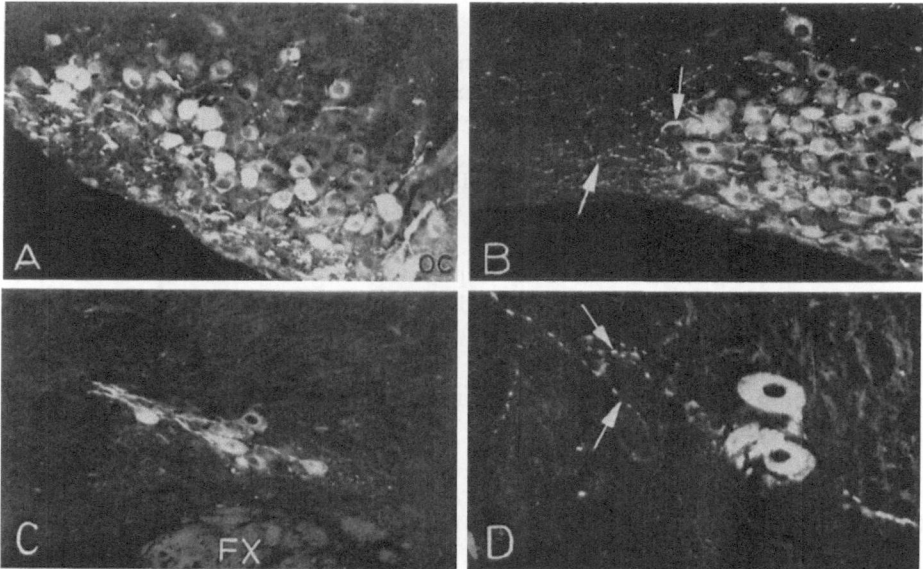

Fig. 2. Frontal section of a normal rat hypothalamus. A: supraoptic nucleus ($\times$ 180), B: paraventricular nucleus ($\times$ 180), C: anterior fornical nucleus ($\times$ 180), D: isolated cells ($\times$ 500) (OC: optic chiasma, FX: fornix)

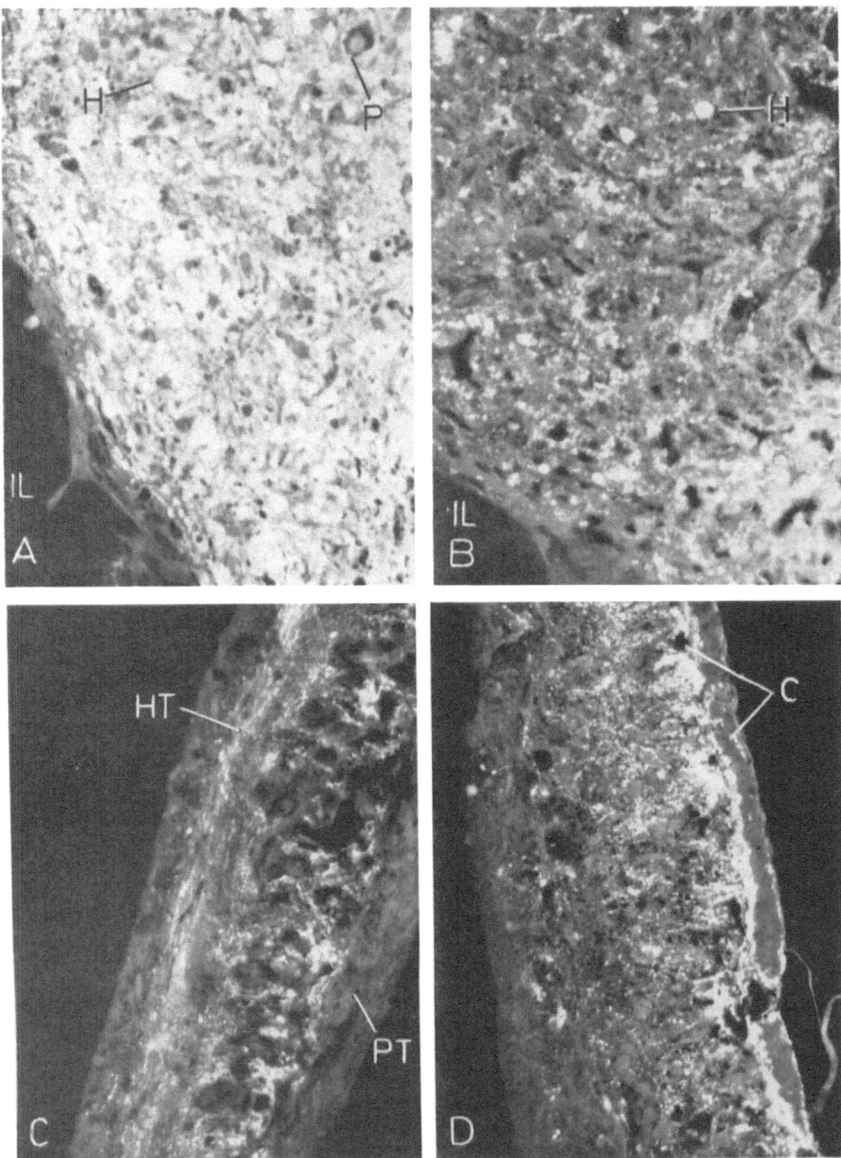

Fig. 3. The neurohypophysis (horizontal section, × 180). A: normal rat, B: dehydrated rat, after one week (P: pituicyte, H: Herring body, IL: intermediate lobe).

The median eminence of hypophysectomized rat: (parasagittal section, × 200). C: after one week; the pericapillary endings loaded with vasopressin, D: after two months: the hypothalamo-neurohypophysial tract is not visible (PT: pars tuberalis, HT: hypothalamo-hypophysial tract, C: portal vessels)

seem totally independent. Fluorescence extends to dendrites of paraventricular neurons oriented toward the ependymal lining of the third ventricle and to dendrites of the SON latero-external zones (Fig. 1). The intra-hypothalamic axonal paths are easily observed (Fig. 2). The fibres of the hypothalamo-neurohypophysial tract can be followed in the ventral and dorsal lips of the infundibulum right to the neurohypophysis. A small number of axons extend from this principal fibrous stem of the median eminence and terminate upon contact with the primary capillary loops of the portal system. Herring bodies are very rich in reactive material. The neurohypophysis exhibits a high fluorescent staining, shown neither by the anterior hypophysis nor by the intermediate lobe.

While in normal animals the two techniques for preparing histological sections yielded comparable results, we had to avoid embedding in paraffin for the samples obtained during dehydration. Under these conditions, the fluorescence of the hypothalamic cells undergoes little change throughout the test. The reactivity of the retro-chiasmatic supraoptic neurons is particularly high and the axons identified in this area are rather numerous. Frequently, after 3 days of dehydration, dendrites swollen with fluorescent material can be localized in the PVN; the vasopressin pericapillary endings of the median eminence's external layer are rich in the hormone and the depletion of neurophysial reactive material begins. This hormonal release becomes more and more pronounced as the experiment continues (Fig. 3) but, even on the 12th day of the test, some of the Herring bodies remain reactive. Paraffin embedding partially inhibits the reactions of supraoptic neurons whereas the results obtained on PVN, accessory nuclei, isolated neurons and the neurohypophysis are unchanged.

Hypophysectomy induces simultaneous cytological modifications in SON and PVN vasopressin neurons. Twenty-four hours after the operation, the specific fluorescence of neurons is very intense and the uneven staining frequently found in the normal animal becomes more homogeneous. In the median eminence, the accumulation above the section is obvious. Between the 3rd and 7th post-operative days, this distal accumulation is accompanied by a massive load of the pericapillary endings (Fig. 3); two and three weeks after the operation the fluorescence of SON and PVN neurons is still visible; the fibres of the HNH tract are practically no longer identifiable in their peri-infundibulary paths, whereas the peri-vascular load increases. These different aspects are pronounced up until the 3rd month following hypophysectomy: fluorescent SON and PVN neurons are very rare, while the isolated neurons in the anterior and median hypothalamus maintain high reactivity.

Discussion

The proposed immunofluorescence technique permits specific localization of vasopressin in SON and PVN. These results are similar to those obtained by various authors using antibodies against different neurophysins (Watkins and Evans, 1972; Alvarez-Buylla et al., Zimmermann et al., Evans and Watkins, 1973). Besides hypothalamic nuclei, the hormone is present in numerous isolated cells; Hayward and Jennings (1973), using electrophysiological data, demonstrated the presence of osmosensitive neurosecretory cells situated outside SON and PVN. Our findings seem to confirm this observation.

During dehydration, neurohypophysial fluorescent material depletion correlates with hormonal assays described by Diamond (1956), and Jones and Pickering (1969). We wish, however, to emphasize the remarkable stability of the Herring bodies' content; even after a long test, the neurohypophysial AVP is never totally depleted. The assays made on SON indicate that the hormonal contents remain unchanged for the first week and significantly decrease after ten days' dehydration (Vilhard, 1971).

The immunochemical stains gave consistent results when particular technical precautions were taken; we think that during the experiments, the hormone in the tissue may be easily destroyed during preparation of the material.

Morphological, histoautoradiographical and enzymological observations prove that hypothalamic neurons remaining intact after hypophysectomy, show signs of secretory hyper-activity (Stutinsky, 1957; Moll and De Wied, 1962; Flament-Durand, 1966; Klein et al., 1969; Burlet, 1971). Our findings demonstrate that vasopressin is present only in some of them. Therefore, we must assume that either the remaining neurons do not synthetise AVP, or that their synthetic and releasing activities are continued in such a way that the hormonal accumulation in the perikaryon is no longer visible. The latter hypothesis appears unlikely, for during this period the functional reorganization of HNHS is incomplete (Moll and De Wied, 1962). The loading of pericapillary endings in the median eminence strengthens the hypothesis of vasopressin release into the portal hypophysial system. The multiplication of these fibres during the second and third post-operative months cannot be explained only by the activity of rare SON and PVN intact neurons but should be related to the activivity of isolated cells which maintain a high hormonal content.

References

Alvarez-Buylla, R., Livett, B. G., Uttenthal, L. O., Hope, D. B., Milton, S. H.: Immunochemical evidence for the transport of neurophysin in the hypothalamo-neurohypophyseal system of the dog. Z. Zellforsch. **137**, 435—450 (1973).

Bargmann, W.: Über die neurosekretorische Verknüpfung von Hypothalamus und Neurohypophyse. Z. Zellforsch. **34**, 610—634 (1949).

Burlet, A.: Mise en évidence de zones fonctionnelles différentes dans le noyau supra-optique du Rat après déshydratation, surrénalectomie et hypophysectomie. C. R. Ass. Anat. **151**, 276—283 (1971).

Burlet, A., Marchetti, J., Duheille, J.: Preliminary research on the detection of vasopressin by immunofluorescence. Lille méd. **17**, 1415 (1972).

Burlet, A., Marchetti, J., Duheille, J.: Etude par immunofluorescence de la répartition de la vasopressine au niveau du système hypothalamo-neurohypophysaire du Rat. C. R. Soc. Biol. (Paris) **167**, 924—927 (1973).

Diamond, M. C.: The effect of hypophysectomy, removal of the posterior pituitary, adrenalectomy and dehydration on the antidiuretic activity of the rat hypothalamic-neurohypophyseal system. Endocrinology **58**, 461—470 (1956).

Evans, J. J., Watkins, W. B.: Localization of neurophysins in the neurosecretory elements of the hypothalamus and neurohypophysis of the normal and osmotically stimulated guinea-pig as demonstrated by immunofluorescence histochemical techniques. Z. Zellforsch. **145**, 39—55 (1973).

Flament-Durand, J.: Contribution à l'étude de la neurosécrétion chez le Rat par la méthode autoradiographique. In: Neurosecretion (F. Stutinsky, Ed.), p. 60—76. Berlin-Heidelberg-New York: Springer 1966.

Gabe, M.: Neurosecretion, p. 13—21. Oxford: Pergamon press 1966.

Gutierrez, M., Sloper, J. C.: Reaction *in vitro* of synthetic oxyctocin and lysine-vasopressin with pseudoisocyaninchloride technique used for the demonstration of neurophysial neurosecretory material. Histochemie 17, 73—77 (1969).

Hayward, J. N., Jennings, D. P.: Activity of the magnocellular neuroendocrine cells in the hypothalamus of unanesthetized monkeys. J. Physiol. (Lond.) 232, 515—543 (1973).

Hild, W., Zetler, G.: Über die Funktion des Neurosekrets im Zwischenhirn-Neurohypophysen-system als Trägersubstanz für Vasopressin, Adiuretin und Oxytocin. Z. ges. exp. Med. 120, 236—243 (1953).

Jones, C. W., Pickering, B. T.: Comparison of the effects of water deprivation and sodium chloride inhibition on the hormone content of the neurohypophysis of the rat. J. Physiol. (Lond.) 203, 449—458 (1969).

Klein, M. J., Stoeckel, M. E., Porte, A., Stutinsky, F. S.: Etude ultrastructurale des noyaux neurosécréteurs hypothalamiques chez le Rat hypophysectomisé. C. R. Soc. Biol. (Paris) 163, 2698—2700 (1969).

Marchetti, J.: Immunoassay for LVP: comparison of biological and immunological activity of lysine-vasopressin and some of its synthetic analogues. Experientia (Basel) 29, 351—353 (1973).

Moll, J., De Wied, D.: Observations on the hypothalamo-posthypophyseal system of the posterior lobectomized rat. Gen. comp. Endocr. 2, 215—218 (1962).

Moses, A. M., Leveque, T. F., Giambatista, M., Lloyd, C. W.: Dissociation between the content of vasopressin and neurosecretory material in the rat neurohypophysis. J. Endocr. 26, 273—278 (1963).

Peterson, R. P.: Magnocellular neurosecretory centers in the rat hypothalamus. J. comp. Neurol. 128, 181—185 (1966).

Rinne, U. K.: Neurosecretory material around the hypophysial portal vessels in the median eminence of the rat. Acta endocr. (Kbh.) 35, suppl. 57, 1—108 (1960).

Sawyer, W. H.: Neurohypophysial hormones. Pharmac. Rev. 13, 225—277 (1961).

Stutinsky, F. S.: Recherches expérimentales sur le complexe hypothalamoneurohypophysaire. Arch. Anat. micr. Morph. exp. 46, 93—158 (1957).

Vilhard, H.: Vasopressin content and neurosecretory material in the hypothalamo-neurohypophyseal system of rats under different states of water metabolism. Acta Endocr. (Kbh.) 63, 585—594 (1970).

Watkins, W. B., Evans, J. J.: Demonstration of neurophysin in the hypothalamo-neurohypophysial system of the normal and dehydrated rat by use of cross-species reactive anti-neurophysins. Z. Zellforsch. 131, 149—170 (1972).

Zamboni, L., De Martino, C. D.: Buffered picric-acid formaldehyde: a new rapid fixative for electron microscopy. J. Cell Biol. 35, 148A (1967).

Zimmerman, E. A., Hsu, C. C., Robinson, A. G., Carmel, P. W., Frantz, A. G., Tannenbaum, M.: Studies of neurophysin secreting neurons with immunoperoxidase techniques employing antibody to bovine neurophysin. I. Light microscopic findings in monkey and bovine tissues. Endocrinology 92, 931—940 (1973).

Exo-Endocytosis in the Neurohypophysis as Revealed by Freeze-Fracturing

J. J. Dreifuss[1], J. J. Nordmann*[1], K. Akert[2], C. Sandri[2], and H. Moor[3]

Department of Physiology, University of Geneva[1]; Brain Research Institute, University of Zürich[2], and Institute of General Botany, Federal Institute of Technology, Zürich[3] (Switzerland)

Evidence has accumulated to indicate that the release of the neurohypophysial hormones occurs by exocytosis (emiocytosis, and reverse pinocytosis, are synonyms). During this process, the secretory granule-limiting membrane fuses with the plasma membrane, and an opening is formed which allows passage of the soluble content of the neurosecretory granules to the extracellular environment.

Although unequivocal evidence that such a process occurs in the vertebrate neurohypophysis is now available, a clear correlation between the frequency of exocytotic events in neurosecretory cells, and hormone release, has only been demonstrated in invertebrates (Norman and Duve, 1969), where exocytosis in neuroendocrine cells had been first reported. On the basis of a highly significant, positive correlation between the frequency of exocytosis, and the occurrence of clusters of microvesicles ("synaptic vesicles") seen in corpora cardiaca in the insect *Calliphora*, Norman (1970) proposed that these two phenomena must be causally related, and has suggested that microvesicles are formed by endocytosis (pinocytosis) in a process which allows the neurosecretory endings to keep their volume constant in the face of ongoing exocytosis.

Douglas et al. (1971a) have published electron micrographs which indicate that exocytosis occurs also in hamster and rat neurohypophyses. Moreover, evidence consistent with the view that microvesicles arise by endocytosis in a process serving to recapture excess membrane is available: first, coated vesicles characteristic of micropinocytosis are found predominantly in stimulated preparations, and secondly, microvesicles filled with extra-cellular marker substances that do not traverse the intact cell membrane have been reported in actively secreting neurosecretory endings (Bunt, 1969; Douglas et al., 1971b; Nagasawa et al., 1971; Smith, 1970).

The rarity of exo-endocytotic images seen with the transmission electron microscope, even in strongly stimulated preparations, has been emphasized. This may be a reflection of the fleeting nature of exocytotic processes, and of the shortcoming of the viewing technique. Direct evidence for exocytosis in a thin section from a neurohypophysis may be obtained only if the plane of section pas-

---

* Present address: Department of Pharmacology, Medical School, Cambridge, England.

ses through an exocytotic opening, or if electron dense material is present between the basement membrane and a pit in the plasma membrane. Since exocytotic openings may well have a small diameter, and since the core of neurosecretory granules apparently dissolves rapidly once it has made contact with the extra-cellular environment, the probability of seeing a granule undergoing exocytosis is exceedingly small. To investigate the importance of exocytosis in stimulated hormone release, we used the freeze-fracturing technique, which gives views of large areas of cell membrane, and this facilitates the analysis of events occurring at the level of the plasma membrane.

Isolated rat neurohypophyses were immersed in oxygenated Locke solution, and hormone secretion was evoked by one of the following means: electrical stimulation, exposure to excess KCl, to lanthanum, or to cold. The preparations were fixed for 2 hours at room temperature in 3 % glutaraldehyde. Freeze-fracturing was performed on tiny blocks after soaking them for 30 min in a 25 % glycerol/Ringer solution. They were then rapidly frozen in liquid Freon, fractured, and briefly etched.

The freeze-fracture procedure results either in a fracture through the intra- and extra-cellular compartments, or in a split occurring within membranes, thereby revealing the internal membrane structure. The splitting of membranes is believed to run through the middle of the lipid bilayer, and to expose either the internal, or the external, leaflet of the membrane (Branton, 1966). The fracture face which is associated with the cytoplasmic half of the membrane (face A) contains a larger number of 8—10 nm particles than the external fracture face (face B).

The plasma membrane of actively secreting neurosecretory endings displays numerous membrane modulations (cf. Pfenninger et al., 1972), approximately 20—40 nm in diameter; they are seen as pits when viewed from the extra-cellular space (face A), and as protuberances when viewed from the cytoplasm (face B). The frequency with which they were encountered was much higher in stimulated preparations than in unstimulated controls. We interpret them as indicative of an ongoing exo-endocytotic process, and believe that variations in their size and form might represent different stages of this process. Representative examples of modulations are illustrated in Fig. 1. Figures 1A and 1B show an A and a B face, respectively, from preparations depolarized for 10 min in a high K, low Na Locke solution (cf. Dreifuss et al., 1971); Figs. 1C and 1D show membrane faces from neurohypophyses exposed to cold. Numerous membrane pits are seen on the A faces, which correspond in all likelihood to the protuberances seen on the B faces. Some of the protuberances are open to the extra-cellular space by a narrow channel lying in their center.

Larger (i.e. ≧ 50 nm), circular openings in the plasma membrane, were seen more rarely some distance away from the neuro-vascular contact area (Fig. 2A).

When the limiting membrane of a neurosecretory granule was split, its internal fracture face B was generally found to be rather smooth. In some granules, however, possibly in those lying close to the plasma membrane, an array of membrane-associated particles was found at the pole of the granule facing the plasma membrane (Fig. 2B). Since aggregates of particles were detected on neighbouring areas of the plasma membrane, we envisage that the array of particles on the granule-

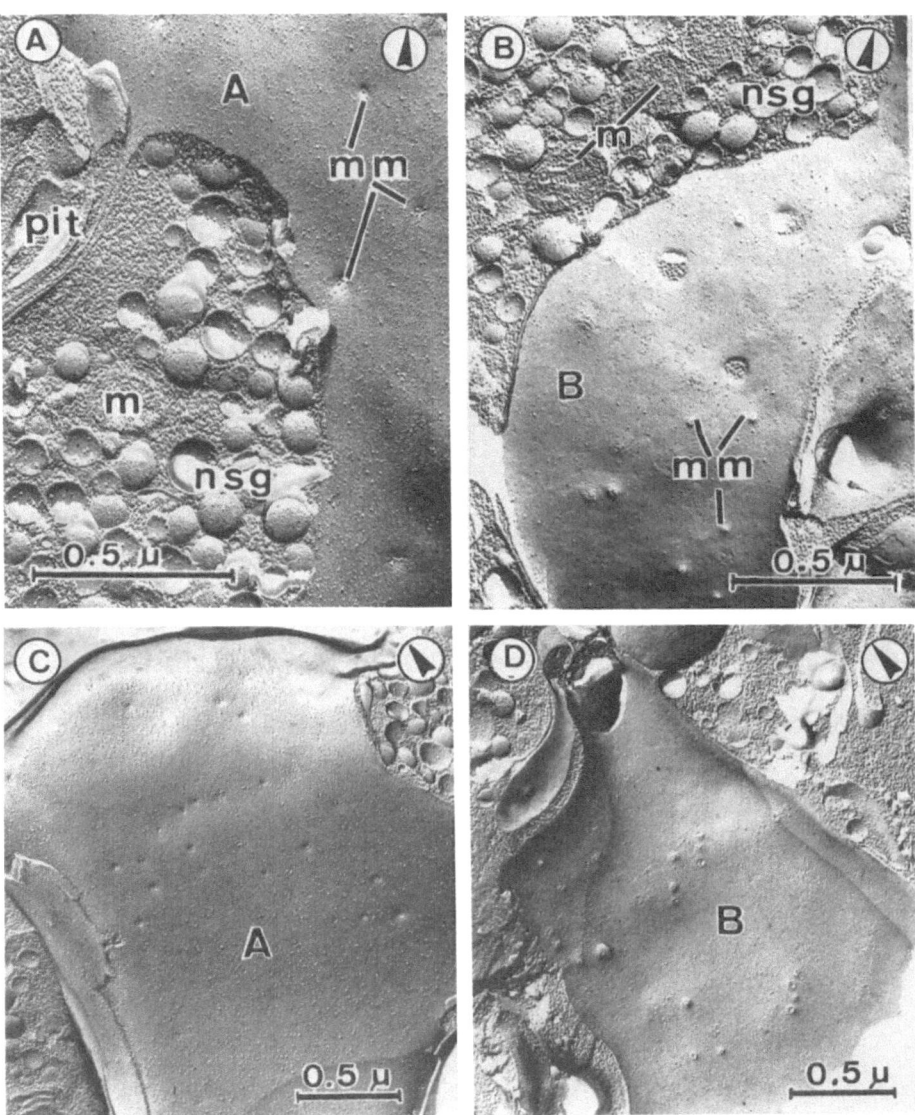

Fig. 1 A—D. Freeze-fracture replicas of stimulated neurosecretory nerve terminals. Isolated neurohypophyses were fixed after 10 min of incubation in a high K, low Na medium (1 A, 1 B), or following 7 min at 4° C in 0.2 M phosphate-buffered saccharose solution (1 C, 1 D). A and B refer also to membrane fracture-faces respectively (see text). The fractures run through part of the plasma membranes, and through cytoplasm, therein exposing mitochondria (m) and neurosecretory granules (nsg). Membrane modulations (mm) appear as pits of variable depth on the A-faces, and as protuberances on the B-faces. Note that some protuberances are crater-like. Glutaraldehyde fixation. Encircled arrowheads indicate orientation of shadow casting. Primary magnification 20000 ×

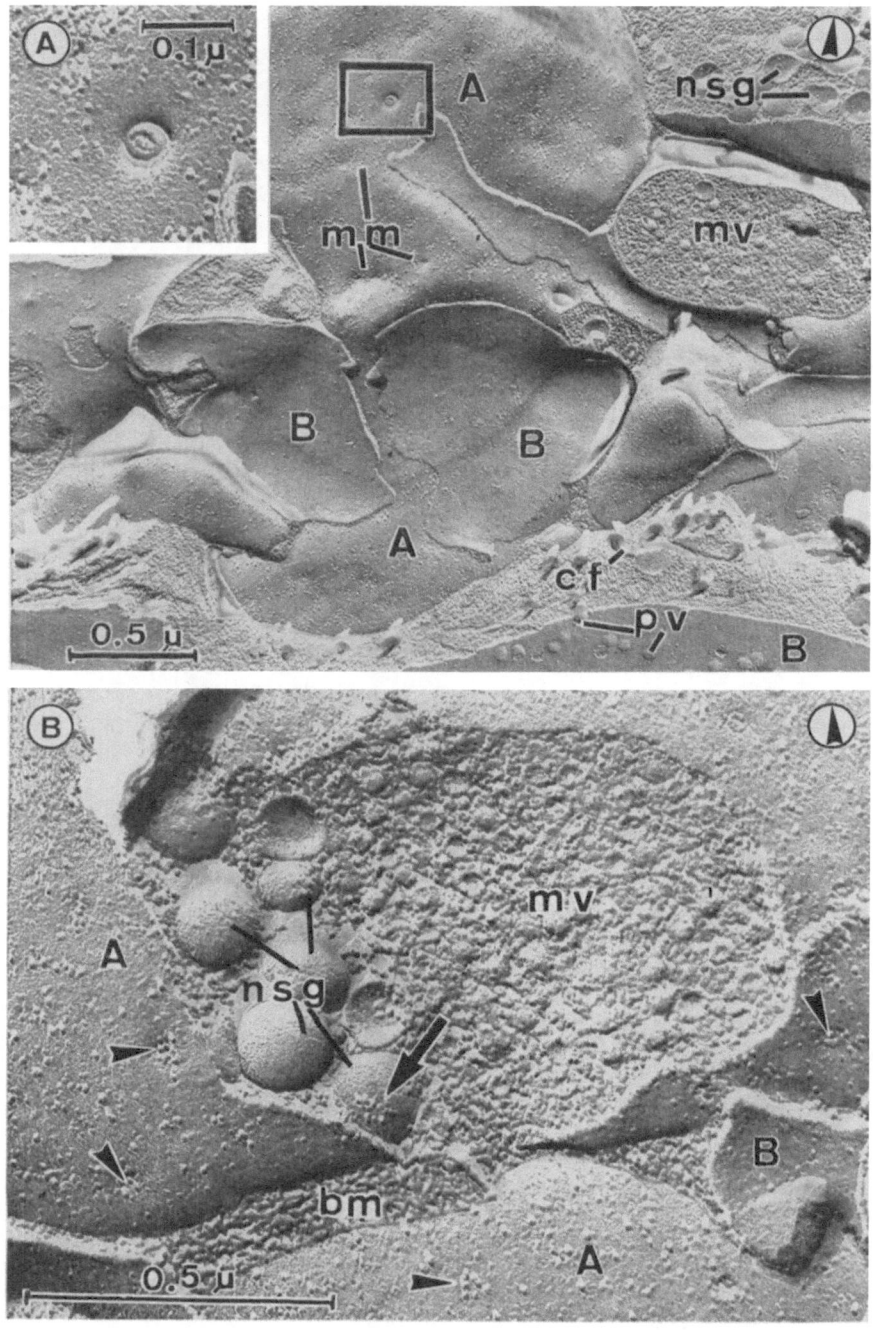

Fig. 2 A and B (Legend see p. 35)

limiting membrane may fuse during exocytosis with the particles located on the plasma membrane. Particles present on fracture faces probably represent protein molecules which penetrate into, or even traverse, the membrane. The particle aggregates seen in neurosecretory granule and plasma membranes thus represent an orderly arrangement of proteins within the lipid matrix of the membrane. If particles which have aggregated at one pole of a neurosecretory granule were to fit exactly onto a complementary array of membrane-bound particles associated with the plasma membrane, it is possible that ions and small molecules might diffuse through such a membrane apposition from the interior of the granule to the extra-cellular space, or *vice-versa*.

In this study, a high density of membrane modulations was found in actively secreting neurosecretory endings. We are unable to decide whether they correspond to early stages of exocytosis, ones in which neurosecretory granules have fused with the plasma membrane, and are open to the extra-cellular space through a narrow channel (Douglas et al., 1971a; Krisch et al., 1972), or to micropinocytotic activity. Assuming that endocytosis following exocytosis results solely in the formation of microvesicles, Douglas et al. (1971a) have estimated that endocytosis may outnumber exocytosis up to 20 times. Some further evidence showing that endocytosis in the rat neurohypophysis is secretion-dependent has been recently obtained. Nordmann et al. (1974) have shown that actively secreting neurohypophyses retain (following thorough washing of the extra-cellular spaces) more radioactive inulin, mannitol or albumin than do unstimulated controls. This extra uptake of extra-cellular tracer substance was shown not to be dependent on membrane depolarization alone, since it was not seen in neurohypophyses depolarized in presence of manganese ions of D 600 (a methoxy-derivative of verapamil which powerfully reduces the calcium permeability of excitable cells) at concentrations which abolish the secretory response (Dreifuss et al., 1973).

Maybe because the exo-endocytotic process is slowed at low temperature, particularly valuable information was obtained from neurohypophyses stimulated by cold. The stimulatory effect of cold on neurohypophysial hormone secretion is well established (Douglas and Ishida, 1965), but it has been questioned whether lowering the temperature causes secretion by exocytosis, because cold-induced secretion occurs also when neurohypophyses are kept in a Ca-free solution. We have, however, seen images of exocytosis in cold-stimulated preparations viewed by transmission electron microscopy. We thus believe that one likely interpretation of the independence of cold-induced hormone secretion on extra-cellular

---

Fig. 2A and B. Freeze-fracture replicas of cold stimulated neurohypophyses. *Upper figure:* Neuro-vascular contact zone characterized by a neurosecretory nerve ending abutting an extracellular space filled with collagen fibrils (cf), and the B-face of an endothelial membrane displaying pinocytotic activity (pv). Numerous membrane modulations (mm) are present on the exposed A-face of the membrane of the neurosecretory nerve terminal, as well as one larger circular opening, which is illustrated at higher magnification in the inset. *Lower figure:* Neurosecretory granules (nsg) and microvesicles (mv) in nerve terminal. Note the presence of particle aggregations (arrowheads) on the A-face of the plasma membrane, and an annulus of particles (arrow) bound to the inner membrane leaflet (B-face) of a neurosecretory granule. bm, basement membrane. Glutaraldehyde fixation. Encircled arrowheads indicate orientation of shadow casting. Primary magnifications A) 20000 ×, B) 40000 ×

calcium is that low temperature may stimulate exocytosis by causing a redistribution of intra-cellular calcium.

In summary, the freeze-fracture data presented here, as well as others published recently (Dempsey et al., 1973; Dreifuss et al., 1973), indicate that hormone release from actively secreting neurohypophyses is accompanied by membrane phenomena which would be unnecessary if secretion occurred by simple diffusion of hormone molecules through the plasma membrane; rather, they strongly favour the view that hormones (and neurophysins) contained within the neurosecretory granules are expelled to the extra-cellular space in an exo-endocytotic process.

Acknowledgments. This work was supported by Swiss National Science Foundation grants 3.133.69, 3.134.69 and 3.712.72. The skilful assistance of Miss C. Berger in preparing the replicas is greatfully acknowledged.

References

Branton, D.: Fracture faces of frozen membranes. Proc. nat. Acad. Sci. (Wash.) **55**, 1048—1056 (1966).

Bunt, A. H.: Formation of coated and "synaptic" vesicles within neurosecretory axon terminals of the crustacean sinus gland. J. Ultrastruct. Res. **28**, 411—421 (1969).

Dempsey, G. P., Bullivant, S., Watkins, W. B.: Ultrastructure of the rat posterior pituitary gland and evidence of hormone release by exocytosis as revealed by freeze-fracturing. Z. Zellforsch., in press.

Douglas, W. W., Ishida, A.: The stimulant effect of cold on vasopressin release from the neurohypophysis in vitro. J. Physiol. (Lond.) **179**, 185—191 (1965).

Douglas, W. W., Nagasawa, J., Schulz, R.: Electron microscopic studies on the mechanism of secretion of posterior pituitary hormones and significance of microvesicles ("synaptic vesicles") evidence of secretion by exocytosis and formation of microvesicles as a byproduct of this process. In: Subcellular Organization and Function in Endocrine Tissues. Memoirs of the Society for Endocrinology, No. 19 (H. Heller, K. Lederis, Eds.), p. 353—377. Cambridge: University Press 1971 a.

Douglas, W. W., Nagasawa, J., Schulz, R.: Coated microvesicles in neurosecretory terminals of posterior pituitary glands shed their coats to become smooth "synaptic" vesicles. Nature (Lond.) **232**, 340—341 (1971 b).

Dreifuss, J. J., Akert, K., Sandri, C., Moor, H.: The fine structure of freeze-fractured neurosecretory nerve endings in the neurohypophysis. Brain Res., in press.

Dreifuss, J. J., Grau, J. D., Bianchi, R. E.: Antagonism between Ca and Na ions at neurohypophysial nerve terminals. Experientia (Basel) **27**, 1295—1296 (1971).

Dreifuss, J. J., Grau, J. D., Nordmann, J. J.: Effects on the isolated neurohypophysis of agents which affect the membrane permeability to calcium. J. Physiol. (Lond.) **231**, 96—98 P (1973).

Krisch, B., Becker, K., Bargmann, W.: Exocytose am Hinterlappen der Hypophyse. Z. Zellforsch. **123**, 47—54 (1972).

Nagasawa, J., Douglas, W. W., Schulz, R.: Micropinocytotic origin of coated and smooth microvesicles ("synaptic vesicles") in neurosecretory terminals of posterior pituitary glands demonstrated by incorporation of horseradish peroxidase. Nature (Lond.) **232**, 341—342 (1971).

Nordmann, J. J., Dreifuss, J. J., Ravazzola, M., Malaisse-Lagae, F., Orci, L.: Secretion-dependent endocytosis in the rat neurohypophysis. Submitted for publication.

Norman, T. C.: The mechanism of hormone release from neurosecretory axon endings in the insect *Calliphora erythrocephala*. In: Aspects of Neuroendocrinology (W. Bargmann, B. Scharrer, Eds.), p. 30—42. Berlin-Heidelberg-New York: Springer 1970.

Norman, T. C., Duve, H.: Experimentally induced release of a neurohormone influencing hemolymph trehalose level in *Calliphora erythrocephala* (Diptera). Gen. comp. Endocr. **12**, 449—459 (1969).

Pfenninger, K., Akert, K., Moor, H., Sandri, C.: The fine structure of freeze-fractured pre-synaptic membranes. J. Neurocytol. 1, 129—149 (1972).

Smith, U.: The origin of small vesicles in neurosecretory axons. Tissue and Cell **2**, 427—433 (1970).

Ascending Neurosecretory Pathways of the Peptidergic Type

G. STERBA

Department of Cell Biology and Regulation, Section Biowissenschaften of the Karl-Marx-University, Leipzig (GDR)

In recent years various actions of posterior lobe hormones on the central nervous system have been described: changes in the EEG of rabbits by the administration of oxytocin and vasopressin (Faure et al., 1959; Faure et al., 1960); increase in the readiness of motor reaction and changes in the EEG by intravenous injection of oxytocin in rats (Sterba, 1966; Schäker et al., 1966); changes in the reaction time — interval between an acoustic stimulation and the conditioned motor response for its elimination—in rats; injected oxytocin shortens, and injected vasopressin extends, the reaction time (Schwarzberg, 1968; Schwarzberg and Unger, 1970); vasopressin or related peptides of the neural lobe affect the retention of avoidance behaviour in such a way that there is a long-term preservation of the conditioned responses (De Wied and Bohus, 1966; Bohus, 1971; Bohus et al., 1972). Lysine vasopressin and ACTH restored the impaired avoidance reaction of hypophysectomized rats. ACTH-analogues restore fear motivation while vasopressin is involved in the consolidation of adversely motivated learning processes (De Wied, 1965, 1966; Bohus and De Wied, 1966; Bohus et al., 1973). Under *in vitro* conditions oxytocin increases the glucose uptake by brain cell suspensions by more than 20% (Wolf and Sterba, in press).

These observations suggest that the hormones of the peptidergic neurosecretory nuclei of the hypothalamus not only influence extracerebral peripheral sites of action but also have intracerebral functions, i.e. they take part in information processing in the central nervous system in some way. This hypothesis is based on the presumption that the peptide hormones of the oxytocin type reach target sites in the central nervous system either unchanged or in a modified form. For this to occur there are three possibilities:

1. Neurohormones released in the neurohypophysis might reach their target sites in the central nervous system through the vascular system (blood pathway). A variant of this pathway would occur if the hormones were to be transported from the vascular system via the plexus into the cerebrospinal fluid and then reach their target sites via the c.s.f.

2. From liquor-contacting neurons of the nuclear areas mentioned, neurohormones could be discharged into the c.s.f. and reach target sites near the ventricle via the c.s.f. (liquor pathway).

3. Neurosecretory axons of the Nucleus supraopticus and N. paraventricularis or N. preopticus might, within the hypothalamus, establish relations with other nuclear areas or penetrate into other regions of the brain as extrahypothalamic pathways (nervous or direct pathways).

In the last few years we have studied the morphology of the possible pathways in our laboratory and I should like to report our first findings.

In a large number of older descriptions of the peptidergic neurosecretory system of vertebrates we already find indications of extrahypothalamic neuro- secretory pathways and their target sites. Scharrer (1951) observed an extra- hypothalamic tract to the epithalamus in a garter snake *(Thamnophis)*. Legait and Barry (1954—1961) conducted a great number of tests to study these questions. The fact that a wider attention was not paid to these studies was primarily due to an insufficient specificity and sensitivity of the staining techniques. None of the authors could prove with adequate reliability that the nerve fibres demonstrable outside the hypothalamus by means of the basic component of the chrome-alum- haematoxylin-phloxin method according to Gomori-Bargmann (CAH) or the aldehyde-fuchsin method according to Gabe (AF) actually were part of the

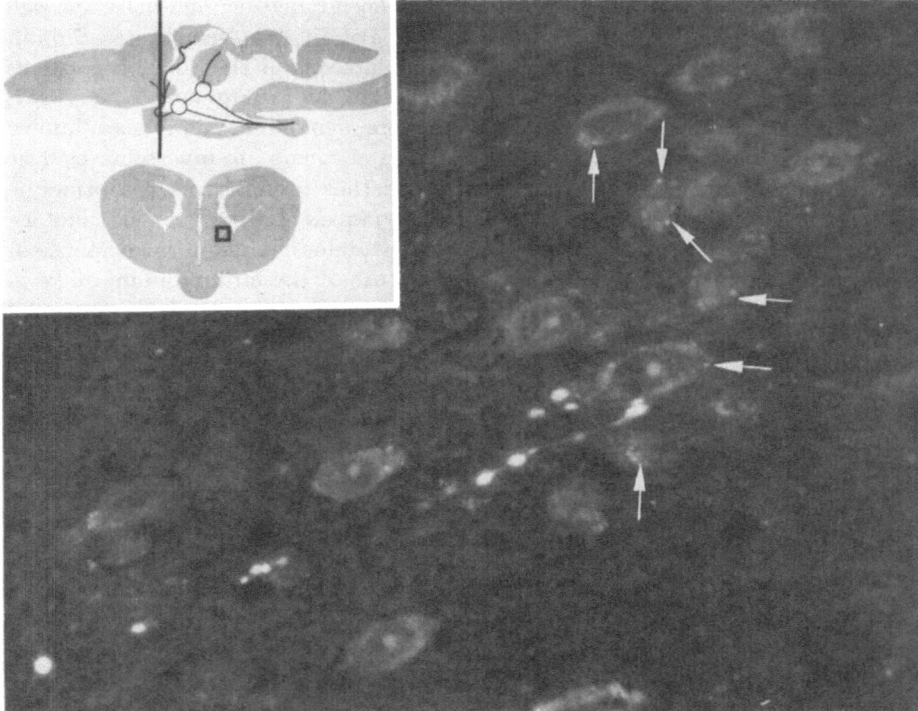

Fig. 1. Septal nucleus of a turtle *(Clemys caspica)* with a neurosecretory fibre. The fluorescent spots at the surface of the cell bodies (denoted by arrows) probably are terminals of the pep- tidergic type. The inset indicates the peptidergic pathways in turtles and the position of the section. Pseudoisocyanine; × 800

peptidergic hypothalamic system. Not until new methods such as the fluorescence techniques and electron-microscopic studies in connection with ultrahistochemical methods were developed was an improved analysis of exohypothalamic peptidergic fibres possible (Figs. 1 and 2). Studies carried out by my co-workers with the help of these more recent methods on various vertebrates were able, as a first result, to confirm the statements made earlier by other authors for lampreys, salamanders, frogs, reptiles (Fig. 1) and mammals.

The extrahypothalamic axons of peptidergic neurons which can be demonstrated by means of light and fluorescence microscopy can also be demonstrated by means of the electron microscope. In regions where peptidergic fibres could be demonstrated by means of the light microscope aminergic axons also occurred, and therefore care should be taken in the evaluation of fibre sections with vesicles. It is essential that statistical evaluations of granule size and analyses of the fine structure as used in the eminentia mediana or neurohypophysis for the classification of granule types should be supplemented by ultrahistochemical methods. The following techniques are suitable (Fig. 2).

The detection of extrahypothalamic fibres and of their target sites poses a question as to how the terminals of these axons are organized and whether there are contact relations with cellular elements in the targets. Synaptoid contacts between peptidergic neurosecretory fibres and ependymal or glial cells are well known in the infundibulum and in the neural lobe of different vertebrates. Similar contacts between peptidergic fibres and glandular cells of the adenohypophysis have been described, especially in the intermediate lobe. Bargmann et al. (1967) termed such contacts "peptidergic". Furthermore, synaptoid contacts are known between peptidergic fibres and other cellular elements in invertebrates (see Scharrer and Weitzman, 1970). The question whether or not axons of peptidergic neurons form axo-dendritic or axo-somatic synapses received no satisfactory answers till recently. In publications we find only an indication of the existence of such synapses. In their study on the fine structure of the infundibulum of *Rana catesbeiana*, Oota and Kobayashi (1963a, b) described axo-dendritic synapses between neurosecretory axons and non-secretory fibres.

In some of our material we have been able to demonstrate by fluorescence microscopy that peptidergic neurosecretory fibres terminate with small knobs at the perikarya of the neurons in the target regions, e.g. in the septum region of the tortoise *Clemmys caspica* (Fig. 1).

After staining with CAH or AF, Barry (1954) observed similar knobs in different target sites of extrahypothalamic pathways in bats and assumed that these were »Synapses neurosécrétoires« of the axo-somatic type. Although Barry could not furnish satisfactory proof for this statement, we must admire his exact observation and his courageous interpretation of the observed phenomena.

Terminals and their synaptic connexions can conclusively only be analysed by means of the electron microscope. Unfortunately, it is a difficult and time consuming task to search for terminals of peptidergic neurosecretory fibres electron microscopically and at the same time characterise them ultrahistochemically. Until now my co-workers succeeded in finding such terminals in a few cases only. Nevertheless, we can say already today that peptidergic neurosecretory neurons indeed form contact points with other neurons.

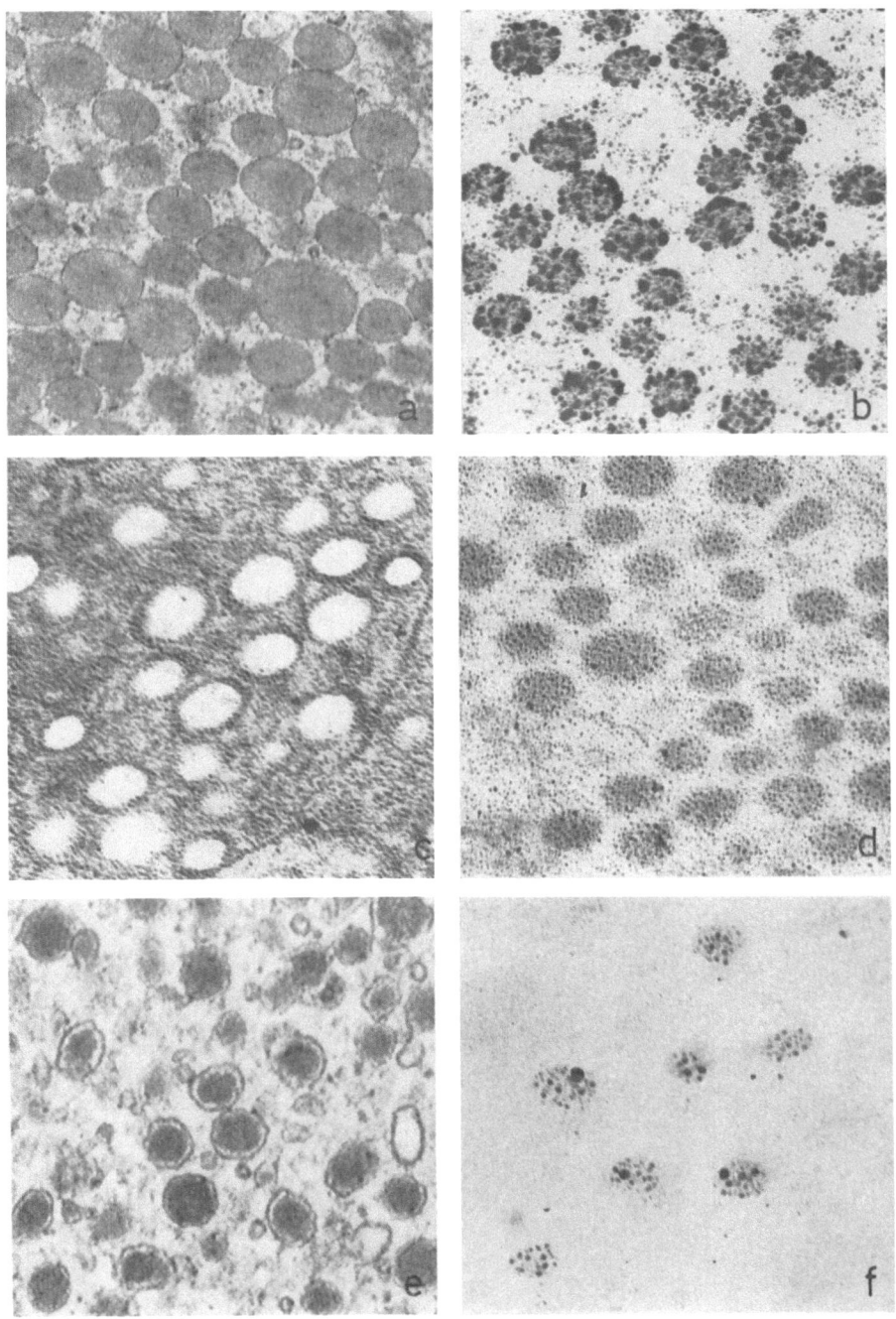

Fig. 2. (a) Neurophysin-containing granules: normal. (b) Neurophysin-containing granules: silver-methenamine technique according to Swift, 1968 (modified). (c) Neurophysin-containing granules: only oxidized with potassium permanganate. (d) Neurophysin-containing granules: oxidation and following treatment with barium chloride according to Blinzinger and Matussek, 1966 (modified). (e) Catecholamine-containing granules: normal. (f) Catecholamine-containing granules: glutaraldehyde-silver technique according to Cannata et al., 1968

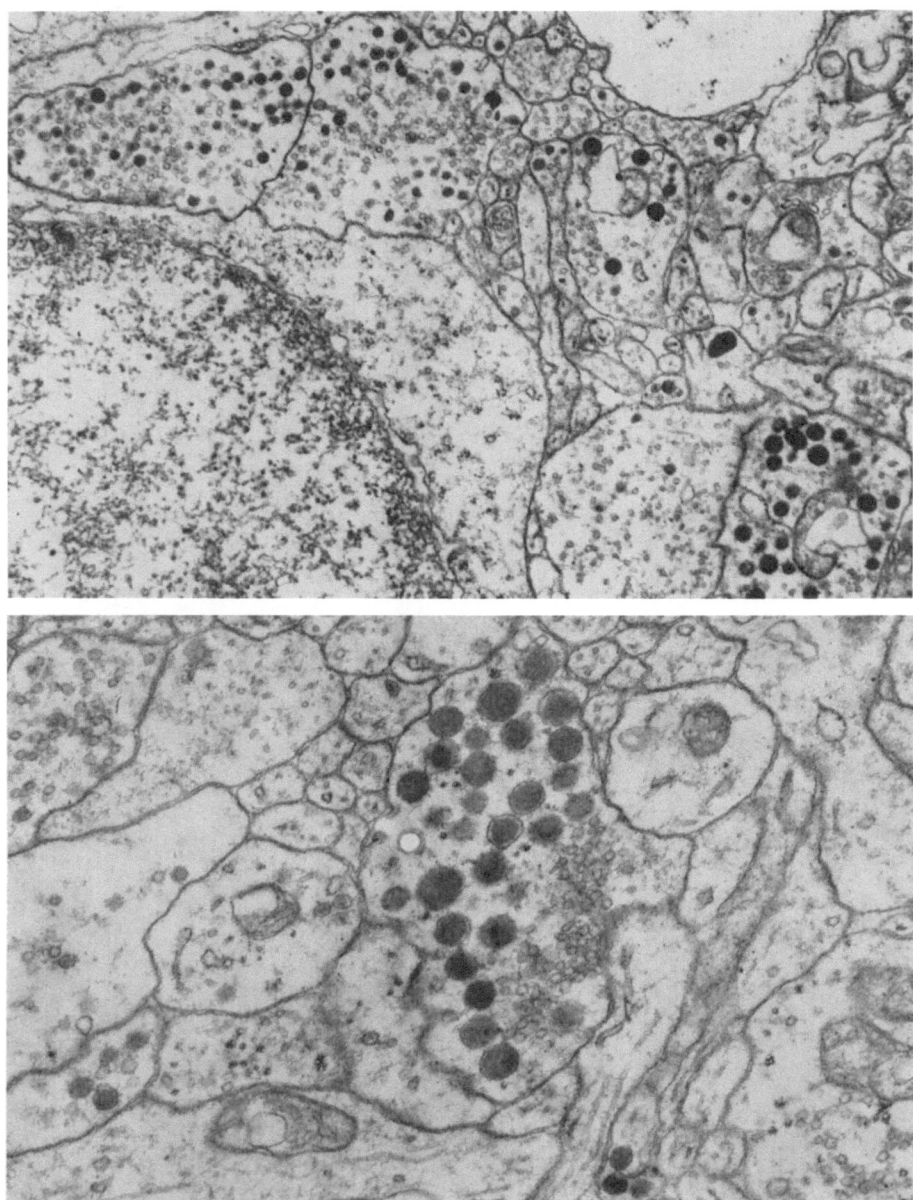

Fig. 3. Neurosecretory fibres in the tectal region of a salamander *(Pleurodeles waltli)*. Above:
Section showing two types of fibre. In the upper left corner fibres with granules 90 nm in
diameter; in the lower right corner a fibre with granules 170 nm in diameter; × 16 000. Below:
Terminal of a peptidergic axon demonstrating features characteristic of a synapse. In addition
to microvesicles, granules, 170—180 nm in diameter, are present: × 35 000

The synapses are distinguished by clouds of synaptic vesicles (30—50 nm) in front of the slightly thickened presynaptic membrane, mitochondria and neurosecretory vesicles of the peptidergic type. The synaptic cleft is narrow and the postsynaptic membrane is slightly thickened (Fig. 3).

The electron-microscopic proof of synapses with vesicles of the peptidergic type does not however give any indication as to the manner of transmission at these contact points. One may postulate that the transmission is effected by known transmitter substances and that the locally released peptide hormones cause regional changes in the milieu, for example by changes in the permeability of neuronal membranes. Calculations regarding the local hormone concentration at such terminals of extrahypothalamic axons made by my co-worker Wolf have shown that these may be of the order of some units/ml and, therefore, must be rated higher than the concentrations detected in the blood (μU/ml). These calculations were based on the assumption that the same amount of hormone can be released from an extrahypothalamic terminal as from a terminal in the neurohypophysis. Here, mention should be made of the fact that the classical transmitter substances also show a higher concentration in the region of the synaptic cleft than in blood.

In this connection, attention should be focussed on an interesting observation made by my co-worker Weiss. In electron microscopic studies on the neural relations between the Nucleus praeopticus (NPO) and the Nucleus lateralis tuberis (NLT) in the trout he showed that axons from the NPO pass through the NLT and make contact with the perikarya of the NLT (see also Stutinsky, this volume p. 15). In such contact zones, the myelin sheaths of these axons are reduced and there is a distinct indication of a local exocytosis. Similar conditions are well known to exist in invertebrates (see Scharrer and Weitzman, 1970). There, areas of this kind are denoted as synaptoid structures and considered as sites of hormone release.

The results obtained in the study of extrahypothalamic pathways cannot yet be finally evaluated, but some generalizations may be attempted: In all vertebrates studied so far, from the primitive lampreys to the mammals, extrahypothalamic axons of the magno-cellular hypothalamic nuclei reach two targets—the septal region and the habenular region (Table 1). They follow known fibre connections of the limbic system. Furthermore, in some other species extrahypothalamic peptidergic neurosecretory pathways have been observed to terminate in limbic structures including the olfactory apparatus or in the Formatio reticularis mesencephali closely associated with the latter (Fig. 4).

The limbic system belongs to the phylogenetically old systems of the vertebrate brain; it shows a distinctly progressive development in mammals. It performs the function of a visceral centre and in addition it plays an important role in emotional reactions (Papez, 1937) such as aggressiveness, rage, placidity and feelings of sexual urge. Not only all sensory modalities but also information of the neuroendocrine hypothalamus gain access to this system (Donovan, 1973). In this system, the amygdaloid nuclei which are connected with the ventral septum, the rostral and ventromedial hypothalamus, the Cortex piriformis, regions of the neocortex and other centres are of a central importance (Goddard, 1964). Efferents of the limbic system to the magno-cellular nuclear regions of the hypothalamus

Table 1. Instances of peptidergic fibres in different regions of the brain of vertebrates (data published up to 1972)

	Cyclostomata	Selachii	Teleostei	Urodela	Anura	Reptilia	Aves	Mammalia	Total
Number of species investigated	3	1	5 (7)	7 (9)	6 (8)	17	5	17 (18)	61 (68)
Telencephalon	1		1	2	4			6	14
lobus olfact.	1			1		1			3
corpus striatum	1								1
hippocampus					3			3	6
septum			2	3	6	5	7	3	26
amygdaloid nuclei								10	10
lamina terminalis							1	9	10
subfornical organ				5	7	10	6	8	36
paraphysis				1	1	10			12
Diencephalon			1		1	1		1	4
thalamus				1					1
habenular region	1		4	3	5	3	5	3	24
epiphysis		1			1				2
subcommissural org.	1		1	2		4			8
mamillary body									0
Mesencephalon	1			1					2
tectum	1			1					2
tegmentum	2			1					3
Cerebellum							4		4
Medulla oblongata	3			1					4

were demonstrated by electrophysiological means some years ago, and thus it was proved that electrical stimulation of the anterior limbic region especially the medial amygdaloid nucleus of the cat (Shealey and Peele, 1957) and the cingulate gyrus of the cat (Beyer et al., 1961) evokes oxytocin release in the neurohypophysis. Recently Losev et al. (1971) reported on probable afferents to the limbic system from the magno-cellular nuclear regions. After stimulating the N. paraventricularis and N. supraopticus in rabbits, they observed a higher impulse activity in the dorsal hippocampus and in the septal region. The same effect was observed after microinjection of oxytocin into the above-mentioned areas. Morphologically, afferents to these limbic centres have not yet been traced. In my view these extra-hypothalamic neurosecretory fibres and their terminals represent such afferents.

This interpretation of the extrahypothalamic peptidergic connections gives the morphological facts a physiological significance which justifies further studies. The assumption that oxytocin or related hormones take part in the modulation of central nervous processes is corroborated by the morphological proof of the existence of efferent axons to various switch points of the limbic system, and also suggests that, among other things, the neurohormones may take part in the

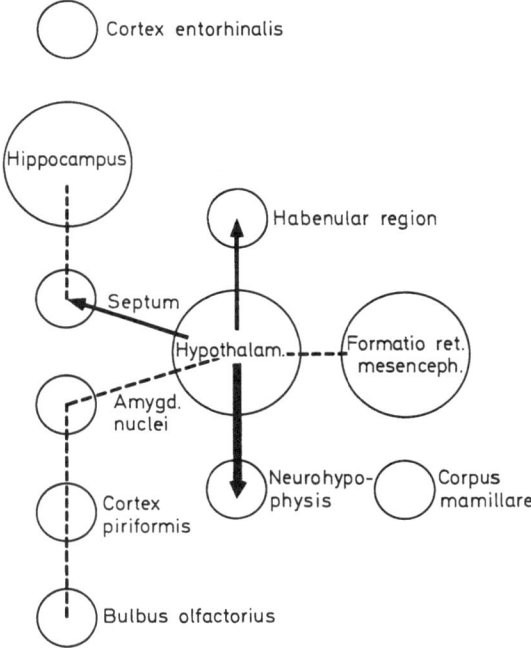

Fig. 4. The peptidergic efferents of the hypothalamic magnocellular nuclei. Besides the descending hypothalamo-hypophysial tract, ascending pathways are present which terminate in different structures of the limbic system. ——— pathways found in all vertebrates. - - - - - - pathways observed in several species only

generation of emotions. Assuming that a signal input to the neurosecretory nuclear area leads to a simultaneous hormone release in the neurohypophysis and in the limbic system, we could expect that an increase of the hormone level in the blood is correlated with changes in activity in the limbic system, for example, changes in the emotional condition. Various studies, for example those conducted by Kihlström and Dannings (1972) have shown in the domestic fowl and the pigeon that neurohormones influence the sexual behaviour in this direction. Such a consideration could in addition give clues why, in the case of administration of neurohormones into the blood, changes in the emotional condition and other central nervous phenomena can be observed.

Summary

1. Most of the axons of the hypothalamic magno-cellular nuclear areas form the well known neurosecretory pathway and terminate in the neurohypophysis. A smaller number of peptidergic secretory axons leave the hypothalamus and terminate at various structures of the limbic system. In many vertebrates, the existence of such extrahypothalamic fibres leading to the septal region and to the habenular region have been demonstrated.

2. The terminals of the peptidergic efferents to the limbic system form contacts with other neurons. It may be assumed that neurohormones are released at the terminals.

3. The hypothalamo-limbic pathway should be considered as an integral subsystem of the main peptidergic neurosecretory system.

4. It is conceivable that neurohormones influence various central nervous processes by means of this subsystem and ensure an adjustment of the emotional condition which is in correlation with the hormone release from the neurohypophysis.

References

Bargmann, W., Lindner, E., Andres, K. H.: Über Synapsen an endokrinen Epithelzellen und die Definition sekretorischer Neurone. Untersuchungen am Zwischenlappen der Katzenhypophyse. Z. Zellforsch. 77, 282—298 (1967).

Barry, J.: Neurocrinie et synapses «neurosécrétoires». Arch. Anat. micr. Morph. exp. 43, 310—320 (1954).

Barry, J.: Recherches morphologiques et expérimentales sur la glande diencéphalique et l'appareil hypothalamo-hypophysaire. Ann. Sci. Univ. Besançon, Zool. Physiol. Sér., 2, 3—133 (1961).

Beyer, C. F., Anguiano, G. L., Mena, F. J.: Oxytocin release in response to stimulation of cingulate gyrus. Amer. J. Physiol. 200, 625—627 (1961).

Blinzinger, K., Matussek, N.: Die Dünnschnittkontrastierung mittels Bariumchlorid: Eine Methode für den topochemischen Nachweis von Stoffen mit unvollständig veresterten Schwefelsäuregruppen im submikroskopischen Bereich. Histochemie 6, 173—184 (1966).

Bohus, B.: Effect of hypophysial peptides on memory functions in rat. In: Biology of memory (G. Adam, Ed.), p. 93. Proc. Symp. Tihany 1969. Budapest: Akadémiai Kiadó 1971.

Bohus, B., Ader, R., De Wied, D.: Effects of vasopressin on active and passive avoidance behavior. Hormones and Behavior 3, 191 (1972).

Bohus, B., De Wied, D.: Inhibitory and facilitatory effect of two related peptides on extinction of avoidance behavior. Science 153, 318—320 (1966).

Bohus, B., Gispen, W. H., De Wied, D.: Effects of lysine vasopressin and ACTH $_{4-10}$ on conditioned avoidance behavior of hypophysectomized rats. Neuroendocrinology 11, 137—143 (1973).

Cannata, M. A., Chiocchio, S.-R., Tramezzani, J. H.: Specificity of the glutaraldehyde silver technique for catecholamines and related compounds. Histochemie 12, 253—264 (1968).

De Wied, D.: The influence of the posterior and intermediate lobe of the pituitary and pituitary peptides on the maintenance of a conditioned avoidance response in rats. Int. J. Neuropharmacol. 4, 157—167 (1965).

De Wied, D.: Inhibitory effect of ACTH and related peptides on extinction of conditioned avoidance behavior in rat. Proc. Soc. exp. Biol. (N.Y.) 122, 28—32 (1966).

De Wied, D., Bohus, B.: Long term and short term effects on retention of a conditioned avoidance response in rats by treatment with long acting pitressin and α-MSH. Nature (Lond.) 212, 1484—1486 (1966).

Donovan, B.: Neuroendokrinologie der Säugetiere. Stuttgart: Thieme 1973.

Faure, J., Loiseau, P., Friconneau, C.: Influence de l'oxytocine sur l'électroencéphalogramme du lapin. Rev. neurol. 101, 302—308 (1959).

Faure, J., Loiseau, P., Vincent, D.: Influence de l'hormone antidiurétique (A.D.H.) sur l'électroencéphalogramme du lapin éveillé et libre. Rev. neurol. 102, 333—338 (1960).

Goddard, G. V.: Functions of the amygdala. Psychol. Bull. 62, 89—109 (1964).

Kihlström, J. E., Dannings, J.: Neurohypophysial hormones and sexual behavior in males of the domestic fowl (Gallus domesticus L.) and the pigeon (Columba livia Gmel.). Gen. comp. Endocr. 18, 115—120 (1972).

Legait, H.: Les voies extra-hypothalamo-neurohypophysaires de la eurosécrétion diencephalique dans la série des vertébrés. In: 2. Internat. Symposion über Neurosekretion, Lund, p. 42—51. Berlin-Göttingen-Heidelberg: Springer 1958.

Legait, H., Legait, E.: Mise en évidence de voies neurosécrétoires extra-hypothalamo-hypophysaires chez quelques Batraciens et Reptiles. C. R. Soc. Biol. (Paris) 150, 1429—1431 (1956).

Legait, H., Legait, E.: Relations entre les noyaux hypothalamiques neurosécrétoires et les régions septale et habénulaire chez quelques Oiseaux. Acta neuroveg. (Wien) 17, 143—147 (1957).

Losev, N. A., Tomilina, J. V., Borodkin, Y. S.: Analysis of interrelations between the anterior hypothalamus and some limbic structures (in Russ.). Fiziol. Zh. (Mosk.) 57, 760—797 (1971).

Oota, Y., Kobayashi, H.: Synapses between neurosecretory axons and the processes of non-neurosecretory neurons (preliminary report). Zool. Magazin 72, 35—39 (1963).

Oota, Y., Kobayashi, H.: Fine structure of the median eminence and the pars nervosa of the bullfrog, Rana catesbeiana. Z. Zellforsch. 60, 667—687 (1963).

Papez, J. W.: A proposed mechanism of emotion. Arch. Neurol. Psychiat. (Chic.) 38, 725—743 (1937).

Schäker, W., Klingberg, F., Sterba, G., Pickenhain, L.: Der Einfluß von Oxytocin auf zentralnervöse Funktionen bei der Ratte im chronischen Experiment. Pflügers Arch. ges. Physiol. 288, 322—351 (1966).

Scharrer, E.: Neurosecretion. 10. A relationship between the paraphysis and the paraventricular nucleus in the garter snake (Thamnophis sp.). Biol. Bull. 101, 106—113 (1951).

Scharrer, B., Weitzman, M.: Current problems in invertebrate neurosecretion. In: Aspects of neuroendocrinology (W. Bargmann, B. Scharrer, Ed.), p. 1—23. Berlin-Heidelberg-New York: Springer 1970.

Schwarzberg, H.: Untersuchungen über den Einfluß des Wasserentzuges auf das periphere und zentralnervöse Geschehen an Ratten. Acta biol. med. germ. 21, 23—49 (1968).

Schwarzberg, H., Unger, H.: Änderung der Reaktionszeit von Ratten nach Applikation von Vasopressin, Oxytocin und Na-Thioglykolat. Acta biol. med. germ. 24, 507—516 (1970).

Shealey, C. N., Peele, T. L.: Studies on amygdaloid nucleus of cat. J. Neurophysiol. 20, 125—139 (1957).

Sterba, G.: Zur cerebrospinalen Neurokrinie der Wirbeltiere. Verh. Dtsch. Zool. Ges. in Jena 1965. Zool. Anz. Suppl. 29, 393—440 (1966).

Swift, J. A.: The electron histochemistry of cystine-containing proteins in thin transverse sections of human hair. J. roy. micr. Soc. 88, 449—460 (1967).

Wolf, G., Sterba, G.: Effect of oxytocin on glucose uptake by brain tissue (in-vitro study). In press.

The Use of the Cobalt Chloride-Ammonium Sulfide Precipitation Technique for the Delineation of Invertebrate and Vertebrate Neurosecretory Systems

CAROL ANN MASON* and RICHARD S. NISHIOKA

Department of Zoology and its Cancer Research Laboratory, University of California, Berkeley (USA)

Since the mid-1960's, neurobiologists, especially those working on invertebrate preparations, have employed intracellular injection of dyes to elucidate the geometry of single neurons responsible for a particular neurophysiological process. Procion yellow was first successfully used for this purpose in conjunction with fluorescence microscopy (Stretton and Kravitz, 1968). The technology of dye injection has advanced considerably with the recent introduction of cobaltous chloride as a dye (Pitman et al., 1972). After filling neurons with cobalt, the preparation is immersed in a solution of ammonium sulfide. A black precipitate, cobaltous sulfide, is formed, and neurons are elegantly delineated when viewed in whole mount. Because cobaltous sulfide is electron dense, tissues can also be examined by electron microscopy, a major advantage of cobalt in comparison with procion yellow.

If the neurosecretory neuron is to be studied as a neuroendocrine unit, it would be useful to know the exact topography of neurosecretory cell groups, patterns of axonal branching and general dendritic morphology, and pathways of neurosecretory axons to areas associated with the neurosecretory complex in question. The conventional staining methods specific for neurosecretion have given incomplete information on these questions, since some neurosecretory neurons do not take up stain, and if certain regions of neurons are devoid of neurosecretion, those regions do not stain. In addition, if there are specific non-neurosecretory neurons involved in neuroendocrine regulation and associated with neurosecretory groups, staining would not delineate them. The cobalt technique provides data on all of these aspects, and although the technique alone does not demonstrate neurosecretion, it can support existing data obtained from staining methods and from physiological experimentation.

This paper will describe three methods by which neurons can be filled with cobalt and their application to several invertebrate and vertebrate neurosecretory systems.

---

* Present address: Department of Anatomy, The Medical School, University of Bristol, Bristol BS8 1TD, England.

A. Axonal Iontophoresis

Originally described by Iles and Mulloney (1970) for use with procion yellow, this method allows neuronal cell bodies and their processes to be filled with dye along the axons of a cut nerve. The tract or nerve containing axons of a particular group of cells is cut, and vaseline is carefully applied to the area and around the cut nerve, which serves as a "wick" (Fig. 1a). A drop of cobaltous chloride is placed on the cut end of the nerve and a current is applied for several hours, with the positive pole in the cobalt solution and the negative pole elsewhere in the preparation. Vaseline is then removed, and the preparation is rinsed in saline. Next, immersion of the preparation in a weak ammonium sulfide solution (0.5 ml 44% ammonium sulfide in 10 ml saline) precipitates the cobalt. Tissues are again rinsed in saline and fixed for conventional light microscopy to be examined in whole mount or in section, or for electron microscopy (see Section D).

Several precautions must be mentioned. The nerve must be cut with sharp scissors or a razor blade and never pinched with forceps, so that the axons do not collapse. Vaseline is most easily applied with a syringe and fine needle. The outer nerve membrane must be thoroughly dry when vaseline is applied; otherwise cobalt will leak and pass between the vaseline and nerve rather than move inside the axons. In the case of the insect system described below, the entire dissection is performed without addition of saline. In the vertebrate preparations tried, however, the greater part of the tissue was placed in a depression in the dissection dish, and saline was added into the depression after preparing the nerve wick. The molarity of the cobalt solution should approximate the osmotic concentration of the animal's blood, and should be made up fresh every week. Melted vaseline was always applied to cover the drop of cobalt to prevent evaporation.

Any source of current, either constant or pulsed, can be used, but current should be monitored throughout the experiment, since the resistance of the preparation will fluctuate. Current strengths used on the systems described varied between 10^{-7} and 10^{-6} amperes, passed for 3—8 h. Some preparations were set up without current; in these instances, the entire preparation was kept in the cold overnight or for one or two days. In the insect, this modification seemed to improve contrast and prevent extracellular leakage. The vaseline cover and exoskeleton of the insect prevented drying out and decay of the tissue, but vertebrate tissues may not be able to withstand such treatment.

Carnoy's fixative gave best results for viewing whole mounts. Tissues were dehydrated, cleared and stored in methyl benzoate or methyl salicylate. Preparations were stored in the dark to prevent fading of cobalt over a period of several months.

Axonal iontophoresis has been employed to elucidate some features of the brain-retrocerebral neuroendocrine complex of the locust *Schistocerca vaga* (Mason, 1973). Some of these results will be discussed again here.

It has been known that the nervi corporis cardiaci I (NCC I) carry the axons of the medial neurosecretory cells (MNC) from the brain to the corpora cardiaca. If one NCC I is cut and cobalt iontophoresed through the nerve toward the brain, the MNC in the pars intercerebralis of the protocerebrum will fill (Fig. 2a). Viewed from the anterior face of the brain, about 400 cells are visible. No extensive branch-

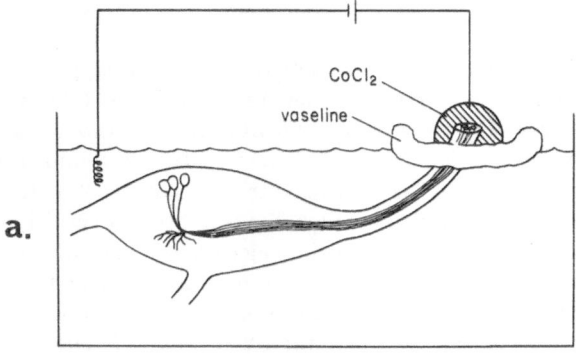

Axonal Iontophoresis ("Wick Technique")

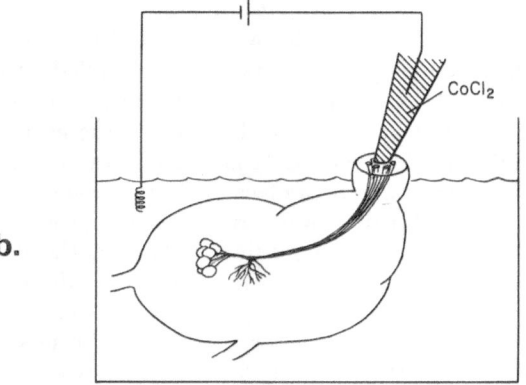

Suction-electrode Iontophoresis

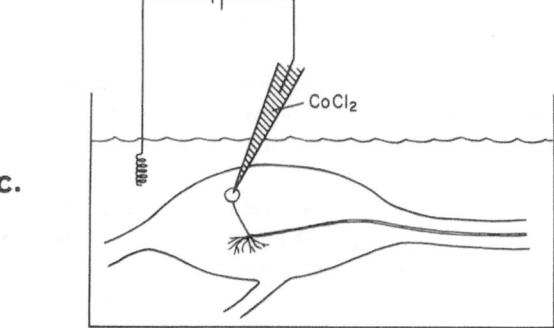

Single-cell (Microelectrode) Iontophoresis

Fig. 1 a—c. Three methods by which neurons can be filled with cobalt (see text)

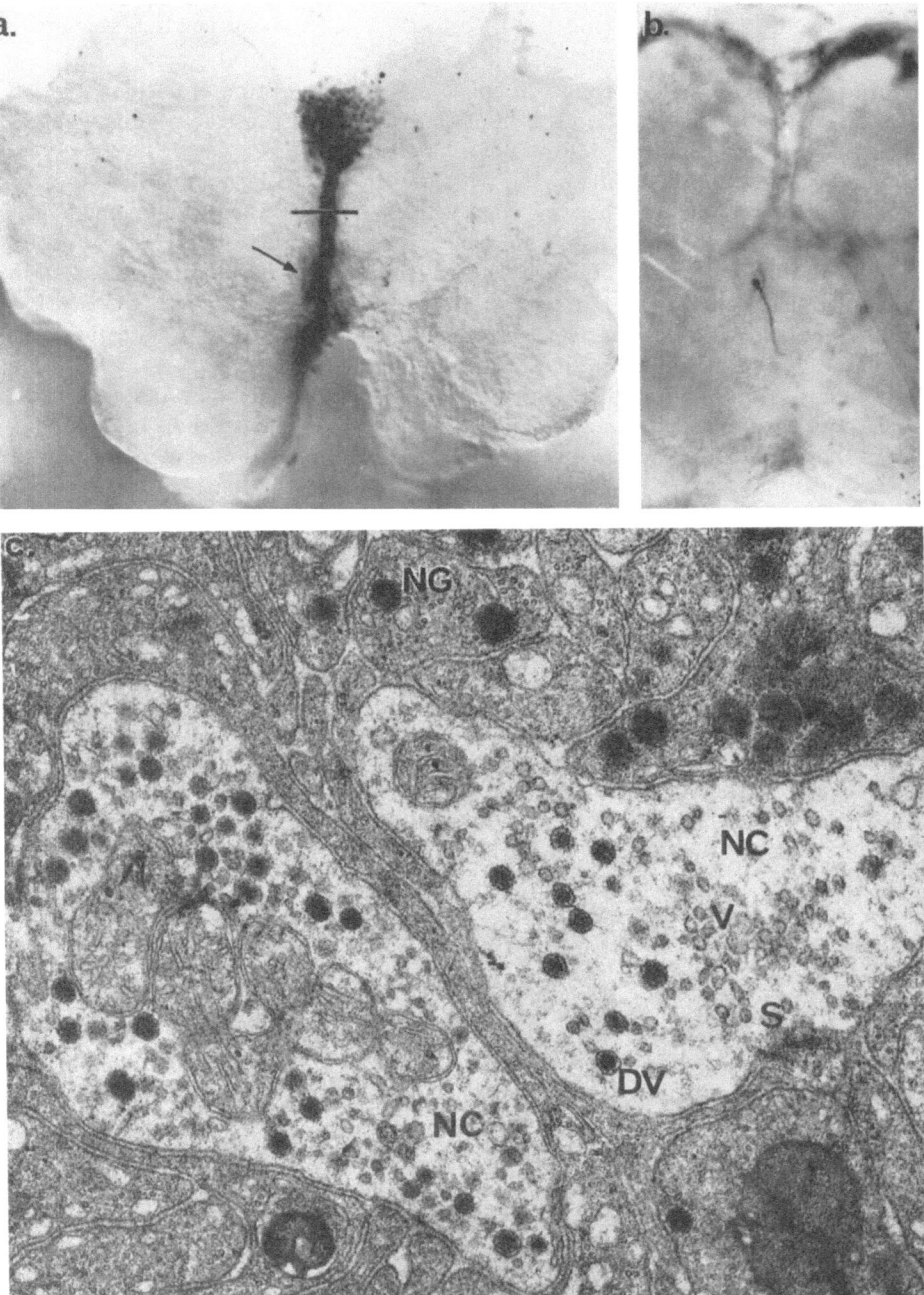

Fig. 2. (a) Medial neurosecretory cells in the pars intercerebralis of the locust *S. vaga* (anterior view), filled by axonal iontophoresis of the NCC I. Note loop (arrow) extending laterally from the axon tract. Line refers to plane of section in c. × 66. (b) A single medial neurosecretory cell filled with cobalt by microelectrode iontophoresis. Three fine branches projecting from the initial portion of the axon are in view. This cell is in the pars intercerebralis contralateral to the cells in a. × 75. (c) Electron micrograph of the medial neurosecretory cell axon tract which has been filled with cobalt by means of axonal iontophoresis (see a.). All profiles contain cobalt except for two (NC). Note preservation of neurosecretory granules (NG), dense core vesicles (DV), and electron-lucent vesicles (V). A possible synaptic thickening (S) is also seen. × 38 500

ing of neurons is seen along the axon tract, with the exception of a "loop" which occurs in many fills, about two-thirds of the way down the tract. Thus, general topography of this well-known group can be observed.

A second group of cells fills in the tritocerebrum (see Mason, 1973). Its axons are carried in the NCC I (otherwise they would not have filled), and some axons contact the axons of the MNC within the brain as well. The tritocerebral group does not take up conventional neurosecretory stains. This is the first indication in any insect that cells in the tritocerebrum are associated with the MNC, so that even if they prove to be non-neurosecretory neurons, they remain as candidates for neuronal units involved in neuroendocrine regulation.

If cobalt is iontophoresed through the NCC I away from the brain and toward the corpora cardiaca, the neurohemal area for the MNC, a pattern of branching is seen in the corpora cardiaca as well as in the hypocerebral ganglion (Fig. 3a). Since cobalt does not cross conventional chemical synapses, this pattern can be considered to reflect axonal terminations of the MNC. No fibers are seen in the corpora allata. However, when the NCC II, which carry axons of the lateral neurosecretory cells, are filled with cobalt, fibers do appear in the corpora allata. Thus, the presence of fibers in such neurohemal, neural, and non-neural structures can be correlated precisely with their origins.

The technique of axonal iontophoresis has also been employed to delineate the caudal neurosecretory cells in the teleost spinal cord. If the urophysis, the neurohemal organ for these cells, is cut in a posterior location, the cut urophysis and last segments of the spinal cord can serve as the wick. In the mudsucker *Gillichthys mirabilis*, the Dahlgren cells fill with cobalt and their position and size are confirmed (Bern, 1969). In addition, some axons pass anteriorly in the cord before curving posteriorly toward the urophysis.

B. Suction-Electrode Iontophoresis

If the tract containing the axons of the cells of interest is not contained in nerve which can easily be isolated, a modification of the axonal iontophoresis method can be employed. A tissue which contains fibers or nerve terminals can be cut in such a way that axons are opened to the cut surface (Fig. 1b). A length of fine glass tubing with an opening approximately the diameter of the tract is cut with a diamond scriber to insure a smooth ending; the ending may be firepolished. The tubing can be filled with cobalt chloride of the appropriate concentration and a silver wire inserted into it. If the electrode is placed on the cut surface of the tissue and slight suction applied to the electrode via plastic tubing and a syringe, a tight seal can be formed. Vaseline could also be applied to the remaining area to guard against any leakage of the cobalt from the electrode and to prevent drying of the tissue. Current is passed in the same fashion as above, again for three to six hours, depending on the size of the tissue and suspected diameter of the axons. Smaller diameter axons fill more slowly.

Suction-electrode iontophoresis was used on the teleost hypothalamo-hypophysial system to distinguish between the origins of the neurosecretory peptidergic and aminergic fibers observed in the pituitary by conventional electron microscopy

(Zambrano, 1970a, b; Bern et al., 1971; Nishioka et al., 1972; Zambrano et al., 1972). The fish *Tilapia mossambica* was studied, and the pituitary was cut to expose the neurohypophysis as well as a portion of the adenohypophysis (Fig. 3b). A current of approximately 2×10^{-6} amperes was passed in a pulsed fashion (2 pulses/sec) for 4—6 h.

Fibers project to the preoptic nucleus, the suspected source of neurosecretory cells terminating in the neurohypophysis. The somata of these cells have not yet been filled by this method, but work is still in progress. Small cells were also filled lateral and dorsal to the pituitary. These may be the aminergic cells seen in this area with electron microscopy, and part of the source of aminergic endings seen in contact with cells of the adenohypophysis. No fibers were observed proceeding to the nucleus lateralis tuberis, considered to be an additional source of fibers ending in the neurohypophysis.

The method was also applied to the optic gland of the cephalopod *Octopus bimaculatus* again to ascertain the origin of aminergic fibers seen to contact cells of the gland (Nishioka et al., 1970). The origin of these fibers was thought to be neurons in the subpedunculate lobe of the brain. If the optic gland is cut and cobalt passed into it anywhere along the cut surface, fibers which fill with cobalt exit from the gland, travel in the large optic nerve, enter the brain, and pass toward the region of the subpedunculate lobe. As in the case of the fish hypothalamus, somata have not yet been filled.

C. Single-Cell Iontophoresis

The first two methods primarily indicate topography of cell groups and correlate precisely presence of fibers with their origins. To observe finer features such as geometry of dendritic or axonal branching of an individual neuron, or morphological differences between neurons of a given group, iontophoresis of cobalt through a microelectrode into single cells can be performed. The original paper by Pitman et al. (1972) was based on this method as applied to motor neurons in the cockroach. Here the method will be discussed with reference to the medial neurosecretory cells (MNC) of the locust *S. vaga*.

Conventional glass microelectrodes (tip diameter about 0.5 mμ) were filled with distilled water, backfilled with a 1.5 M cobaltous chloride solution with a fine three-inch needle and syringe, and placed in a dish of cobaltous chloride for 15 min to allow diffusion of the dye into the tip. The resistance of these electrodes was between 25 and 60 megohms. The brain was exposed frontally, and its sheath kept intact. The electrode was advanced toward the pars intercerebralis, and tapped sharply to ensure penetration through the sheath. A second tap would generally result in penetration of a cell. Since each group of MNC contains about 400 cells, a wide latitude in electrode placement was possible. Cobalt was passed into those cells showing both a drop in resting potential (40—70 mv) and electrical activity. Activity most often seen were EPSP's of 1—3 mv in amplitude, occasionally occurring with regular rhythmicity. Spikes were seen in a few cases (Fig. 3c). These were of unusually long duration, and appeared to be similar to those in other insect neurosecretory cells (Gosbee et al. 1968; Wilkens and Mote, 1970;

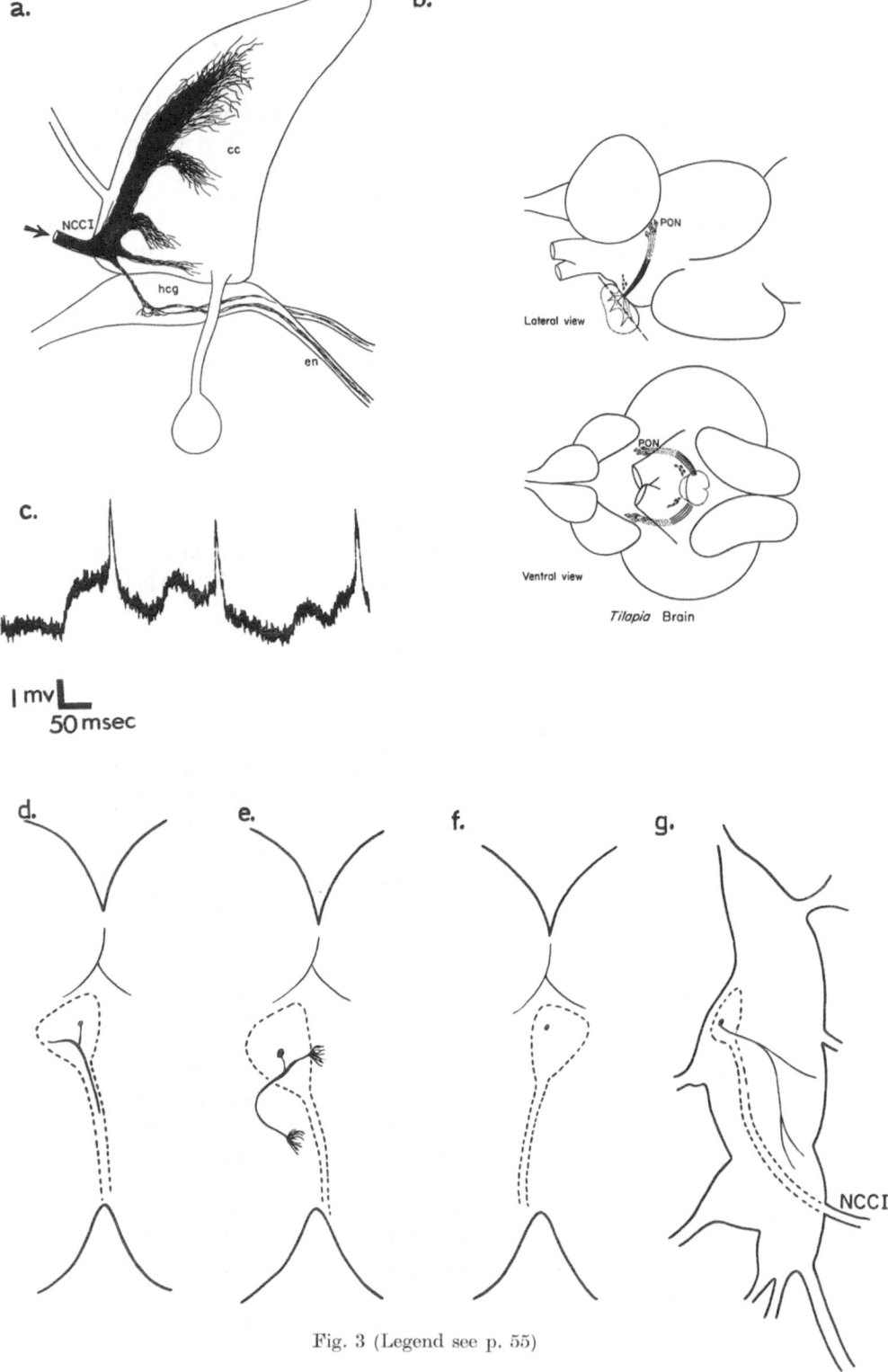

a.

cc

NCCI

hcg

en

b.

PON

Lateral view

PON

Ventral view

Tilapia Brain

c.

1 mv

50 msec

d.

e.

f.

g.

NCCI

Fig. 3 (Legend see p. 55)

Cook and Milligan, 1972). Cobalt was injected into the cell by passing a depolarizing current of 2.5×10^{-9} amperes through the recording microelectrode, using conventional bridge circuitry. Current was passed for 20—30 min, and the brain was immediately immersed in ammonium sulfide and fixed as described above for viewing in whole mount.

Figure 2b shows a single MNC filled with cobalt. The soma is about $15\,\mu$ in diameter and the axon passes ventrally in the expected direction of the MNC axon tract. Fine branches project from the initial segments of the axon for $60\,\mu$ in each direction. This is the first observation of such a nature in a single neurosecretory cell, although axon collaterals on neurosecretory cells have been described in the MNC of the cockroach as seen in Victoria blue-stained whole mounts (Adiyodi and Bern, 1968) and in silverstained preparations of the vertebrate hypothalamus (Christ, 1966) and of the locust brain (pars intercerebralis) (Williams, 1971). The conformation of the axon and branches is typical of invertebrate neurons. Of five successfully filled cells, two others also displayed axons running in the direction of the MNC tract.

The additional two cells are shown in Fig. 3e and f. In Fig. 3e, the cell soma is in the expected location in the pars intercerebralis, but the axon leaves the MNC tract and sends one branch to the region of the tract, while the other curves laterally and then returns to the path of the tract. Both ends of the axon branches display fine ramifications. In Fig. 3f, the axon runs directly transversely in the brain and the axon divides. One branch continues in this direction, while the other ramifies into two. One of the finer subdivisions approaches the path of the MNC tract as it leaves the brain in the NCC I.

At this point, it is necessary to establish the neurosecretory nature of these varied morphological types of cells. The major basis for proposing that these are neurosecretory cells is the location of their somata. Only one of the five filled cells displayed activity typical of a neurosecretory cell. Therefore, additional electrophysiological and ultrastructural criteria must be correlated with this sort of anatomical information.

Nonetheless, if this range of morphology is found after filling a random selection of so few putative neurosecretory neurons, an even greater range probably exists. Further, the emerging morphological differences may reflect distinct electrophysiological and biochemical ones, the latter already indicated by histochemistry (Girardie and Girardie, 1966). Rowell (manuscript in preparation) compares invertebrate neurosecretory neurons to other recently identified single cells in

---

Fig. 3. (a) Diagram of fibers projecting into corpus cardiacum (cc), hypocerebral ganglion (hcg), and esophageal nerves (en), after NCC I is filled posteriorly (arrow). (b) Diagram of *Tilapia* brain. Pituitary was cut (broken line, lateral view) and cobalt passed into axons by suction-electrode iontophoresis. Fibers project toward the preoptic nucleus (PON) (solid lines), but not as far as putative location of somata (dotted lines). Small somata suspected to be aminergic cells have also been filled dorsal and lateral to pituitary. (c) Action potentials recorded from the single cell shown in Fig. 2b, prior to injection of cobalt. (d, e, f) Three cell types delineated by microelectrode iontophoresis of cobalt into cells of the pars intercerebralis of the locust *S. vaga*. Their geometry is compared to the topography of the medial neurosecretory cell group (dashed line). (d, e) anterior view of brain; (f) anterior and lateral view

well-known invertebrate nervous systems, arguing that a single insect neuro-secretory cell may comprise a morphological and physiological unit, rather than the entire group. By this hypothesis, each neurosecretory cell should have a defined morphology and unique set of input connections, repeatable from individual to individual.

D. Examination of Cobalt-Filled Neurons by Electron Microscopy

Preliminary ultrastructural examination of cobalt-filled preparations has been performed on the brain of *S. vaga* after the NCC I has been iontophoresed with cobalt (Fig. 2a), as described in Part A.

Cobalt was precipitated with ammonium sulfide solution for only one to two minutes rather than the thirty minutes prescribed by Pitman et al. (1972). A freshly-made solution was always used, to ensure as rapid precipitation as possible. Since the ammonium sulfide causes general precipitation of protein and destroys ultrastructure, this step has been considered the most troublesome in the preparation of specimens for electron microscopy. Brains were then rinsed very briefly in saline and fixed in Karnovsky's fixative (Karnovsky, 1965), washed in 0.1 M cacodylate buffer, and post-fixed in 2% osmium tetroxide. The last step was not included in the Pitman procedure, since osmium blackens the tissue and prevents visualization of the filled neuron after it is dehydrated and embedded. If a diagram is made of the neuron and its general projections before osmication, if it can be seen through the glutaraldehyde-fixed block, then osmication can follow. Post-fixation in osmium greatly improves preservation of membranes and synaptic vesicles, the most important structures to be observed in this type of study. Tissues are then dehydrated in ethanols, infused with propylene oxide, and embedded in Spurr's medium. The brain was sectioned about half-way down the MNC axon tract. Thick sections (1 mμ) were cut and stained with toluidine blue. Cobalt cannot be too well-disinguished at the light microscope level; however, cobalt-filled neurons appear to stain more intensely. Thin sections (100 nm) were cut and stained with aqueous uranyl acetate and lead citrate (Reynolds, 1963) and examined in a Siemens Elmiskop I.

Figure 2c shows an example of a section through the MNC axon tract filled with cobalt. Most axons in the micrograph contain cobalt, which appears as dark grey particles, similar to ground substance. Two large profiles do not contain cobalt. A presynaptic thickening can be seen in one of the unfilled axons. and generally membranes appear to be well-fixed. Neurosecretory granules are visible, though poorly preserved in cobalt-filled axons.

It is difficult to determine precisely why some profiles are not filled with cobalt. Some axons in the NCC I may have collapsed during preparation of the nerve for axonal iontophoresis. This is unlikely since the unfilled ones are large, and some smaller ones, which collapse more easily, contain cobalt. More satisfactory explanations are that they derive from a) neurons outside of the pars intercerebralis, coming into the MNC tract to synapse with the MNC; b) neurosecretory neurons in the contralateral pars intercerebralis which are synapsing with those of the bilateral group; c) neurosecretory neurons from the ipsilateral pars intercerebralis which, like the cell pictured in Fig. 3e, leave the main MNC tract and return to synapse on other elements, and do not exit in the NCC I.

In summary, these techniques can elucidate the fine anatomy of nerve cells irrespective of their contents and correlate precisely the presence of fibers with their origins. Ultrastructural examination of preparations in which a single neurosecretory cell is iontophoresed with cobalt will give the much needed information on the synaptic relations among neurosecretory neurons and between neurosecretory and non-neurosecretory neurons. Such analysis will indicate the nature of synapses mediating the electrophysiological phenomena observed so far in neurosecretory cells (simultaneous bursting of cells in a group; recurrent inhibition), the structural basis of inhibitory and excitatory transmitters controlling neurosecretory cell function, and whether dendrites contain neurosecretory granules. These techniques are presently being applied to single cells of the hypothalamc-neurohypophysial system of the rat in an attempt to answer such questions.

Acknowledgements. The generous advice and cooperation of Dr. Mick O'Shea is acknowledged, especially on the single-cell iontophoresis experiments. Mrs. Emily Reid prepared the figures, and Mr. John Underhill assisted with photography. Aided by NSF Grant GB-35239X and NIH Grant CA-05045 to H.A. Bern and NIH Grant NS-09404 to C.H.F. Rowell.

References

Adiyodi, K.G., Bern, H.A.: Neuronal appearance of neurosecretory cells in the pars intercerebralis of *Periplaneta americana*. Gen. comp. Endocr. 11, 88—91 (1968).

Bern, H.A.: Urophysis and caudal neurosecretory system. In: Fish Physiology (W.S.Hoar, D.J.Randell Eds.), Vol. 1, p. 399—418. New York: Academic Press 1969.

Bern, H.A., Zambrano, D., Nishioka, R.S.: Comparison of the innervation of the pituitary of two euryhaline teleost fishes, *Gillichthys mirabilis* and *Tilapia mossambica*, with special reference to the origin and nature of type "B" fibres. Mem. Soc. Endocr. 19, 817—822 (1971).

Christ, J.F.: Nerve supply, blood supply and cytology of the neurohyophysis. In: The Pituitary Gland (G.W.Harris, B.T.Donovan, Eds.), Vol. 3, p. 62—130. London: Butterworths 1966.

Cook, D.J., Milligan, J.V.: Electrophysiology and histology of the medial neurosecretory cells in adult male cockroaches, *Periplaneta americana*. J. Insect. Physiol. 18, 1197—1215 (1972).

Girardie, A., Girardie, J.: Etude histologique, histochimique, et ultrastructurale de la pars intercerebralis chez *Locusta migratoria* L. (Orthoptère). Z. Zellforsch. 78, 54—75 (1966).

Gosbee, J.L., Milligan, J.V., Smallman, B.N.: Neural properties of the protocerebral neurosecretory cells of the adult cockroach, *Periplaneta americana*. J. Insect Physiol. 14, 1785—1792 (1968).

Iles, J.F., Mulloney, B.: Procion yellow staining of cockroach motor neurons without the use of microelectrodes. Brain Res. 30, 397—400 (1971).

Karnovsky, M.J.: A formaldehyde-glutaraldehyde fixative of high osmolarity for use in electron microscopy. J. Cell Biol. 27, 137a (1965).

Mason, C.A.: New features of the brain-retrocerebral neuroendocrine complex of the locust *Schistocerca vaga* (Scudder). Z. Zellforsch. 141, 19—32 (1973).

Nishioka, R.S., Bern, H.A., Golding, D.W.: Innervation of the cephalopod optic gland. In: Aspects of Neuroendocrinology (W.Bargmann, B.Scharrer, Eds.), p. 47—54. Berlin-Heidelberg-New York: Springer 1970.

Nishioka, R.S., Bern, H.A., Nagahama, Y.: Innervation of the pituitary of the teleost *Tilapia mossambica*. Amer. Zool. 12, 678a (1972).

Pitman, R.M., Tweedle, C.D., Cohen, M.J.: Branching of central neurons: intracellular cobalt injection for light and electron microscopy. Science 176, 412—414 (1972).

Reynolds, E. S.: The use of lead citrate at high pH as an electron-opaque stain in electron
    microscopy. J. Cell Biol. **17**, 208—212 (1963).
Stretton, A. O. W., Kravitz, E. A.: Neuronal geometry: delineation with a technique of intra-
    cellular dye injection. Science **162**, 132—134 (1968).
Wilkens, J. L., Mote, M. I.: Neuronal properties of the neurosecretory cells in the fly *Sarcophaga
    bullata*. Experientia (Basel) **26**, 275—276 (1970).
Williams, J. L. D.: Some observations on the neuronal organisation of the supraoesophageal
    ganglion in *Schistocerca gregaria* Forskål with particular reference to the central complex.
    Ph.D. thesis, University of Wales 1971.
Zambrano, D.: The nucleus lateralis tuberis system of the gobiid fish *Gillichthys mirabilis*.
    I. Ultrastructural and histochemical characterization of the nucleus. Z. Zellforsch. **110**,
    9—26 (1970a).
Zambrano, D.: The nucleus lateralis tuberis system of the gobiid fish *Gillichthys mirabilis*.
    II. Innervation of the pituitary. Z. Zellforsch. **110**, 496—516 (1970b).
Zambrano, D., Nishioka, R. S., Bern, H. A.: The innervation of the pituitary gland of teleost
    fishes. In: Brain-Endocrine Interaction. Median Eminence: Structure and Function
    (K. M. Knigge, D. E. Scott, A. Weindl, Eds.) p. 50—66. Basel: S. Karger 1972.

The Perisympathetic Organs of Insects

M. Raabe, N. Baudry, J. P. Grillot, and A. Provansal

Equipe de Neuroendocrinologie des Insectes, Laboratoire de Zoologie, Paris (France)

The neurosecretory cells of the insect brain were described many years ago and we know that their secretions are stored in the *corpora cardiaca*. Neurosecretion is not, however, limited to the cephalic region. Various ganglia of the ventral nerve cord also possess neurosecretory elements controlling various functions. Associated with these ganglia are neurohaemal organs which present a structural resemblance to the *corpora cardiaca* and appear to be neurosecretory storage and release centres.

The perisympathetic organs (PO) were so-named by reason of their association with the fibres of the posterior sympathetic nervous system. Such a link, which one finds also in the *corpora cardiaca* which are connected to the hypocerebral ganglion of the anterior sympathetic nervous system, has certainly a physiological significance.

First discovered in phasmids (Raabe, 1965), the PO were subsequently found in the major orders of the Pterygota (Raabe et al., 1971). They are characterized by a basically metameric distribution. They sometimes fuse however, when the first or the last abdominal neuromeres coalesce. In the abdominal region of certain Diptera (Grillot and Raabe, 1973), Homoptera and Heteroptera (Baudry, 1971, 1972) fusion is specially pronounced, one organ corresponding to all the abdominal ganglia joined to form a single mass.

The perisympathetic organs seem to be absent from the thoracic region of certain orders, notably Coleoptera, despite the individuality of the neuromeres at this level. In other orders they are well developed all along the ventral nerve cord, particularly near the head between the prothoracic and sub-oesophageal ganglia (Ensifera, Dermaptera). The significance of these anatomical differences is not clear.

Types

In primitive orders, the perisympathetic organs have a relatively uniform disposition and are situated along the course of the median and transverse nerves. They form slight thickenings or small spindle-shaped swellings, which were first noticed by Lyonet in 1762.

In the most evolved groups (Coleoptera, Diptera, Hymenoptera, Homoptera, and Heteroptera) there is considerable diversity. The PO divide or associate themselves closely with ganglia or somatic nerves. These features are related to the degree of concentration of the central nervous system and to the lack of a distinct posterior sympathetic system. They may also be related to general insect anatomy.

The PO thus present a large number of morphological types for which a nomenclature has been proposed (Grillot et al., 1971).

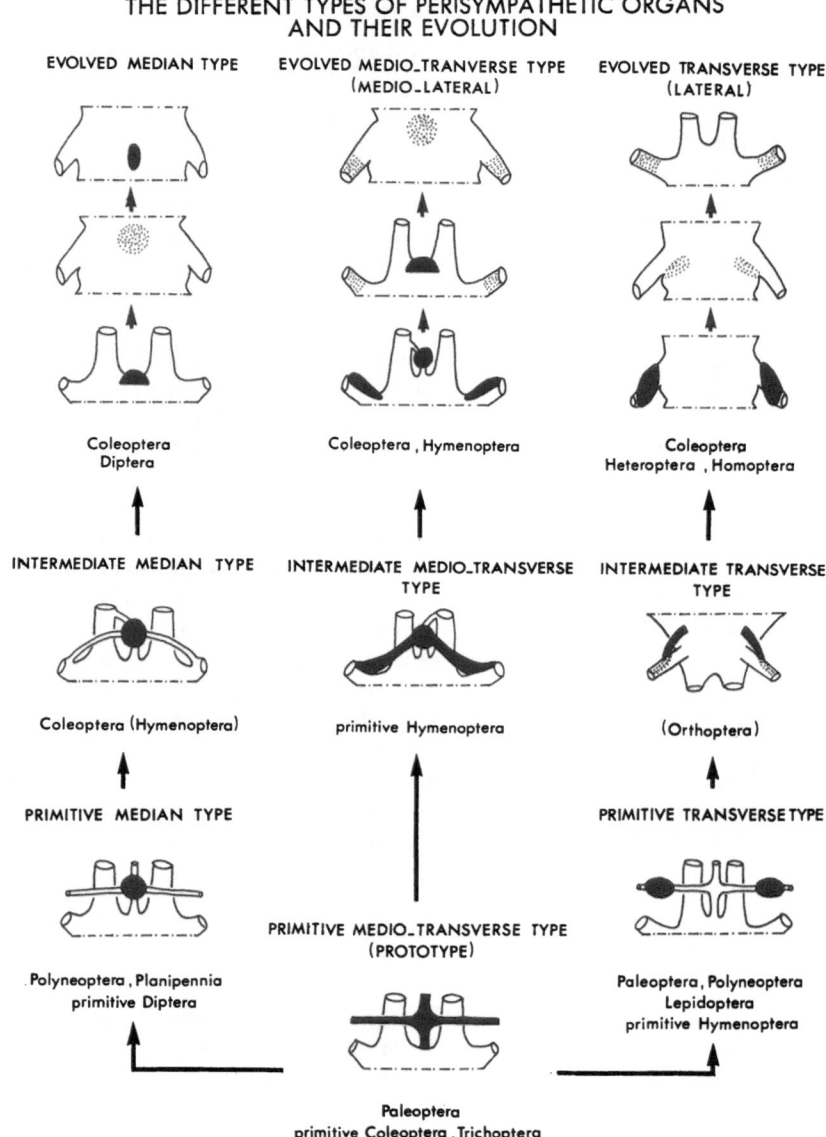

THE DIFFERENT TYPES OF PERISYMPATHETIC ORGANS
AND THEIR EVOLUTION

EVOLVED MEDIAN TYPE

EVOLVED MEDIO-TRANVERSE TYPE
(MEDIO-LATERAL)

EVOLVED TRANSVERSE TYPE
(LATERAL)

Coleoptera
Diptera

Coleoptera , Hymenoptera

Coleoptera
Heteroptera , Homoptera

INTERMEDIATE MEDIAN TYPE

INTERMEDIATE MEDIO-TRANSVERSE
TYPE

INTERMEDIATE TRANSVERSE
TYPE

Coleoptera (Hymenoptera)

primitive Hymenoptera

(Orthoptera)

PRIMITIVE MEDIAN TYPE

PRIMITIVE TRANSVERSE TYPE

Polyneoptera , Planipennia
primitive Diptera

PRIMITIVE MEDIO-TRANSVERSE TYPE
(PROTOTYPE)

Paleoptera, Polyneoptera
Lepidoptera
primitive Hymenoptera

Paleoptera
primitive Coleoptera , Trichoptera

Fig. 1

Three main categories of PO can be distinguished according to their positions on the median and transverse nerves: median, transverse and medio-transverse. In addition various evolutionary steps exist in each of these categories. The prototype (see Fig. 1) consists of organs distributed over a length of median and transverse nerves. In the medio-transverse, median and transverse forms, primitive, intermediate and advanced positions may be recognised.

Phylogeny

The direct relationship between the primitive and more evolved forms is clearly evident in certain cases. In the *Gryllidae* we can observe the different stages in the evolution of the transverse organs. From the primitive type found in abdominal segments 3—7, the PO assume, in the first segment, the intermediate or evolved form depending upon their degree of coalescence with the somatic nerve (Thomas and Raabe, 1973).

In the larva of the Hymenopteran *Diprion*, the median and transverse neurohaemal organs are contiguous (intermediate medio-transverse form), whereas in the adult they are clearly separated into one median organ and two lateral organs adjacent to the somatic nerves (evolved medio-transverse form) (Provansal, 1971).

The phylogeny of evolved median organs can be seen in the Coleopteran *Dytiscus*, at the metamere level. Primitively lying external to the ganglia, and adjacent to them, the PO become internal when there is partial fusion between the neuromeres and re-appear externally on the dorsal side in the case of complete fusion (Grillot, 1970). The evolution of evolved transverse organs becomes apparent from the study of various families of Heteroptera (Baudry, 1971, 1972). External to the ganglia, they comprise a single mass next to the abdominal nerves in the *Belostomatidae*; this mass is found on the interior of the fused nerve ganglia in the *Nepidae*. In the *Coreidae* and the *Pyrrhocoridae*, they split into fragments which migrate in the somatic nerves, either in part (in the *Pentatomidae*) or as a whole (in the *Reduviidae*).

Type Distribution

We may consider the most primitive organs, those at the origin of the various evolutionary lines, to be the primitive medio-transverse organs, found principally in the Paleoptera.

The primitive median and transverse organs seem to originate directly from this prototypic medio-transverse form. They coexist with these in several species. They are characteristic of the Polyneoptera and are also found in few Coleptera, primitive Diptera, the Planipennia and Lepidoptera.

The most evolved organs are present only in the Oligoneoptera and the Paraneoptera studied. Several types are found together in the Coleoptera, a fairly diversified order, while one type of PO predominates in other orders (Hymenoptera, Homoptera, Heteroptera).

Structure

The PO have a characteristic neurohaemal structure which appears with methylene-blue staining, in histological sections and under the electron microscope.

They contain highly branched nerve fibres, often loaded with neurosecretion. The fibres are surrounded by numerous glial cells and terminate on the organ's thin boundary membrane which is often deeply invaginated. The large number of tracheae in these organs indicates a considerable metabolic activity.

However, according to their anatomical position and their form, the PO present a number of structural differences. These differences may be correlated with modifications in the release of neurosecretory material.

In numerous species, in which the PO are short and thick, the passage of neurohormones into the blood stream takes place at the periphery, but above all through the numerous internal sinuses. These sinuses were clearly seen in phasmids using the electron microscope (Raabe and Ramade, 1967) and in the lateral organs of the Hymenoptera, *Vespula germanica* (Raabe et al., 1970).

In species in which the PO are slim and diffuse, release of neurosecretory products takes place mostly at the surface which presents a relatively large area of contact with the internal environment. This is the case in primitive groups like the Paleoptera where the neurohaemal structures form a fine sheath over a great distance of the sympathetic nerves (Raabe and Provansal, 1972). It is also the case for more evolved groups. Sometimes the neurohaemal structures appear as neurosecretory endings spread along the somatic nerves forming the evolved transverse organs of certain Coleoptera (Grillot in Provansal and Grillot, 1972) and Heteroptera (Maddrell, 1966). Sometimes they are associated with numerous somatic nerve branches and make up a fine distal neurohaemal network (evolved transverse organs in Homoptera and Heteroptera; Baudry, 1972). Sometimes intermingling with the ventral diaphragm which serves as a support, they make up a very thin lamina (primitive transverse organs of Dermaptera; Raabe, 1972; and Lepidoptera; Provansal, 1972).

Globular perisympathetic organs, apparently less adapted for a neurohaemal function, are found among the median-type organs. Ultrastructural studies show that they are generally formed of two zones: a central zone mostly of nerve fibres and a peripheral zone with few sinuses, where the neurosecretory terminals are most often surrounded by glial cells (Provansal et al., 1970).

Neurosecretion can thus occur in two distinct ways: directly across the connective tissue or after passage through the glial layer, as Scharrer suggested in 1968.

As in various other neurohaemal organs the PO contain synaptoid sites characterized by a thickening of the axolemma and an accumulation of electron-transparent vesicles of 400—500 Å, probably representing sites of neurosecretory release. This feature seems to occur by exocytosis of electron-dense granules as shown in some other species.

Few current data are available on the mechanisms governing the discharge of the neurosecretory products contained in the PO. A search for amines using the Falck and Hillarp technique gave no positive data for phasmids (Raabe and Monjo, 1970). Past efforts on the *corpora cardiaca* led to conflicting results. Recently, however, Lafon-Cazal et al. (1973) showed an uptake of tritiated

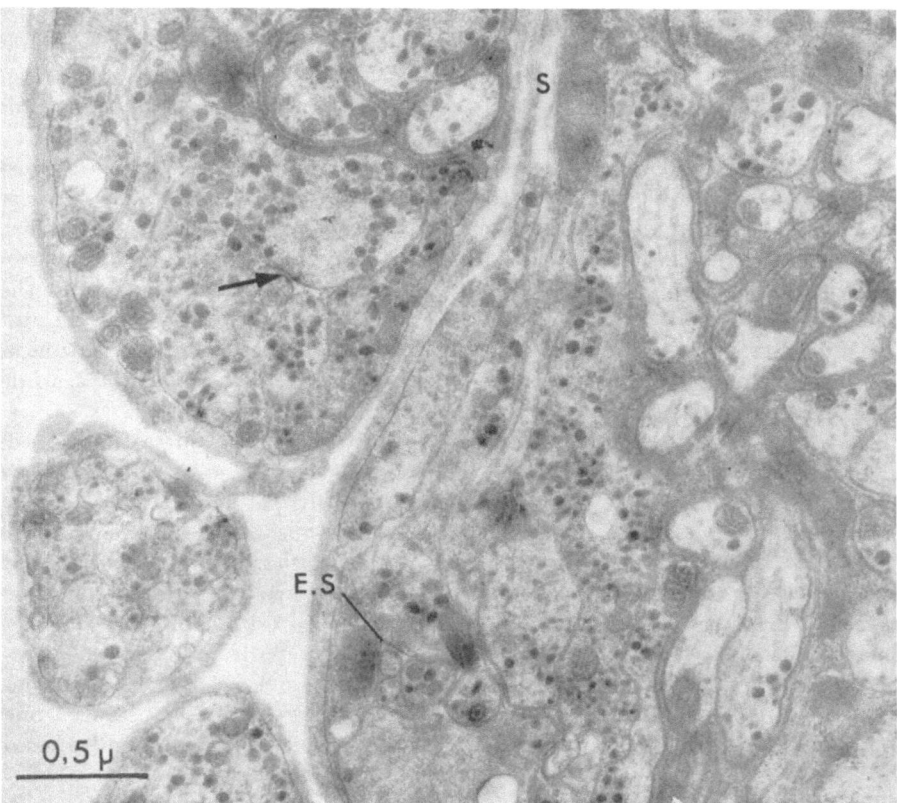

Plate I. Lateral perisympathetic organ of *Vespula germanica*. Note the lack of glial processes between the axons at the outer part of the organ and synaptoid structure (arrow) with an electron-dense deposit below the plasma membrane. ES: extracellular space, S: sinus (× 52000)

monoamines by the axons of the *corpora cardiaca* in the locust. The discharge mechanism in these organs may thus involve monoamines.

The PO of the Paleoptera, Polyneoptera and most Coleoptera do not seem to contain neurosecretory cells. On the other hand those of several Hymenoptera, other Coleoptera (Provansal and Grillot, 1972) and Homoptera (Baudry, 1972) do possess a few. Numerous neurons occur in distal PO associated with the ventral diaphragm of *Locusta* (Thomas and Raabe, 1973). The neurons present in the PO frequently contain secretory products which can be seen with both the light and electron microscopes. They may be neurosecretory sensory cells whose association with the PO could be more or less direct. In some species sensory neurons have been observed along nerves and near the PO (Phasmids; Finlayson and Osborne, 1968; Heteroptera; Baudry, personal communication).

In the *corpora cardiaca*, an association between intrinsic cells and the neurohaemal zone is usually the rule; however, there is complete dissociation in some Heteroptera.

One might ask, in the case of the PO, what may be the physiological significance of a relationship between neurohaemal areas and nerve cells which may be sensory. That these cells play a role in the discharge mechanism seems possible and brings to mind relationships existing in the vertebrates at the level of hypothalamic osmoreceptors.

The neurosecretory products stored in the PO originate entirely or for the most part in the neurosecretory cells of the ventral nerve cord. The axons of these neurons pass within the sympathetic nerves alongside non-neurosecretory fibres. In some cases, it is possible to follow the complete course of the neuro-secretory products, starting from cell bodies, through the neuromeres and the nerves leading to the PO.

A short time after sectioning of the sympathetic nerves, an accumulation of neurosecretory products can be observed at the proximal ends of the fibres, while the distal ends and the PO empty progressively (Raabe, 1965).

There are several types of neurosecretory cells in the insect ventral nerve cord. They have been classified according to their affinity for different stains and their location (cf. Raabe, 1971). As in the brain three principal types are frequently encountered. Types A and B have been described for many species and the authors' terminology is relatively uniform. However, the term type "C" is not always used for comparable elements. We use it here to designate those secretions which stain intensely with azocarmin of azan, but not with chrome-haematoxylin or paraldehyde-fuchsin and irregularly with phloxine or picro-indigo-carmine. These irregularities may result either from differences in concen-tration of stainable material, or from the existence of two distinct substances, one staining only with azocarmin and the other staining with azocarmin and several acid stains.

The neurosecretory nature of type C material has sometimes been disputed. However, its neurosecretory role now seems well established, as it is stored in neurohaemal organs, shows up under the electron microscope as classical electron-dense granules and possesses several physiological activities.

Type C cells have recently been found in the *pars intercerebralis* of phasmids. Their secretory products are very abundant in the *corpora cardiaca* (Raabe and Monjo, 1970).

Phasmids type C secretions are destroyed by proteolytic enzymes; they stain intensely with Mazia, Brewer and Alfert's bromophenol blue, Alfert and Ge-schwind's fast green F.C.F. and have a positive Glenner reaction. It may thus be concluded that type C products are basic proteins, containing indolic and pyrrolic groups. Some assays upon insects belonging to other orders give similar results when using the fast green method (Raabe and Monjo, 1970).

With the electron microscope, the distinction of the types of neurosecretion contained in the PO is more difficult. Electron dense granules of 1000—1800 Å have been frequently observed (Raabe and Ramade, 1967; Scharrer, 1968; Raabe et al.; Provansal et al., 1970). Less electron-dense granules or transparent vesicles, which may possibly represent another type of neurosecretion, have occasionally been described (Brady and Maddrell, 1967).

The most abundant material stored in the PO is of the C type. Type A secre-tions exist in small amounts in the PO of some orders where they are found with type B and C secretions. In such cases, the PO may act as release centres for all neurosecretion from the ventral nerve cord. In other species the problem of the site of release for A and B types remains unsolved, although several hypotheses have been proposed.

The first hypothesis is the possibility of some neurohaemal organs still unknown.

Numerous type A neurosecretion aggregates are to be found in the dorsal neuropile of the ventral ganglia (Stutinsky, 1952, phasmids; Panov, 1962, Orthoptera). Pasteels (1965), Naisse and Mouton (1965) (sub-oesophageal ganglion of phasmids) and Seshan (1968) (ventral ganglia of a bug *Iphita*) consider them to be neurohaemal areas. However, this view can be debated, as these aggregates are not really peripheral. They likely represent neurosecretory material occurring in the dendrites and the collaterals of neurosecretory cells, as suggested by Raabe (1965) and Adiyodi and Bern (1968) in their study of phasmids and cockroaches. Intra-cerebral neurosecretory endings of hypothalamic origin have also been observed in the vertebrates. Neurosecretion may well play a role in the functioning of nervous centres by diffusing through the lacunar glial system.

Various authors have noticed neurosecretory tracts in the ventral nerve cord connectives (Füller, 1960, *Corethra*; Panov, 1962, Orthoptera; Raabe, 1965, stick insects; Chalaye, 1966, locusts). They observed also a neurosecretory supply to various organs: endocrines, luminescent organ, heart, rectum, etc. (Bounhiol et al., 1953; Arvy and Gabe, 1953; Johnson and Bowers, 1963; Smith, 1963; Maddrell, 1965, etc.). Thus, for some neurosecretory cells, migration of material may occur over wide distances: along the ventral nerve cord and somatic nerves.

The occurrence of neurosecretion at the target organ level is of particular interest; it seems characteristic of insects and has never been reported in other groups. One may indeed wonder whether some neurosecretory products are closer to neurotransmitter substances than has previously been considered. The neurosecretory material may have two distinct modes of release. The first one, of minor importance, occurs in the vicinity of the organs themselves and induces a localised effect. The second one, more important, results from the neurohaemal activity, and promotes a very large diffusion of neurosecretory products, mainly from the PO to the whole insect body.

Physiological Activities

Injection of organ extracts has revealed substances in the ganglia of the ventral nerve cord which are able to influence various physiological phenomena: chromatic adaptation, cardiac rhythm, water metabolism, cuticular tanning, diapause, reproduction, etc.. Histophysiological study of neurosecretory cells from these ganglia has also shown the occurrence of substantial variations, associated with the female reproductive cycle.

It is thus not surprising to find similar data for the perisympathetic organs. Their metameric distribution make extirpation experiments practically impossible and limits the methods of investigation. Nonetheless, data have been accumulated through extracts injected to whole animals or added to the perfusion liquid for isolated organs (heart, Malpighian tubules and rectum).

COMPARATIVE PHYSIOLOGICAL ACTIVITIES
COMPARATIVE PHYSIOLOGICAL ACTIVITIES

OF CORPORA CARDIACA AND PERISYMPATHETIC ORGANS

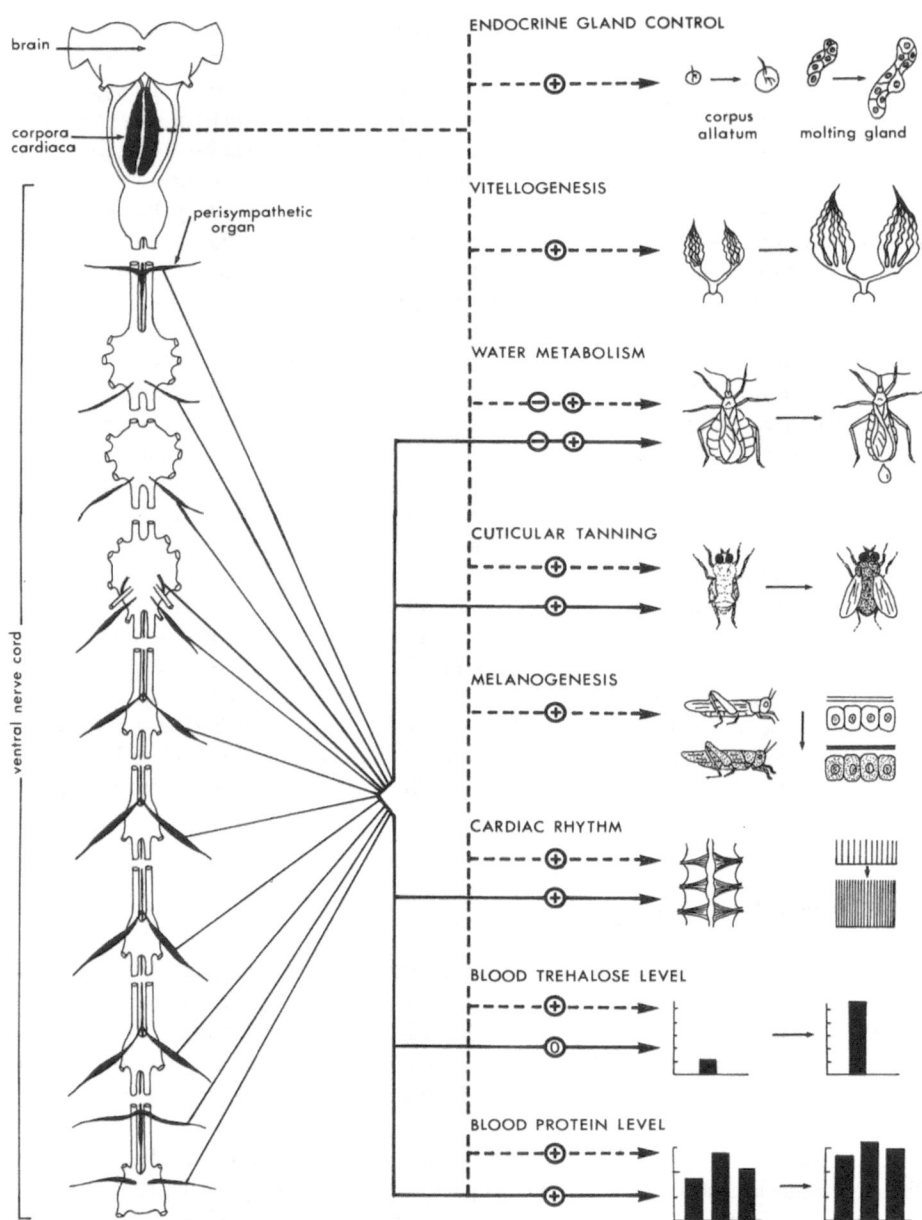

Fig. 2

At present it seems that the perisympathetic organs have no effect on the physiological chromatic adaptation of phasmids and Crustacea (Raabe et al., 1967); phasmids oviposition (Thomas and Mesnier, 1973) and regulation of blood trehalose level in locusts and cockroaches (Chalaye, 1969). On the other hand they do possess several physiological activities.

PO and Heart Rhythm

The PO have an interspecific cardio-accelerating effect similar to that of the *corpora cardiaca* in cockroaches, phasmids and locusts. The concentration of active substance is fairly high: 10 pairs of PO produce about the same effect as 1 to 2 pairs of *corpora cardiaca* (Raabe et al., 1967).

PO and Diuresis

The PO affect diuresis, as do the *corpora cardiaca*, in two opposing ways. This was shown in vitro for the Malpighian tubules of *Rhodnius* (Maddrell, 1966) the Malpighian tubules and the rectum of *Clitumnus*, *Periplaneta*, and *Locusta* (de Bessé and Cazal, 1968). Their action is diuretic in the first species and anti-diuretic in the three others. Histophysiological examination on phasmids confirms experimental data. Under relatively humid conditions corresponding to periods when the antidiuretic factor is not released, the PO are especially full (Raabe, 1965).

PO and Tanning

The role of the PO in the regulation of cuticular tanning in the Coleopteran *Tenebrio molitor* has been established by injecting extracts into ligatured nymphs which have been thus rendered incapable of undergoing imaginal tanning. The activity of nerve ganglia and perisympathetic organs varies significantly during the nymphal stage. The active factor, present in the anterior abdominal ganglia on day three of the pupa, migrates to the corresponding PO on day five and is totally discharged at the end of exuviation (Delachambre et al., 1972). In the Polyneoptera, the definite function of the PO could not be determined but it seems that the PO of the cockroach possess some tanning activity (Vincent, 1972).

PO and Blood Proteins

Using electrophoresis, Demarti (1971), has studied the blood of adult females of various ages in the phasmid *Carausius morosus*: two bands show a very clear variation. During a brief phase, band 5, at first very intense, decreases rapidly; it remains very reduced during the whole of the imaginal period, which makes up the second phase. Band 4 undergoes the inverse process: it appears at the end of the first period and remains subsequently at a constant level.

Injections of PO extracts seem to have no effect on band 4, but they lead to an early decrease of band 5. Thus, the PO accelerate a process which normally appears at the beginning of imaginal life (Raabe and Demarti, 1973).

PO and Moulting Gland

We unfortunately have no experimental data on this subject, but in several species, the innervation of the moulting gland by sympathetic nerves bearing well developed PO has been observed (Orthoptera, Dermaptera). In the cricket, there is close contact between some areas of the anterior large prothoracic PO and the moulting gland (Thomas and Raabe, 1973). In addition, we may note modifications in the PO in relation to moulting: in the phasmids they are almost empty at this time (Raabe, 1965); in the dragonfly, *Aeschna*, permanent larvae obtained by removal of the moulting gland reveal a large storage of neurosecretion at the PO level (Schaller and Charlet, 1970).

The PO thus possess diverse activities related to the regulation of the insect vegetative life and seem to play a role similar to that of the *corpora cardiaca*. Their metameric arrangement assures a great efficiency since the hormone discharge points are distributed over the animal's entire body.

A functional asynchronism between the thoracic and abdominal PO has been noted in an Odonata (Raabe and Provansal, 1972) and a Dermaptera, (Raabe, 1972). These PO may thus have different physiological functions either because of differences in the substances they contain or in the times when these are released.

It is important to note that the PO do not possess all the activities of the ventral nerve cord. This may result from the fact that they contain mostly type C secretions. It is however possible that certain hormones exist in a less stable form in the neurohaemal organs than in nervous centres.

Conclusion

In addition to the cephalic neurohaemal system composed of cerebral neurosecretory cells and the *corpora cardiaca*, insects possess a second, more extensive system consisting of a succession of metameric organs associated with other parts of the nervous system. This arrangement may not be confined to the insects, but could exist in other segmented invertebrates.

Apparently homologous structures have in fact been described in the stomatopod, *Squilla mantis*, few Brachyurans pericardial organs (Alexandrowics, 1952; Maynard, 1961) and in the myriapod *Geophilus longicornis* (Ernst, 1971). They are doubtlessly related to the basic design of a segmented nervous system.

References

Adiyodi,K.G., Bern,H.A.: Neuronal appearance of neurosecretory cells in the *pars inter-cerebralis* of *Periplaneta americana* (L.). Gen. comp. Endocr. 11, 88—91 (1968).

Alexandrowicz,J.S.: Notes on the nervous system in the Stomatopoda. I. The system of median connectives. Pubbl. Staz. Zool. (Napoli) 23, 201—214 (1952).

Arvy,L., Gabe,M.: Particularités histophysiologiques des glandes endocrines céphaliques chez *Tenebrio molitor* L. C. R. Acad. Sci. (Paris) 237, 844—846 (1953).

Baudry,N.: Recherches sur la localisation et la structure des organes neurohémaux métamériques des *Belostomatidae* (Hétéroptères). C. R. Acad. Sci. (Paris) 272, 2946—2949 (1971).

Baudry,N.: Comparaison des différents types d'organes périsympathiques de quelques familles d'Hétéroptères *(Nepidae, Pyrrhocoridae, Coreidae et Pentatomidae)*. C. R. Acad. Sci. (Paris) 275, 1535—1538 (1972).

Baudry, N.: Les organes périsympathiques des Homoptères. Localisation et structure chez les *Cicadidae*. C. R. Acad. Sci. (Paris) **275**, 1673—1676 (1972).

de Bessé, N.: Recherches des organes neurohémaux associés à la chaîne nerveuse ventrale de deux blattes, *Leucophaea maderae* et *Periplaneta americana*. C. R. Acad. Sci. (Paris) **263**, 404—407 (1966).

de Bessé, N., Cazal, M.: Action des extraits d'organes périsympathiques et de *corpora cardiaca* sur la diurèse de quelques Insectes. C. R. Acad. Sci. (Paris) **266**, 615—618 (1968).

Bounhiol, J. J., Gabe, M., Arvy, L.: Données histochimiques sur la neurosécrétion chez *Bombyx mori* L. et sur ses rapports avec les glandes endocrines. Bull. Biol. France Belgique **87**, 323—333 (1953).

Brady, J., Maddrell, S. H. P.: Neurohaemal organs in the medial nervous system of insects. Z. Zellforsch. **76**, 389—404 (1967).

Chalaye, D.: Recherches sur la destination des produits de neurosécrétion de la chaîne nerveuse ventrale du Criquet migrateur, *Locusta migratoria*. C. R. Acad. Sci. (Paris) **262**, 161—164 (1966).

Chalaye, D.: La tréhalosémie et son contrôle neuroendocrine chez le Criquet migrateur, *Locusta migratoria migratorioides*. II. Rôle des *corpora cardiaca* et des organes périssympathiques. C. R. Acad. Sci. (Paris) **268**, 3111—3114 (1969).

Delachambre, J., Provansal, A., Grillot, J. P.: Mise en évidence de la libération d'un facteur de tannage assimilable à la bursicon par les organes périsympathiques chez *Tenebrio molitor* L. (Ins. Col.). C. R. Acad. Sci. (Paris) **275**, 2703—2706 (1972).

Demarti, F.: Etude par électrophorèse sur gel d'acrylamide des protéines de l'hémolymphe du phasme *Carausius morosus*. C. R. Acad. Sci. (Paris), **273**, 1844—1846 (1971).

Ernst, A.: Licht- und elektronenmikroskopische Untersuchungen zur Neurosekretion bei *Geophilus longicornis* Leach unter besonderer Berücksichtigung der Neurohämalorgane. Z. wiss. Zool. (Leipzig) **182**, 62—130 (1971).

Finlayson, L. H., Osborne, M. P.: Peripheral neurosecretory cells in the stick insect *(Carausius morosus)* and the blowfly larva *(Phormia terrae-novae)*. J. Insect Physiol. **14**, 1793—1802 (1968).

Füller, H. B.: Morphologische und experimentelle Untersuchungen über die neurosekretorischen Verhältnisse im Zentralnervensystem von Blattiden und Culiciden. Zool. Jahrbücher **69**, 223—250 (1960).

Grillot, J. P.: Description d'organes neurohémaux métamériques associés à la chaîne nerveuse ventrale chez deux Coléoptères: *Chrysocarabus auronitens* Fabr. *(Carabidae)* et *Oryctes rhinoceros* L. *(Scarabaeidae)*. C. R. Acad. Sci. (Paris) **267**, 772—775 (1968).

Grillot, J. P.: Considérations sur la diversité des organes neurohémaux métamériques associés à la chaîne nerveuse ventrale de l'imago de *Dytiscus marginalis* L. (Coléoptère, *Dytiscidae*). C. R. Acad. Sci. (Paris) **270**, 403—406 (1970).

Grillot, J. P.: Recherches sur la localisation et la structure des organes neurohémaux métamériques associés à la chaîne nerveuse ventrale chez les Coléoptères. C. R. Acad. Sci. (Paris) **270**, 847—850 (1970).

Grillot, J. P., Provansal, A., Baudry, N., Raabe, M.: Les organes périsympathiques des Insectes Ptérygotes. Les principaux types morphologiques. C. R. Acad. Sci. (Paris) **273**, 2126—2129 (1971).

Grillot, J. P., Raabe, M.: Recherches préliminaires sur les organes périsympathiques des Diptères. C. R. Acad. Sci. (Paris) **277**, 425—428 (1973).

Johnson, B., Bowers, B.: Transport of neurohormones from the *corpora cardiaca* in Insects. Science **141**, 263—266 (1963).

Lafon-Cazal, M., Calas, A., Bosc, S.: Capture et rétention de monoamines tritiées dans les *corpora cardiaca* de *Locusta migratoria* L. Etude *in vitro* par radioautographie à haute résolution. J. Microscopie **17**, 223—226 (1973).

Lyonet, P.: Traité anatomique de la chenille qui ronge le bois de saule. La Haye: Gosse and Pinet 1762.

Maddrell, S. H. P.: Neurosecretory supply to the epidermis of an insect. Science **150**, 1033—1034 (1965).

Maddrell, S. H. P.: The site of release of the diuretic hormone in *Rhodnius*. A new neurohaemal system in insects. J. exp. Biol. **45**, 499—508 (1966).

Maynard, D. M.: Thoracic neurosecretory structures in Brachyura. I. Gross Anatomy. Biol. Bull. **121**, 316—329 (1961).

Naisse, J., Mouton, J.: Phénomènes neuro-endocrines au niveau de la chaîne nerveuse ventrale de *Carausius morosus* (Phasmides-Orhoptères). C. R. Acad. Sci. (Paris) **261**, 3887—3890 (1965).

Panov, A. A.: Distribution of neurosecretory cells in the abdominal section of the nerve cord of the Orthoptera. Dokl. Akad. Nauk. SSSR, **145**, 1409—1412 (1962).

Pasteels, J. M.: Description d'un système neuroendocrinien dans le ganglion infraoesophagien du Phasme *Carausius morosus* (Insecte, Orthoptère). C. R. Acad. Sci. (Paris) **261**, 3884—3886 (1965).

Provansal, A.: Mise en évidence d'organes neurohémaux métamériques associés à la chaîne nerveuse ventrale chez *Vespa crabro* L. et *Vespula germanica* Fabr. (Hyménoptères *Vespidae*). C. R. Acad. Sci. (Paris) **267**, 864—867 (1968).

Provansal, A.: Caractères particuliers des organes périsympathiques de la larve de *Diprion pini* L. (Hyménoptères, Symphyte, *Diprionidae*). C. R. Acad. Sci. (Paris) **272**, 855—858 (1971).

Provansal, A.: Les organes périsympathiques des Lépidoptères. C. R. Acad. Sci. (Paris) **274**, 97—100 (1972).

Provansal, A., Baudry, N., Raabe, M.: Recherches sur l'ultrastructure des organes neurohémaux périsympathiques des *Vespidae* (Hyménoptères). Les organes médians sphériques. C. R. Acad. Sci. (Paris) **271**, 1115—1118 (1970).

Provansal, A., Grillot, J. P.: Les organes périsympathiques des Insectes Holométaboles. I. Coléoptères. Ann. Soc. entomol. France (Paris) (N. S.) 8, 863—913 (1972).

Provansal, A., Grillot, J. P.: Les organes périsympathiques des Insectes Holométaboles. II. Hyménoptères. (Sous presse.)

Raabe, M.: Etude des phénomènes de neurosécrétion au niveau de la chaîne nerveuse ventrale des Phasmides. Bull. Soc. Zool. France **90**, 631—654 (1965).

Raabe, M.: Neurosécrétion dans la chaîne nerveuse ventrale des Insectes et organes neurohémaux métamériques. Arch. Zool. exp. gén. **112**, 679—694 (1971).

Raabe, M.: Les organes périsympathiques des Dermaptères. C. R. Acad. Sci. (Paris) **275**, 2925—2928 (1972).

Raabe, M., Baudry, N., Grillot, J. P., Provansal, A.: Les organes périsympathiques des Insectes. Distribution. Caractères généraux. C. R. Acad. Sci. (Paris) **273**, 2324—2427 (1971).

Raabe, M., Baudry, N., Provansal, A.: Recherches sur l'ultrastructure des organes neurohémaux périsympathiques des *Vespidae* (Hyménoptères). Les organes latéraux longitudinaux. C. R. Acad. Sci. (Paris) **271**, 1210—1213 (1970).

Raabe, M., Cazal, M., Chalaye, D., de Bessé, N.: Action cardioaccélératrice des organes neurohémaux périsympathiques ventraux de quelques Insectes. C. R. Acad. Sci. (Paris) **263**, 2002—2005 (1967).

Raabe, M., Demarti, F.: Etude de l'action des organes périsympathiques sur la protéinémie du Phasme, *Carausius morosus*. C. R. Acad. Sci. (Paris) (sous presse) (1973).

Raabe, M., Monjo, D.: Recherches histologiques et histochimiques sur la neurosécrétion chez le Phasme, *Clitumnus extradentatus*: les neurosécrétions de type C. C. R. Acad. Sci. (Paris) **270**, 2021—2024 (1970).

Raabe, M., Provansal, A.: Les organes périsympathiques des Paléoptères. C. R. Acad. Sci. (Paris) **275**, 925—928 (1972).

Raabe, M., Ramade, F.: Observations sur l'ultrastructure des organes périsympathiques des Phasmides. C. R. Acad. Sci. (Paris) **264**, 77—80 (1967).

Schaller, F., Charlet, M.: Evolution du système neurosécréteur de larves d'*Aeschna cyanea* Müll. (Insecte, Odonate) privées d'ecdysone. C. R. Acad. Sci. (Paris) **271**, 2004—2007 (1970).

Scharrer, B.: Neurosecretion. XIV. Ultrastructural study of sites or release of neurosecretory material in blattarian insects. Z. Zellforsch. **89**, 1—16 (1968).

Seshan, M. K. R.: Les phénomènes de neurosécrétion dans la chaîne nerveuse ventrale d'*Iphita limbata*. C. R. Acad. Sci. (Paris) **266**, 619—622 (1968).

Smith, D. S.: The organization and innervation of the luminescent organ in a firefly *Photuris pennsylvanica* (Coleoptera). J. Cell Biol. **16**, 323—359 (1963).

Stutinsky, F.: Etude du complexe rétro-cérébral de quelques insectes avec l'hématoxyline chromique. Bull. Soc. Zool. France **127**, 61—67 (1952).

Thomas, A., Mesnier, M.: Le rôle du système nerveux central sur les mécanismes de l'oviposition chez *Carausius morosus* et *Clitumnus extradentatus*. J. Insect Physiol. **19**, 383—396 (1973).

Thomas, A., Raabe, M.: Les organes périsympathiques des Orthoptères Ensifères. Bull. Soc. Zool. France (sous presse) (1974).

Vincent, J. F. V.: The dynamics of release and the possible identity of bursicon in *Locusta migratoria migratorioides*. J. Insect Physiol. **18**, 757—780 (1972).

b) Biochemistry and General Physiology

Biochemical Aspects of the Hypothalamo-Neurohypophysial Neurone

B. T. PICKERING, C. W. JONES, and G. D. BURFORD*

Department of Anatomy, University of Bristol, Bristol (Great Britain)

Many of our current ideas of the dynamics of neurosecretory neurones come from contributions by microscopists who have studied their structure in animals in different physiological conditions. These findings have provided the basis for discussion at each of the previous Symposia on Neurosecretion and the purpose of this paper is to review the extent of biochemical support that exists for these current concepts, although rather more examples will be drawn from the work of our own laboratory than its importance might warrant.

That the mammalian hypothalamus is indeed capable of synthesising the neurohypophysial hormones, was first demonstrated biochemically when Sachs (1960) isolated radioactive vasopressin from the hypothalami of dogs which had received intraventricular infusions of [^{35}S]cysteine. Since these original experiments on the biosynthesis of a neurosecretory product, Sachs and his co-workers have continued to study the mechanism of biosynthesis and release of vasopressin and their results are discussed in several reviews (Sachs et al., 1967a; Sachs, 1969; Sachs et al., 1969; Sachs et al., 1971). Perhaps one of their most significant contributions was the discovery that vasopressin is synthesised by way of a protein precursor which "matures" to yield the free hormone by a process which is unaffected by inhibitors of protein-synthesis and which takes about 1—1$^1/_2$ h in the guinea-pig (Sachs and Takabatake, 1964; Takabatake and Sachs, 1964).

Transport and Turnover of Oxytocin and Vasopressin

Evidence that the neurosecretory products of the supraoptic and paraventricular nuclei are transported along the hypothalamo-neurohypophysial tract for storage in the neural lobe was discussed at the 1st Symposium in Naples in 1953 (e.g. Scharrer, 1954; Bargmann, 1954; Zetler and Hild, 1954) and the first attempt at measuring the rate of transport along the axons was described by Sloper (1958a) to the 2nd Symposium in Lund in 1957. Using Sloper's method of subarachnoid injection of [^{35}S]cysteine several attempts have been made to determine the intra-axonal transport velocity with autoradiographic techniques (Sloper et al., 1960;

---

* Present address: Division of Pharmacology, University of Calgary, Calgary Alta. (Canada).

Sloper, 1966; Flament-Durand, 1961, 1967; Nishioka et al., 1970; Flament-Durand and Dustin, 1972). In the past few years we have extended this approach and have measured the incorporation of radioactivity into various chemically identified neurosecretory products. Isotopically pure preparations of radioactive oxytocin and vasopressin can be prepared from the pooled neural lobes of 4—5 rats which have received injections of radioactive amino acid into the cisterna magna (Pickering and Jones, 1971a). Using this technique we have been able to show that radioactive hormone begins to arrive in the gland between one and two hours after injection of the label, reaches a peak some 12 h after injection and then slowly declines over the next few weeks (Jones and Pickering, 1970; 1972; Pickering and Jones, 1971b). Taking the average length of the axons in the hypothalamo-neurohypophysial tract of the rat to be 2—3 mm (Sloper, 1958b) these results mean that the minimum velocity of the neurosecretory granules along these axons must be 1—3 mm/h. This calculation has allowed the whole of the 1—2 h lag period to be used for transport, but synthesis of the precursor and its "maturation" must also occur within this time, so that the actual velocity could be a good deal higher. Indeed, if "maturation" must be completed before transport can commence the velocity could be greater than 6 mm/h since Sachs and Takabatake (1964) showed that synthesis and "maturation" takes $1—1^{1}/_{2}$ h in the guinea-pig. There are however a number of pieces of evidence (e.g. see Sachs et al., 1969 and the Discussion after Pickering et al., 1971) which suggest that "maturation" is completed after the packaging of the precursor, and during the transport of the granules towards the neurohypophysis. It seems, therefore, that the lower estimate of intra-axonal transport rate may be the more likely one but, even so, this puts neurosecretory products in the class of substances which are rapidly transported in neurons. Discussion of the mechanisms involved in such rapid transport occurs elsewhere in this volume (Flament-Durand and Dustin, 1974; Grainger and Sloper, 1974).

It was found (Jones and Pickering, 1972) that, after reaching peaks at about 12 h after injection, the specific activities of the radioactive oxytocin and vasopressin declined exponentially and gave highly significant log-linear relationships with time. These curves describe the total rate of disappearance of hormone from the gland. Since this may possibly include a component from enzymic degradation within the neural lobe this rate cannot necessarily be equated with release. However, since the gland content of hormone remains constant (Heller, 1966) the rate of disappearance of hormone must be balanced by the arrival of newly synthesised hormone. Thus the slopes of these regression lines can be used to calculate the rates of synthesis of each hormone in the male rat in water balance, and give values of about 20 mU/day for oxytocin and 30 mU/day for vasopressin (Jones and Pickering, 1972). If the breakdown of hormone in the gland is ignored, and these values taken to represent hormone release, then, knowing the volume of distribution and the half-lives of the hormones in the blood, an estimate of plasma concentration can be made. Making these assumptions and substituting the necessary values from the literature the plasma concentration of both oxytocin and vasopressin was calculated to be about 3 µU/ml (Jones and Pickering, 1972) which is at the lower end of the range of values determined by direct assay.

The Role of Neurophysin

As Acher (1958) pointed out at the 2nd Symposium in Lund, the hormones oxytocin and vasopressin occur in the neural lobe as a complex with a cysteine-rich protein which he and his colleagues (Acher et al., 1955) named neurophysin(e). Neurophysin occurs in the same elementary neurosecretory granules as the hormones (Ginsburg and Ireland, 1963, 1966; Dean and Hope, 1966, 1967) and was accepted to be the carrier protein necessary for the intraneuronal transport of the hormones, and to be largely responsible for the stainability of neurosecretion in the hypothalamo-neurohypophysial system (Acher, 1958).

The chemical properties of the neurophysins have been studied most extensively with bovine (Rauch et al., 1969) and porcine (Uttenthal and Hope, 1970; Burford et al., 1971a; Coy and Wuu, 1971) material, and in each of these species two major and one minor neurophysin components have been characterized. Multiple forms of neurophysin have also been found in other species (Cheng and Friesen, 1972; Watkins, 1972a).

By convention, the different neurophysins have been designated according to their electrophoretic mobility, so that, for example, porcine Neurophysin I has a higher mobility than porcine Neurophysin II. It cannot be overstressed that this nomenclature is purely on the basis of electrophoretic differences within a species, and may have no functional significance. Indeed, it seems that, functionally, porcine Neurophysin I may be similar to bovine Neurophysin II and porcine Neurophysin II to bovine Neurophysin I (Pickup et al., 1973), an observation which is in keeping with the fact that a large portion of the amino acid sequence of bovine Neurophysin II is identical with that of porcine Neurophysin I (Walter et al., 1971; Wuu, Cramm and Saffran, 1971) and that the homology between the sequences of these two proteins is greater than that between bovine I and II (Capra et al., 1972).

Do the neurophysins occur simply as carrier proteins to bind the hormones and keep them within the neurosecretory granule, or is the association of a more intimate nature? One possibility which has been raised by Sachs and his colleagues (e.g. see Sachs et al., 1969; Sachs et al., 1971) is that neurophysin might be part of the same precursor which they had implicated in the biosynthesis of vasopressin; i.e. that hormones and neurophysins may be the products of the same prohormone. If this were so, the turnover of hormones could be studied by measuring neurophysin changes and, since rat neurophysins can be separated by a single polyacrylamide-gel electrophoresis run (Burford and Pickering, 1971), neurophysin data can be more easily accumulated. The two major and one minor neurophysin(s) of the rat can be labelled by intracisternal injection of [^{35}S]cysteine and, as shown in Fig. 1, more than 90% of the radioactivity recovered after electrophoresis of the extract of the neural lobe of a treated rat could be recovered in association with these components. It might be of interest to point out that the band labelled G in Fig. 1 contains a glycoprotein (e.g. stains with periodic acid—Schiff reagent), is labelled after intracisternal injection of [^{3}H]glucose (M. A. Abrahams and B. T. Pickering, unpublished observations) and seems to be associated with neurosecretory granules prepared by differential centrifugation (R. W. Swann and B. T. Pickering, unpublished observations). It is tempting to speculate that this component may represent the glycoprotein that Picard et al. (1974) have shown (this volume, p. 318) to be located in the periphery of neurosecretory granules and/or the glycoprotein which is the origin of the hexosamine which Thorn and his colleagues (personal communication) have isolated from granule membrane frac-

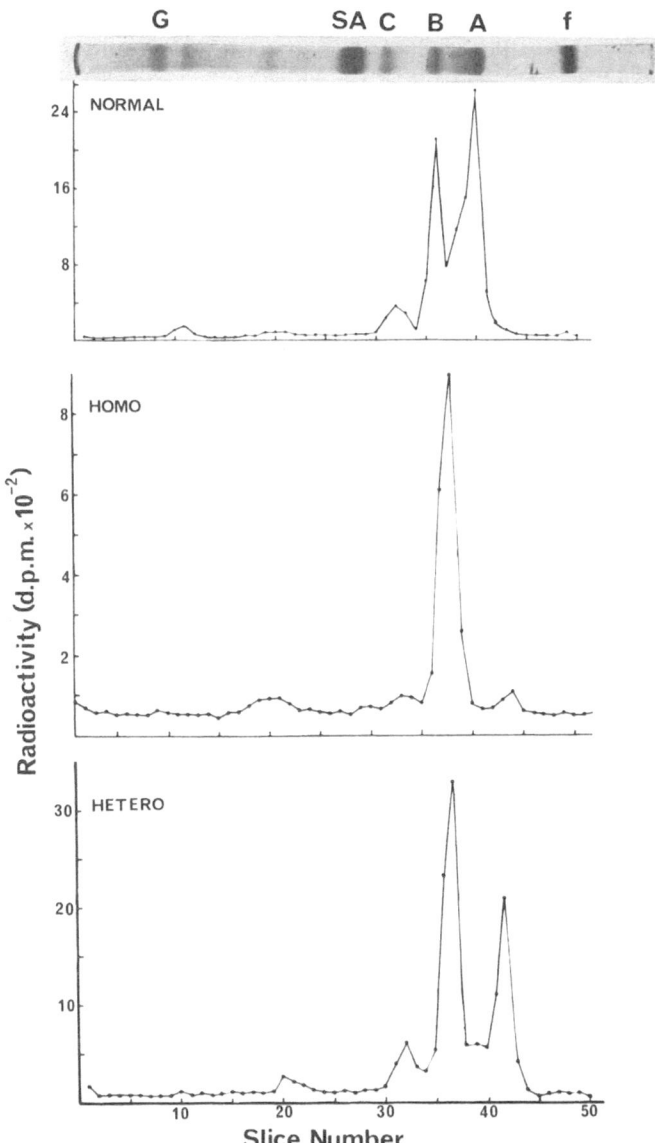

Fig. 1. Polyacrylamide gel electrophoresis of extracts of rat neural lobes. The distribution of radioactivity along the gel is shown for normal, homozygous Brattleboro and heterozygous Brattleboro rats. All rats received 50 μCi [³⁵S] cysteine intracisternally 24 h before death. f, solvent front; A, B, and C, rat neurophysins; SA, rat serum albumin; G, glycoprotein

tions. The origin and function of the glycoprotein component of neurosecretory granules will no doubt be the subject of discussion at future Symposia.

Separate Neurophysins for Oxytocin and Vasopressin

In our early studies of the incorporation of radioactivity into rat neurophysins, we found that the ratio of radioactivity associated with Neurophysin "A" to that with Neurophysin "B" was constant at 1.5 which is the same as the ratio of vasopressin to oxytocin in the gland. The rats in these experiments were all killed within 24 h of injection which, as we shall see later, was fortuitous, but these results gave the first indication that Neurophysin "A" might be related to vasopressin and Neurophysin "B" to oxytocin (Burford et al., 1971 b). This hypothesis received support from the observation that Neurophysin "A" is absent from rats with hereditary hypothalamic diabetes insipidus (Brattleboro) which are unable to synthesize vasopressin. As can be seen in Fig. 1 the neural lobe of a homozygous Brattleboro rat, which is devoid of vasopressin, shows only one major radioactive band after intracisternal injection of [^{35}S]cysteine whereas the heterozygote produces two bands but with more radioactivity in Neurophysin "B" than in Neurophysin "A", and the glands of these animals contain more oxytocin than vasopressin. Thus we propose that "B" is oxytocin-neurophysin and "A", vasopressin-neurophysin. This is not to suggest that these proteins will preferentially bind one or other hormone *in vitro* but that each hormone is biosynthetically linked to its specific neurophysin. Further evidence for this association is afforded by the observation that relatively more oxytocin-neurophysin than vasopressin-neurophysin is synthesised in the paraventricular nucleus whereas the converse is true for the supraoptic nucleus, although both proteins are synthesised in both nuclei (Burford et al., 1972, 1974). Several workers (Norström and Sjöstrand, 1971 a, b; Coy and Wuu, 1972; Watkins 1972 b) were unable to resolve the two major neurophysins of the rat but this was because insufficient bromophenol blue was used in their electrophoretic systems. Bromophenol blue is added to the running buffer in polyacrylamide-gel electrophoresis ostensibly as a marker for the ion-front (Davis, 1964) but, in the electrophoresis of rat neurohypophysial proteins, the dye forms a complex with vasopressin-neurophysin and allows its resolution from oxytocin-neurophysin; this only occurs if the dye is present at a concentration greater than 0.5 µg/ml and is optimal with a dye concentration of 1 µg/ml (Burford and Pickering, 1972).

Transport and Turnover of the Neurophysins

Radioactive vasopressin-neurophysin and oxytocin-neurophysin begin to arrive in the neural lobe between one and two hours after an intracisternal injection of [^{35}S]cysteine, reach a peak 12 h after the injection and gradually decline during the next 5 weeks (Burford and Pickering, 1973). In other words, the time course of labelling of the major neurophysin components is very similar to that of the hormones. Norström and Sjöstrand (1971 a, b) found very similar kinetics for a single component which cross-reacted with antibodies to porcine neurophysin

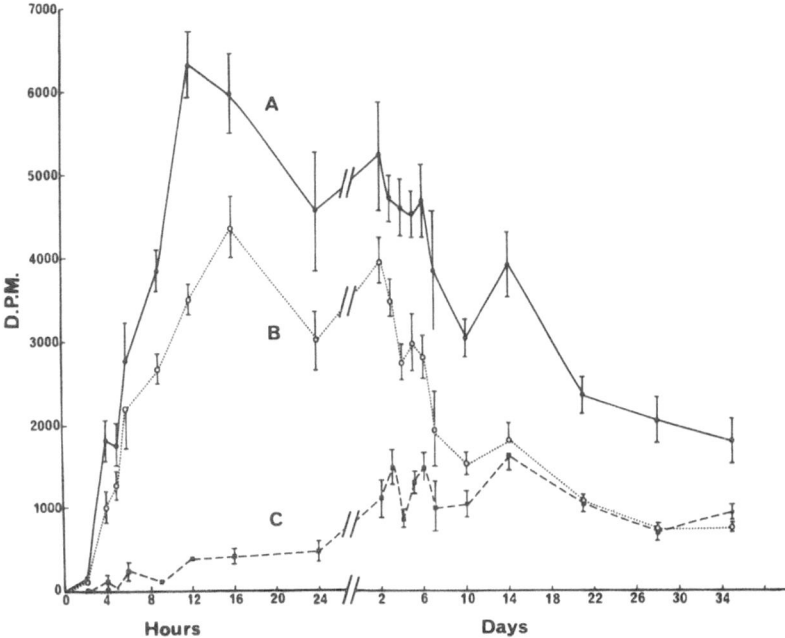

Fig. 2. The radioactivity associated with each rat neurophysin at various times after an intracisternal injection of $50\,\mu$Ci [^{35}S] cysteine. The points shown are means ($\pm$ S.E.M.) for 5—11 rats. Note the change in time scale after 24 h and that the rate of labelling of Neurophysin "C" is quite different from those of the major neurophysins

(Norström et al., 1971) and which was almost certainly an unresolved mixture of oxytocin- and vasopressin-neurophysins. The Swedish workers interpreted their time course to indicate that neurophysin had at least two intra-axonal transport rates. Such an interpretation from our data (Fig. 2) would not be justified. Individual points (e.g. 14 days after injection) may differ significantly (by simple t-test) from their neighbours but it is questionable whether one can make deductions about trends from single points. In fact, the data shown in Fig. 2 give highly significant log-linear regressions (Fig. 3a) for the decline in radioactivity of both major neurophysins from 12 h to 5 weeks after injection; i.e. the fall-off curves do not deviate from simple exponentials, and provide no support for additional radioactive protein arriving later by a slower transport process. From the decay curves it can be shown that the half-life for oxytocin-neurophysin in the gland is 13.3 days and that for vasopressin-neurophysin, 19.8 days. The difference in the slopes of the decay curves for the two neurophysins gives additional support to the contention that they are discrete proteins but raises problems in connection with the designation of "A" and "B" as vasopressin- and oxytocin-neurophysins on the basis of their ratio being equal to the V/O ratio since, clearly, the ratio of radioactivities increases with time. How can this problem be rationalized with the original hypothesis ?

The Significance of the Minor Neurophysin

As pointed out by Norström and Sjöstrand (1971 b), and can be seen from Fig. 2, the labelling of the minor neurophysin component ("C") follows an entirely different time-course from that of the major proteins. It does not become noticeably labelled until 24 h after injection and is still close to its peak value 5 weeks after injection. This raises the possibility that this component arises within the neurosecretory granule after it has arrived in the gland. Could it be that "C" is a metabolic product of oxytocin-neurophysin and is formed *in granulo?* If this were so the combined radioactivity of "B" and "C" should represent the radioactivity of the oxytocin-granule neurophysin and the important ratio would be $\dfrac{\text{radioactivity A}}{\text{radioactivity B + C}}$. In fact this ratio is close to the V/O ratio for all times and the decay curve for "B" and "C" taken together is not significantly different from

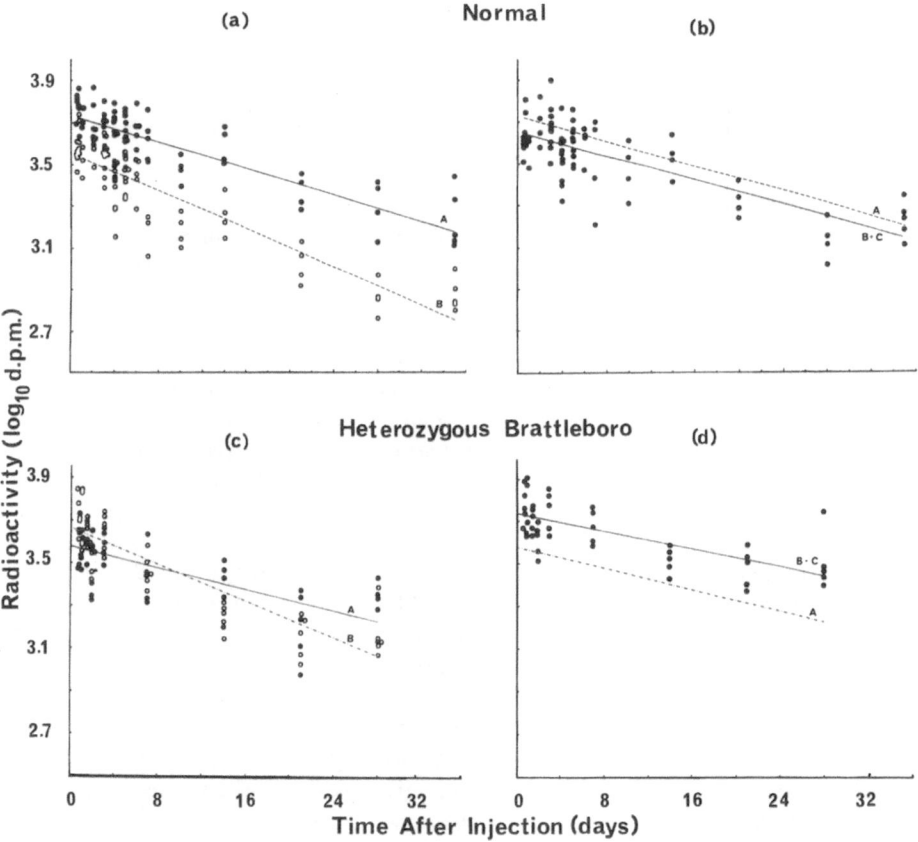

Fig. 3a—d. Decline of radioactivity in the major neurophysins in (a) normal rats and (c) heterozygous Brattleboros. When the radioactivity in Neurophysin "C" was added to that in Neurophysin "B", the combined fall-off curves were parallel to those of the respective vasopressin-neurophysins for both normals (b) and heterozygotes (d)

that for "A" (Fig. 3). This also holds true for heterozygous Brattleboro rats where the ratio is 0.6 (Mallam and Jones, 1974). These results allow the working hypothesis that the rat synthesises *two* hormones and *two* neurophysins and that the minor neurophysin component arises *in granulo*, and one can speculate that the minor components seen in other species have similar origins. Certainly there is evidence that one of the two major neurophysins may be associated with oxytocin and the other with vasopressin in both bovine (Dean et al., 1968) and porcine (Pickup et al., 1973) glands. We can therefore revise our modification (Pickering et al., 1971) of Sachs' original hypothesis (e.g. see Sachs et al., 1969) that the vasopressin precursor (provasopressin) is packaged into granules by the Golgi apparatus of the vasopressin neurone and that provasopressin is proteolytically cleaved to vasopressin and vasopressin-neurophysin ("A") during its passage to the neural lobe. We would now suggest that, in the oxytocin neurone, pro-oxytocin gives rise to oxytocin and oxytocin-neurophysin ("B") but that continued action of the hypothetical proteolytic enzyme on a sensitive bond in the latter leads to the slow appearance of the minor neurophysin component ("C"). There is no evidence to justify the suggestion that the minor neurophysin is associated with coherin— a peptide affecting gastrointestinal activity—which has been isolated (Goodman and Hiatt, 1972) from bovine neurohypophyses. The possibility that the origin of coherin involves one or other components of the neurophysin-neurohypophysial hormone system exists, however, but cannot be deduced from the evidence available at present.

The Origin of the "Readily-Releasable" Pool of Neurohypophysial Hormones

It is well established that the hormone in the neural lobe is distributed between a small "readily releasable" pool, from which hormone is easily released in response to a stimulus, and a larger storage pool the contents of which are much less accessible (Thorn, 1966; Sachs et al., 1967b; Sachs and Haller, 1968; Sachs, 1971). Sachs also has evidence that newly synthesised hormone enters the "readily releasable" pool before it equilibrates with the larger storage pool (Sachs and Haller, 1968) and Norström (1974) reaches similar conclusions from the results of the double labelling experiments which he presented to this Symposium. We have examined a number of mathematical models describing the passage of hormone through the gland and found that our data for the change in radioactivity of vasopressin-neurophysin gave a significantly better fit to the model based on the Sachs hypothesis than to any simpler model (Burford et al., 1973). What could be the morphological correlation of the "readily releasable" pool? An early suggestion was that it might represent extragranular hormone (e.g. see Ginsburg, 1968) and there is evidence for changes in the distribution of radioactive neurophysin between sedimentable and non-sedimentable fractions according to the time that it has spent in the gland (Norström, 1973), although we have been unable to confirm this (R. W. Swann and B. T. Pickering unpublished observations) and believe that the evidence is compatible with all neurophysin being intragranular and that the non-sedimentable fraction arises during homogenisation. There is mounting evidence that hormone is released by exocytosis of the whole granule contents (e.g. Douglas, 1974; Dreifuss et al., 1974; Dempsey et al., 1974) leading to a parallel release of neurophysin and hormone (Fawcett et al., 1968; McNeilly et al., 1972; Matthews et al., 1973). One of the possible explanations of the "readily releasable" pool considered by Sachs and Haller (1968) was that it may arise from the "spatial orientation (of hormone) within the axon (e.g. only those neurosecretory granules in close apposition to the neuronal membranes in the nerve terminals can discharge their contents into the perivascular space)". This would mean that neurosecretory granules entering the gland would have to travel to the terminal membrane and then move deeper into the nerve swelling. We have attempted to test this hypothesis using E. M. autoradiography (Heap et al., 1973, and unpublished observations). Intracisternal injections of [^{35}S]cysteine (50 μCi) were given to rats which were then killed and their glands prepared for E. M. autoradiography at intervals of up to 4 weeks after the injection. In the preliminary

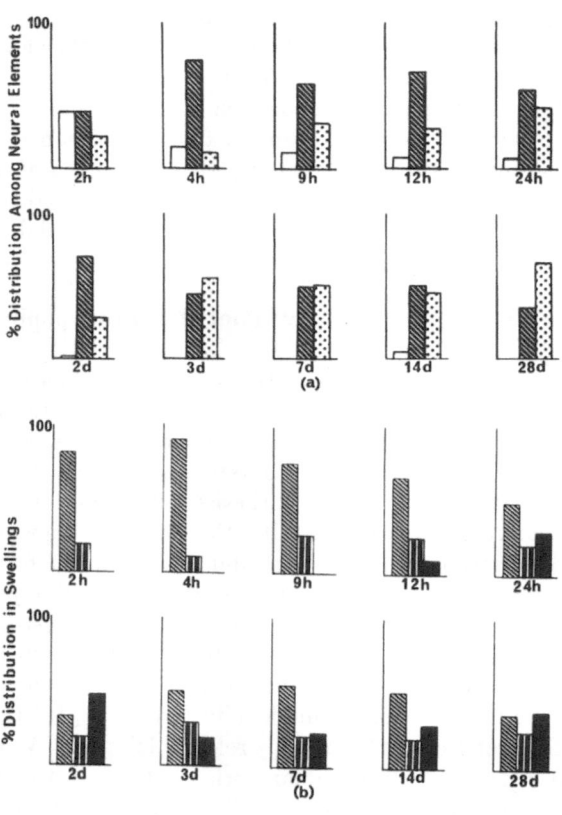

Fig. 4a and b. Distribution of radioactive figures seen in electron microscope autoradiographs of rat neural lobes removed at various times after an intracisternal injection of 50 μCi [^{35}S] cysteine. (a), Distribution among axons, ☐; "nerve endings" ▓, "nerve swellings" ▒. (b), Proportion of radioactive images in swellings which were seen 2 granule diameters, ▨; 4 granule diameters, ▥; more than 6 granule diameters ■; from the pituitary membrane (1 granule diameter is taken as 140 nm which is also the "half diameter" (HD) calculated for ^{35}S under these conditions)

analysis (Fig. 4a) the number of radioactive images corresponding with axons, nerve swellings in which microvesicles could be seen (endings) and those in which no microvesicles could be seen (swellings) were recorded. Figure 4a shows that the proportion of radioactive figures associated with axons fell dramatically within the first day. Moreover, there was a clear indication that radioactive images were more likely to be found in what we arbitrarily classified as nerve "endings" early after injection and in "swellings" at later time periods. This movement from "endings" to "swellings" is probably even more pronounced than the results indicate since some of the profiles which we classified as "swellings" undoubtedly came from nerve swellings which, if the plane of section had been different, would have been shown to contain microvesicles and therefore to be endings. When the radioactive figures were classified according to their proximity to the neuronal membrane, it was found (Fig. 4b) that they tended to occur deeper and deeper inside the profile with longer time intervals after injection of the labelled amino acid. Moreover the mean diameter of the profiles in which radioactive figures could be seen also increased with time, so that 4 weeks after injection 40% of them were found in profiles with a mean diameter greater than 3 μm and thus classifyable as Herring bodies (Dellman and Rodriguez, 1970). Thus the experimental evidence suggests that neurosecretory granules first enter nerve endings in which the presence of microvesicles suggests that release may be occurring (Douglas et al., 1971) and then move back deeper and deeper into larger and larger swellings. This is compatible with the idea that non-released granules are stored and may be finally destroyed in Herring bodies (Dellman and Rodriguez, 1970). It also implies that there must be two-way transport in the hypothalamo-neurohypophysial neurone with granules first being transported to the nerve ending, then back to larger nerve swellings for storage and, under conditions of extreme need, e.g. osmotic stress, back once more to the nerve ending for release. The mechanism by which granules move to and fro is intriguing as also is the question of whether this two-way transport is a special property of neurosecretory granules or a more general phenomenon in secretory cells.

Acknowledgments. The experimental work presented in this paper was supported in part by grants from the Royal Society and the Medical Research Council. We are also grateful for the expert technical assistance of Mrs. Janet Mallam and Mrs. Hazel Searle.

References

Acher, R.: État natural des principes ocytocique et vasopressique de la neurohypophyse. In: Proc. 2nd Int. Symposium on Neurosecretion (W. Bargmann, B. Hanström, B. Scharrer, E. Scharrer, Hrsg.), p. 71—78. Berlin-Göttingen-Heidelberg: Springer 1958.

Acher, R., Manoussos, G., Olivry, G.: Sur les relations entre l'ocytocine et la vasopressine d'une part et la proteine de van Dyke d'autre part. Biochim. biophys. Acta (Amst.) **16**, 155—156 (1955).

Bargmann, W.: Die endokrine Funktion neurosekretorischer Zellen bei Wirbeltieren. Pubb. Staz. Zool. Nap. **24** (Suppl.) 11—14 (1954).

Burford, G. D., Clifford, P., Jones, C. W., Pickering, B. T.: A model for the passage of the neurohypophysial hormones and their related proteins through the rat neurohypophysis. Biochem. J. **136**, 1053—1058 (1973).

Burford, G. D., Dyball, R. E. J., Moss, R. L., Pickering, B. T.: Preferential labelling of "oxytocin-neurophysin" by injection of [^{35}S] cysteine into the paraventricular nucleus of the rat. J. Physiol. (Lond.) **222**, 156—157 P (1972).

Burford, G. D., Dyball, R. E. J., Moss, R. L., Pickering, B. T.: Synthesis of both neurohypophysial hormones in both the paraventricular and supraoptic nuclei of the rat. J. Anat. (Lond.) **117**, 261—269 (1974).

Burford, G. D., Ginsburg, M., Thomas, P. J.: The effect of denaturants and Ca^{2+} on the molecular weight and polymerisation of neurophysin. Biochim. biophys. Acta (Amst.) **229**, 730—738 (1971 a).

Burford, G. D., Jones, C. W., Pickering, B. T.: Tentative identification of a vasopressin-neurophysin and oxytocin-neurophysin in the rat. Biochem. J. **124**, 809—813 (1971 b).

Burford, G. D., Pickering, B. T.: Polyacrylamide gel electrophoresis in the investigation of rat neurophysins. J. Endocr. **51**, 14—15 (1971).

Burford, G. D., Pickering, B. T.: The number of neurophysins in the rat. Influence of the concentration of bromophenol blue, used as a tracking dye, on the resolution of proteins by polyacrylamide-gel electrophoresis. Biochem. J. **128**, 941—944 (1972).

Burford, G. D., Pickering, B. T.: Intra-axonal transport and turnover of neurophysins in the rat. A proposal for a possible origin of the minor neurophysin component. Biochem. J. **136**, 1047—1052 (1973).

Capra, J. D., Kehoe, J. M., Kotelchuck, D., Walter, R., Breslow, E.: Evolution of neurophysin proteins: the partial sequence of bovine Neurophysin I. Proc. nat. Acad. Sci. (Wash.) **69**, 431—434 (1972).

Cheng, K. W., Friesen, H. G.: The isolation and characterisation of human neurophysin. J. clin. Endocr. **34**, 165—176 (1972).

Coy, D. H., Wuu, T. C.: Convenient apparatus for preparative polyacrylamide gel electrophoresis and its use in purification of three porcine neurophysins. Analyt. Biochem. **44**, 174—181 (1971).

Coy, D. H., Wuu, T. C.: Purification and amino acid composition of constituents of rat neurophysin. Biochim. biophys. Acta (Amst.) **263**, 125—132 (1972).

Davis, B. T.: Disc electrophoresis II, Method and application to human serum proteins. Ann. N. Y. Acad. Sci. **121**, 404—436 (1964).

Dean, C. R., Hope, D. B.: Protein constituents of neurosecretory granules isolated from the posterior lobes of bovine pituitary glands. Biochem J. **101**, 17—18 P (1966).

Dean, C. R., Hope, D. B.: The isolation of purified neurosecretory granules from bovine pituitary posterior lobes. Comparison of granule protein constituents with those of neurophysin. Biochem. J. **104**, 1082—1088 (1967).

Dean, C. R., Hope, D. B., Kazic, T.: Evidence for the storage of oxytocin with neurophysin-I and of vasopressin with neurophysin-II in separate neurosecretory granules. Brit. J. Pharmac. **34**, 192 P (1968).

Dellman, H. D., Rodriguez, E. M.: Herring bodies; an electron microscopic study of local degeneration and regeneration of neurosecretory axons. Z. Zellforsch. **111**, 293—315 (1970).

Dempsey, G. P., Bullivant, S., Watkins, W. B.: Exocytosis in the rat neurophypophysis — a freeze-fracture study. In: Neurosecretion — The Final Neuroendocrine Pathway (VI. Int. Symposium on Neurosecretion), p. 301. (F. Knowles, L. Vollrath, Eds.). Berlin-Heidelberg-New York: Springer 1974.

Douglas, W. W.: The Calcium-influx hypothesis and the exocytosis-vesiculation sequence: an interpretation of the mode of secretion of neurohypophysial hormones and significance of microvesicles (synaptic vesicles). In: Neurosecretion — The Final Neuroendocrine Pathway (VI. Int. Symposium on Neurosecretion), p. 302. (F. Knowles, L. Vollrath, Eds.). Berlin-Heidelberg-New York: Springer 1974.

Douglas, W. W., Nagasawa, J., Schulz, R.: Electron microscopic studies on the mechanism of secretion of posterior pituitary hormones and significance of microvesicles (synaptic vesicles): evidence of secretion by exocytosis and formation of microvesicles as a by-product of this process. Mem. Soc. Endocr. **19**, 353—378 (1971).

Dreifuss, J. J., Nordmann, J. J., Akert, K., Sandri, C., Moor, H.: Ultrastructure of the rat neuro-hypophysis as revealed by freeze-etching. In: Neurosecretion — The Final Neuroendocrine Pathway (VI. Int. Symposium on Neurosecretion), p. 31. (F. Knowles, L. Vollrath, Eds.). Berlin-Heidelberg-New York: Springer 1974.

Fawcett, C. P., Powell, A., Sachs, H.: Biosynthesis and release of neurophysin. Endocrinology 83, 1299—1310 (1968).

Flament-Durand, J.: Étude des relations hypothalamo-neurohypophysaires à l'aide de radio-isotopes marqué au Soufre 35. C. R. Hebd. Seanc. Acad. Sci. (Paris) 252, 3476—3500 (1961).

Flament-Durand, J.: Contribution à l'étude de la neurosécrétion chez le rat par la méthode autoradiographique. In: Neurosecretion (F. Stutinsky, Ed.)., p. 60—76. Berlin-Heidelberg-New York: Springer 1967.

Flament-Durand, J., Dustin, P.: Studies on the transport of secretory granules in the magno-cellular hypothalamic neurons. I. Action of colchicine on axonal flow and neurotubules in the paraventricular nuclei. Z. Zellforsch. 130, 440—454 (1972).

Flament-Durand, J., Dustin, P.: Further observations on the action of colchicine on the neuro-secretory paraventricular neurons in the rat. In: Neurosecretion — The Final Neuroendo-crine Pathway (VI. Int. Symposium on Neurosecretion), p. 304. (F. Knowles, L. Vollrath, Eds.). Berlin-Heidelberg-New York: Springer 1974.

Ginsburg, M.: Production, release, transportation and elimination of the neurohypophysial hormones. In: Handbook of Experimental Pharmacology (B. Berde, Ed.), Vol. 23, p. 286—371. Berlin-Heidelberg-New York: Springer 1968.

Ginsburg, M., Ireland, M.: Isolation, hormone-binding capacity and sub-cellular distribution of neurophysin. J. Physiol. (Lond.) 169, 114—115 P (1963).

Ginsburg, M., Ireland, M.: The role of neurophysin in the transport and release of neuro-hypophysial hormones. J. Endocr. 35, 289—298 (1966).

Goodman, I., Hiatt, R. B.: Coherin: a new peptide of the bovine neurohypophysis with activity on gastrointestinal motility. Science 178, 419—421 (1972).

Grainger, F., Sloper, J. C.: Overactivity of the hypothalamo-neurohypophysial neurosecretory system and the problem of the mechanisms of transporting neurosecretory material. In: Neurosecretion — The Final Neuroendocrine Pathway (VI. Int. Symposium on Neuro-secretion), p. 307. (F. Knowles, L. Vollrath, Eds.). Berlin-Heidelberg-New York: Springer 1974.

Heap, P. F., Jones, C. W., Morris, J. F., Pickering, B. T.: Transport and storage pools in the neurohypophysis — an autoradiographic approach. J. Endocr. 57, XVI—XVII (1973).

Heller, H.: The hormone content of the vertebrate hypothalamo-neurohypophysial system. Brit. med. Bull. 22, 227—236. (1966).

Jones, C. W., Pickering, B. T.: Rapid transport of neurohypophysial hormones in the hypo-thalamo-neurohypophysial tract. J. Physiol. (Lond.) 208, 73—74 P (1970).

Jones, C. W., Pickering, B. T.: Intra-axonal transport and turnover of neurohypophysial hormones in the rat. J. Physiol. (Lond.) 227, 553—564 (1972).

Mallam, J. B., Jones, C. W.: Turnover of radioactive neurophysins in the male heterozygous Brattleboro rat. Gen. comp. Endocr. 22, 337 (1974).

Matthews, E. K., Legros, J. J., Grau, J. D., Nordmann, J. J., Dreifuss, J. J.: Release of neuro-hypophysial hormones by exocytosis. Nature New Biology 241, 86—88 (1973).

McNeilly, A. S., Legros, J. J., Forsling, M. L.: Release of oxytocin, vasopressin and neurophysin in the goat. J. Endocr. 52, 209—210 (1972).

Nishioka, R. S., Zambrano, D., Bern, H. A.: Electron microscope radioautography of amino acid incorporation by supraoptic neurons of the rat. Gen. comp. Endocr. 15, 477—483 (1970).

Norström, A.: Subcellular distribution of neurophysin in rats subjected to haemorrhage, salt-loading and lactation and in rats with hereditary diabetes insipidus (Brattleboro strain). Z. Zellforsch. 140, 413—424 (1973).

Norström, A.: The heterogeneity of the neurohypophysial pool of neurophysin. In: Neuro-secretion — The Final Neuroendocrine Pathway (VI. Int. Symposium on Neurosecretion), p. 86. (F. Knowles, L. Vollrath, Eds.). Berlin-Heidelberg-New York: Springer 1974.

Norström, A., Sjöstrand, J.: Axonal transport of proteins in the hypothalamoneurohypophysial system of the rat. J. Neurochem. **18**, 29—39 (1971 a).

Norström, A., Sjöstrand, J.: Transport and turnover of neurohypophysial proteins of the rat. J. Neurochem. **18**, 2007—2016 (1971 b).

Norström, A., Sjöstrand, J., L ivett, B. G., Uttenthal, L. O., Hope, D. B.: Electrophoretic and immunological characterizat ion of rat neurophysin. Biochem. J. **122**, 671—676 (1971).

Picard, D., Michel-Bechet, M., Tasso, F.: Ultrastructural cytochemical observations on the hypothalamo-neu rohypophysial system in the rat. In: Neurosecretion — The Final Neuro-endocrine Pathway (VI. Int. Symposium on Neurosecretion), p. 318. (F. Knowles, L. Voll-rath, Eds.). Berlin-Heidelberg-New York: Springer 1974.

Pickering, B. T., Jones, C. W.: Isolation of radioactive oxytocin and vasopressin from the posterior pituitary gland of the rat after the injection of labelled tyrosine into the cerebro-spinal fluid. J. Endocr. **49**, 93—103 (1971 a).

Pickering, B. T., Jones, C. W.: The biosynthesis and intraneuronal transport of neurohypo-physial hormones: preliminary studies in the rat. Mem. Soc. Endocr. **19**, 337—351 (1971 b).

Pickering, B. T., Jones, C. W., Burford, G. D.: Biosynthesis and intra-neuronal transport of neurosecretory products in the hypothalamo-neurohypophysial system. In: Neuro-hypophysial Hormones, Ciba Fnd. Study Grp., no. 39 (Wolstenholme, G. E. W., Birch, J., Ed.), p. 58—74. London:Livingstone; Churchill 1971.

Pickup, J. C., Johnston, C. I., Nakamura, S., Uttenthal, L. O., Hope, D. B.: Subcellular organi-zation of neurophysins, oxytocin, [8-lysine]-vasopressin and adenosine triphosphatase in porcine posterior pituitary lobes. Biochem. J. **132**, 361—371 (1973).

Rauch, R., Hollenberg, M. D., Hope, D. B.: Isolation of a third bovine neurophysin. Biochem. J. **115**, 473—479 (1969).

Sachs, H.: Vasopressin biosynthesis 1. *in vivo* studies. J. Neurochem. **5**, 297—303 (1960).

Sachs, H.: Neurosecretion. Adv. Enzymol. **32**, 327—372 (1969).

Sachs, H.: Secretion of neurohypophysial hormones. Mem. Soc. Endocr. **19**, 965—973 (1971).

Sachs, H., Fawcett, C. P., Takabatake, Y., Portanova, R.: Biosynthesis and release of vasopres-sin and neurophysin. Recent. Prog. Hormone Res. **25**, 447—491 (1969).

Sachs, H., Haller, E. W.: Further studies on the capacity of the neurohypophysis to release vasopressin. Endocrinology **83**, 251—262 (1968).

Sachs, H., Portanova, R., Haller, E. W., Share, L.: Cellular processes concerned with vasopressin biosynthesis, storage and release. In: Neurosecretion (F. Stutinsky, Ed.), p. 46—154. Berlin-Heidelberg-New York: Springer 1967 a.

Sachs, H., Saito, S., Sunde, D.: Biochemical studies on the neurosecretory and neuroglial cells of the hypothalamo-neurohypophysial complex. Mem. Soc. Endocr. **19**, 325—336 (1971).

Sachs, H., Share, L., Osinchak, J., Carpi, A.: Capacity of the neurohypophysis to release vaso-pressin. Endocrinology **81**, 755—770 (1967 b).

Sachs, H., Takabatake, Y.: Evidence for a precursor in vasopressin biosynthesis. Endocrinology **75**, 943—948 (1964).

Scharrer, E.: Neurosecretion in the vertebrates: a survey. Pubb. Staz. Zool. Nap. **24** (Suppl.), 8—10 (1954).

Sloper, J. C.: The application of newer histochemical and isotope techniques for the localization of protein-bound cystine or cysteine to the study of hypothalamic neurosecretion in normal and pathological conditions. In: Proc. II. Int. Symposium on Neurosecretion (W. Barg-mann, B. Hanström, B. Scharrer, E. Scharrer, Eds.), p. 20—25. Berlin-Heidelberg-New York: Springer 1958 a.

Sloper, J. C.: Hypothalamo-neurohypophysial neurosecretion. Int. Rev. Cytol. **7**, 337—389 (1958 b).

Sloper, J. C.: The experimental and cytopathological investigation of neurosecretion in the hypothalamus and pituitary. The Pituitary Gland (3) p. 131—239. G. W. Harris, B. T. Donovan. London: Butterworths 1966.

Sloper, J. C., Arnott, D. J., King, B. C.: Sulphur metabolism in the pituitary and hypothalamus of the rat: a study of radioisotope-uptake after the injection of ^{35}S dl-cysteine, methionine, and sodium sulphate. J. Endocr. **20**, 9—23 (1960).

Takabatake, Y., Sachs, H.: Vasopressin biosynthesis III *in vitro* studies. Endocrinology **75**, 934—942 (1964).

Thorn, N. A.: In vitro studies of the release mechanism for vasopressin in rats. Acta. Endocr. (Kbh.) **53**, 644—654 (1966).

Uttenthal, L. O., Hope, D. B.: The isolation of three neurophysins from porcine posterior pituitary lobes. Biochem. J. **116**, 899—909 (1970).

Walter, R., Schlesinger, D. H., Schwarz, I. L., Capra, J. D.: Complete amino acid sequence of bovine Neurophysin II. Biochem. biophys. Res. Commun. **44**, 293—298 (1971).

Watkins, W. B.: Neurophysins of the sheep. Biochem. J. **126**, 759—760 (1972a).

Watkins, W. B.: The tentative identification of three neurophysins from the rat posterior pituitary gland. J. Endocr. **55**, 577—589 (1972b).

Wuu, T. C., Crumm, S., Saffran, M.: Amino acid sequence of porcine Neurophysin I. J. biol. Chem. **246**, 6043—6063 (1971).

Zetler, G., Hild, W.: Über die neurosekretorische Tätigkeit des hypothalamisch-neurohypophysären Systems der Säugetiere. Pubb. Staz. Zool. Nap. **24** (Suppl.), 15—17 (1954).

The Heterogeneity of the Neurohypophysial Pool of Neurophysin

ANDERS NORSTRÖM

Institute of Neurobiology, University of Göteborg, Göteborg (Sweden)

The axonal flow of neurosecretory material (NSM) along the hypothalamo-neurohypophysial system (HNS) was demonstrated by histochemical techniques more than two decades ago by Bargmann (1949). Sloper and colleagues (Sloper, 1958; Sloper et al., 1960) introduced radioisotope methods for studies on axonal transport of NSM, preparing autoradiographs of sections of the HNS after intra-cisternal injection of (^{35}S) cysteine. Nine hours after isotope injection and onward, the number of grains over the posterior pituitary exceeded that over the hypothalamus. Flament-Durand (1961), using the same technique, confirmed and extended this finding by showing that the pituitary NSM of dehydrated animals was more heavily labelled and had a more rapid turnover compared with controls. Recently, the axonal transport of NSM, i.e. neurophysin (Acher et al., 1955) and neurohypophysial hormones was characterized with the use of biochemical methods by two independent groups. Sulphur-labelled cysteine was injected either intracisternally or locally into the supraoptic nucleus (SON), and the accumulation of radioactive hormones and/or neurophysin in the neural lobe was measured at various time intervals after isotope injection. As judged from the start of arrival of radioactive products, it was concluded that hormones (Pickering and Jones, 1971), as well as neurophysin (Norström and Sjöstrand, 1971a) are transported in a rapid phase of axonal transport at a rate of approximately 190 mm per day, taking into regard a time period of 1.5 h before newly synthesized NSM becomes available for transport (Sachs and Takabatake, 1964; Norström and Sjöstrand, 1971c). In addition to a maximal net accumulation of radioactive neurophysin 2 days after isotope injection, we found another net increase of radioactivity 7.5 days after injection (Fig. 1, Norström and Sjöstrand, 1971b). The existence of a slow phase of axonal transport of proteins (1 mm per day; Weiss, 1944) has been documented in quite different neurons (cf. reviews by Barondes, 1969; Dahlström, 1971). In accordance with that notion we considered the second peak of neurophysin-bound radioactivity as representing a slow phase of axonal transport (0.5 mm per day) in the HNS. As judged from the rate of decrease of neurophysin-bound radioactivity, approximate half-lives of 12—24 h and 10 days were calculated for the rapidly and slowly transported neurophysin, respectively.

The neurohypophysial hormones and neurophysins are synthesized, transported and stored in neurosecretory granules (NSG) (Palay, 1955; Heller and Lederis, 1961; LaBella et al., 1962; Ginsburg and Ireland, 1966; Dean and Hope,

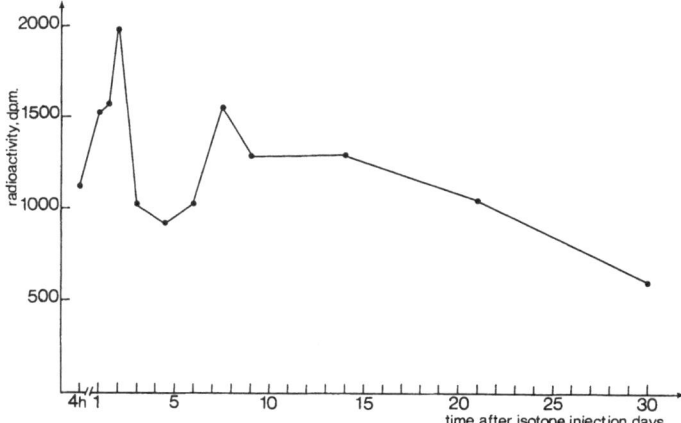

Fig. 1. Net accumulation of radioactive neurophysin in the posterior pituitary gland at various time intervals after injection of (^{35}S) cysteine into the supraoptic nucleus. Radioactivity expressed as d.p.m. (from Norström and Sjöstrand, 1971a)

1967; Dean et al., 1968; Nishioka et al., 1970). A substantial proportion of the neural lobe contents of hormones and neurophysin is not bound to NSG, and is recovered in the supernatant following centrifugation of neural lobe sucrose homogenates (Barer et al., 1963; Ginsburg and Ireland, 1966). Following physiological stimulation *in vivo* or depolarising stimulation *in vitro* only a fraction of the entire neurohypophysial content of vasopressin is released (Ginsburg and Brown, 1956; Thorn, 1965, 1966; Sachs et al., 1967). It was, therefore, suggested that the pool of vasopressin in the neural lobe is heterogeneous, comprising one major "non-easily releasable" reserve pool and a minor (5—20%) "easily releasable" pool (Thorn, 1965, 1966), and Ginsburg and Ireland (1966) proposed that the extragranular hormone pool is the easily releasable one.

On the other hand, Douglas and colleagues, according to their stimulus-secretion-coupling theory, consider NSG to be the only storing site from where NSM can be released, and thus claim that exocytosis is the mode of release (Douglas and Poisner, 1964; Douglas, 1968; Nagasawa et al., 1971).

In the present communication data are presented in support of the notion that the pituitary content of neurophysin is heterogeneous both with respect to subcellular organization and ease of release.

Materials and Methods

Male Sprague-Dawley rats were used in most experiments. (^{35}S) cysteine or (^{3}H) leucine was injected stereotaxically in the SON under halothane anesthesia, and the rats were killed by decapitation at various time intervals after isotope injection (Norström, 1971; Norström and Sjöstrand, 1971c). Neurophysin was isolated from the posterior pituitary gland (homogenized in 50 mM sodium phosphate buffer,

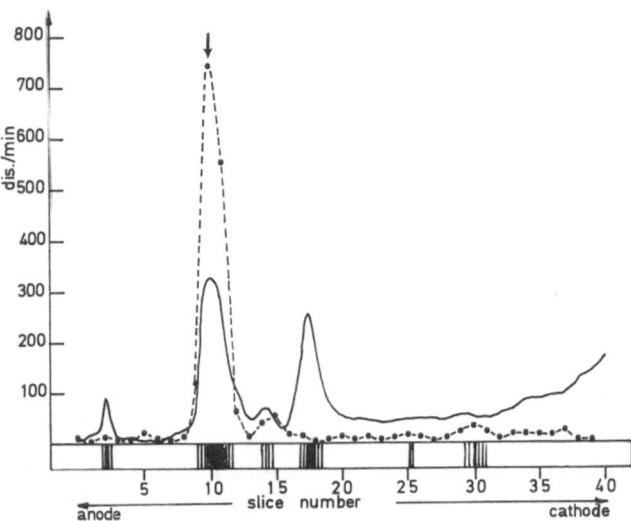

Fig. 2. Separation of neurohypophysial proteins on polyacrylamide gels 6 days after injection of (^{35}S) cysteine into the supraoptic nucleus. Most radioactivity is recovered in the neurophysin band (arrow) and a minor amount is found in a more cathodal protein band (modified from Norström, 1971). ——— optical density, ·········· radioactivity

pH 7.0) by electrophoresis on polyacrylamide gels (Davis, 1964; Ornstein, 1964) (Fig. 2). The total of neurophysin-associated radioactivity in the neural lobe was determined by liquid scintillation (Norström and Sjöstrand, 1971a). For isolation of NSG several posterior pituitary glands were pooled and homogenized in ice-cold 0.44 M sucrose. NSG were obtained by differential centrifugation, mainly according to Barer et al. (1963) (Norström and Hansson, 1972) and isolated as a pellet at 30000 g × 60 min. The final supernatant, containing non-granule bound "free" neurophysin, was recovered at 100000 g × 120 min.

Results and Discussion

Haemorrhage is a stimulus for preferential release of vasopressin (Ginsburg and Smith, 1959) and following acute bleeding about 10—20% of the neural lobe content of vasopressin (the "easily releasable pool") is discharged into the blood stream (Fawcett et al., 1968). In one series of experiments (Norström and Sjöstrand, 1971c) rats were subjected to acute bleeding (5 ml blood, 0.5 ml/min per 100 g body weight) 4 h after injection of (^{35}S) cysteine and killed 15 min later. As judged from optical densitometry estimations of the amount of protein in the stained neurophysin band in polyacrylamide gels, no reduction of neurophysin was found in bled rats compared with controls. Nevertheless, the specific and total radioactivity of neurophysin was reduced in bled animals (Table 1). These results demonstrated that only a minor fraction of neurophysin could have been released following bleeding, and they further indicated to us that the newly synthesized, rapidly transported neurophysin was preferentially released. In order to investigate that possibility, a double-labelling experiment was performed. (^{3}H) leucine was injected into the SON 11 days and (^{35}S) cysteine 5 h before killing. 6 ml blood were withdrawn from the femoral artery before killing by exsanguination (Table 1). The neurophysin-bound radioactivity in the neural lobe was measured and expressed as a (^{35}S): (^{3}H) ratio. Neurohypophyses of control rats contained significantly more (^{35}S) than those of bled rats, giving higher ratio values (Table 1; Norström, 1973, to be published). Thus, the combined results of these experiments suggested that in the neural lobe there exists a minor fraction of the total pool of neurophysin which is easily releasable and contains products which are probably newly synthesized. So far, however, it is not clear what proportion of the total contents of neurophysin this fraction represents.

Table 1. Effect of acute bleeding on the posterior pituitary neurophysin-bound radioactivity. I. Rats weighing 200 g were bled of 5 ml over 5 min, 4 h after injection of (^{35}S) cysteine into the supraoptic nucleus (SON) and killed by decapitation 15 min after start of bleeding. Radioactivity expressed as d.p.m. or d.p.m./μg trichloroacetic acid precipitated protein (parentheses). II. Rats weighing 200 g were injected with (^{3}H) leucine and (^{35}S) cysteine into the SON 11 days and 5 h before killing, respectively. Four ml of blood were withdrawn 2 h before killing, and 2 ml one hour before killing by exsanguination. Radioactivity expressed as a (^{35}S) : (^{3}H) ratio (from Norström and Sjöstrand, 1971c and Norström 1973, to be published)

Animals	Neurophysin-bound radioactivity	
	d.p.m.	(^{35}S): (^{3}H)
I Control	1023 (11.7)	
Acute bleeding	802 (7.7)	
II Control		2.82
Acute bleeding		1.65

Subcellular fractionation of posterior pituitary tissue has shown that there exists an extragranular pool of NSM *(vide supra)*. In addition, there are data favouring the view that there is an exchange of products between intra- and extra-granular compartments. Thus, the supernatant fraction ("extra-granular pool") obtained after centrifugation of pituitary homogenates of control animals contained 20—25% of the total hormone content (Lederis and Heller, 1960; Heller and Lederis, 1961; Barer et al., 1963). Ginsburg and Ireland (1966) claimed that this "free" hormone could not be due to disruption of NSG during preparation. Following physiological stimulation, the non-granule-bound hormone increased proportionally, i.e. the "free" vasopressin represented 50% of total hormone content in dehydrated rabbits (Barer et al., 1963), and more than 80% of the total oxytocin content was recovered extragranularly in lactating rabbits (Lederis, 1967). In order to investigate whether the "free" and granular pools were static, i.e. without exchange of NSM, or dynamic, i.e. with transfer of products between the pools, NSG were prepared from rats which had been injected with (^{35}S) cysteine at various time intervals before killing. The radioactivity associated with neurophysin was measured in NSG and in the supernatant fraction. Eighteen to 24 h after isotope injection, about 20% of the radioactive neurophysin was found extragranularly, and more than 60% was recovered in NSG (Table 2). The amount of "free" radio-active neurophysin increased with time after injection, representing about 40% of the total neurophysin-associated radioactivity 14 days after injection, whereas the labelled neurophysin in NSG correspondingly decreased. These results supported the hypothesis that a redistribution of neurophysin occurs between subcellular compartments in the neural lobe. In order to check the validity of this hypothesis rats were subjected to various kinds of physiological stimulation to see whether such a "transfer" process is influenced by the hormone demand. Acute haemorrhage did not affect the NSG content of (^{35}S) cysteine 24 h after injection, whereas 8.5 or 14 days later increased amounts of radioactive neurophysin were found extragranularly (Table 2). Replacement of drinking water with 2% NaCl

Table 2. Recovery of neurophysin-bound radioactivity in neurosecretory granules and in the cell sap (extragranular neurophysin) of posterior pituitary glands after injection of (^{35}S) cysteine into the supraoptic nucleus. Radioactivity expressed as percentage of the total recovered pituitary radioactivity (from Norström, 1972, 1973)

Animals	Time after isotope injection	Granule-bound neurophysin %	Extragranular neurophysin %
Control	18 hours	64.1	22.8
Thirst 6 days	18 hours	39.5	41.1
Control	24 hours	64.6	20.6
Acute bleeding	24 hours	61.1	22.9
2% NaCl 4 days	24 hours	55.1	35.8
Diabetes insipidus	24 hours	43.2	39.9
Control	8.5 days	55.0	33.8
Acute bleeding	8.5 days	43.8	48.0
Control	14 days	40.8	50.0
Acute bleeding	14 days	34.5	52.6

for 4 days resulted in a slight decrease of radioactive neurophysin in NSG. A more severe osmotic stimulus, i.e. the chronic osmotic stimulus in rats with hereditary hypothalamic diabetes insipidus (Brattleboro strain), or dehydration for 6 days by water deprivation, increased the proportion of extragranular radioactive neurophysin already within 24 h after isotope injection. The data so obtained indicated that the normally occurring subcellular redistribution of neurophysin in secretory terminals, i.e. transfer of neurophysin from NSG to an extragranular space, is dependent on the physiological state of the animal. The differences in the amount of "free" radioactive neurophysin among animals subjected to various kinds of physiological stimulation suggest that the escape of NSM from NSG is dependent on the degree of demand of hormones: the greater the demand, the more extensive is the extrusions of products to an extragranular space. Moreover, since the response to stimulation, as measured by non-granule-bound radioactive neurophysin, was more pronounced at longer time intervals after injection of (^{35}S) cysteine, it appears likely that the NSM has to reach a certain stage of maturity before it can be transferred from NSG. This interpretation is in accordance with the hypothesis advanced by Thorn (1966) who suggested that neurosecretory products undergo a "maturation" process during storage within NSG. At a certain stage of maturity these products are transferred (via an energy-dependent mechanism, Warberg and Thorn, 1969) from the granules to an extragranular pool of hormones.

Further support for the view that "old" NSG and NSG from functionally stimulated rats have a greater maturity, as evidenced by their capacity to extrude neurophysin, was gained when the release of radioactive neurophysin from isolated NSG was studied *in vitro*. Poisner and Douglas (1968) previously demonstrated that the release of vasopressin and proteins from neurosecretory vesicles was energy-dependent and stimulated by ATP. In the present study NSG were incubated in a HEPES-buffered incubation medium, in the absence or presence of an ATP-regenerating system (Norström, 1972, 1973). The spontaneous release in the absence of ATP of neurophysin from NSG of rats injected with (^{35}S) cysteine 14 days before killing ("old" NSG) exceeded that occurring from NSG of rats injected 18 or 24 h before killing (Table 3). In addition, the spontaneous release

Table 3. Release of radioactive neurophysin from isolated neurosecretory granules (NSG) at various time intervals after injection of (^{35}S) cysteine into the supraoptic nucleus. The rats were subjected to various kinds of physiological stimulation. NSG were incubated in the absence ("normal" medium) or presence of an ATP-regenerating system (Poisner and Douglas, 1968). Radioactivity expressed as a ratio of released radioactive neurophysin to that remaining in NSG after incubation. Control values are given within parentheses (from Norström, 1972, 1973)

Experimental group	Time after isotope injection	Normal medium	ATP-regenerating medium
Thirst 6 days	18 hours	3.10 (1.20)	3.40 (2.10)
Acute bleeding	24 hours	1.55 (1.85)	3.45 (3.42)
2% NaCl 4 days	24 hours	2.15 (1.29)	3.00 (2.57)
Diabetes insipidus	24 hours	1.23 (1.29)	1.50 (2.57)
Acute bleeding	8.5 days	3.71 (1.39)	4.27 (3.48)
Acute bleeding	14 days	4.51 (2.79)	4.78 (3.48)

from granules was higher in physiologically stimulated rats as compared with controls. Thus, it appears likely that the capacity of granules to release material increases with time. Further, the time period necessary before neurophysin can be released from NSG seems to be shortened following specific stimulation. This concept was further supported by the fact that exposure of NSG to an ATP-regenerating system was followed by more extensive release of radioactive neurophysin from "old" NSG and NSG of physiologically stimulated rats as compared with controls. In spite of a chronic osmotic stimulus, the spontaneous release of (^{35}S) labelled neurophysin from NSG from *diabetes insipidus*-rats was lower than in control rats, and the response to an ATP-regenerating system was poor. This raises the question as to whether these rats, in addition to being unable to synthesize vasopressin (see Valtin, 1967), are defective in some NSG factor which is essential for the release process.

The results presented in this communication can be interpreted in more than one way. Many objections can be raised to the suggestions made in this study (What are the effects of a traumatic homogenization procedure and exposure to cold ? Are "old" NSG more fragile than "young" NSG ? Are NSG from stimulated

animals more fragile than those from control rats ? etc.). From the results no
conclusions can be drawn about the physiological role of an exchange of NSM to
an extragranular space or its relation to the release process. Neither can any
quantitative estimation be made concerning the proportions of the intra- and
extragranular pools, nor about the subcellular localization of the extragranular
pool, whether it is located inside the nerve ending or in the extraterminal perivascular channels (Barer and Lederis, 1966). Nevertheless, the present results
favour the notion that there exists an exchange of neurophysin between an intragranular and an extragranular pool of neurophysin in the posterior pituitary gland,
and that this exchange is dependent on the age of the NSG and the physiological
state of the animal.

Acknowledgments. I am indebted to Dr. Graham McLean for helpful criticism of my
English and to Miss Gull Grönstedt for careful secretarial work.

References

Acher, R., Manoussos, G., Olivry, G.: Sur les relations entre l'oxytocine et la vasopressine d'une
part et la protéine de Van Dyke d'autrepart. Biochim. biophys. Acta (Amst.) **16**, 155—156
(1955).
Barer, R., Heller, H., Lederis, K.: The isolation, identification and properties of the hormonal
granules of the neurohypophysis. Proc. roy. Soc. B **158**, 388—416 (1963).
Barer, R., Lederis, K.: Ultrastructure of the rabbit neurohypophysis with special reference to
the release of the hormones. Z. Zellforsch. **75**, 201—239 (1966).
Bargmann, W.: Über die neurosekretorische Verknüpfung von Hypothalamus und Neuro-
hypophyse. Z. Zellforsch. **34**, 610—634 (1949).
Barondes, S. H.: Axoplasmic transport. In: A. Lajtha (Ed.): Handbook of neurochemistry,
Vol. II, p. 435—446. New York-London: Plenum Press 1969.
Dahlström, A.: Axoplasmic transport (with particular respect to adrenergic neurons). Phil.
Trans. B **261**, 325—358 (1971).
Davis, B. J.: Disc electrophoresis II. Method and application to human protein. Ann. N. Y.
Acad. Sci. **121**, 404—427 (1964).
Dean, C. R., Hope, D. B.: The isolation of purified neurosecretory granules from bovine pituitary
posterior lobes. Biochem. J. **104**, 1082—1088 (1967).
Dean, C. R., Hope, D. B., Kažić, T.: Evidence for the storage of oxytocin with neurophysin-I
and of vasopressin with neurophysin-II in separate neurosecretory granules. Brit. J.
Pharmac. **34**, 192—193 (1968).
Douglas, W. W.: Stimulus-secretion coupling: the concept and clues from chromoffin and
other cells. Brit. J. Pharmac. **34**, 451—474 (1968).
Douglas, W. W., Poisner, A. M.: Stimulus-secretion coupling in a neurosecretory organ. The
role of calcium in the release of vasopressine from the neurohypophysis. J. Physiol. (Lond.)
172, 1—18 (1964).
Fawcett, C. P., Powell, A. E., Sachs, H.: Biosynthesis and release of neurophysin. Endocrinology **83**, 1299—1310 (1968).
Flament, J.: Étude des relations hypothalamo-neurohypophysaires à l'aide de radioisotopes
marqués au soufre 35. C. R. Acad. Sci. (Paris) **252**, 3487—3489 (1961).
Ginsburg, M., Brown, L. M.: Effect of anesthetics and haemorrhage on release of neurohypophysial antidiuretic hormone. Brit. J. Pharmac. **11**, 236—244 (1956).
Ginsburg, M., Ireland, M.: The role of neurophysin in the transport and release of neurohypophysial hormones. J. Endocr. **35**, 289—298 (1966).
Ginsburg, M., Smith, M. W.: The fate of oxytocin in male and female rats. Brit. J. Pharmac. **14**,
327—333 (1959).
Heller, H., Lederis, K.: Density gradient centrifugation of hormone containing subcellular
granules from rabbit neurohypophysis. J. Physiol. (Lond.) **158**, 27—28 (1961).

LaBella, F. S., Beaulieu, G., Reiffenstein, R. J.: Evidence for the existence of separate vasopressin and oxytocin-containing granules in the neurohypophysis. Nature (Lond.) 193, 172—173 (1962).

Lederis, K.: Beziehung zwischen der Ultrastruktur der Neurohypophyse und der subcellulären Verteilung von biologisch aktiven Substanzen. Naunyn-Schmiedebergs Arch. Pharmak. exp. Path. 257, 53—95 (1967).

Lederis, K., Heller, H.: Intracellular storage of vasopressin and oxytocin in the posterior pituitary lobe. Acta endocr. (Kbh.) Suppl. 51, 115—116 (1960).

Nagasawa, J., Douglas, W. W., Schulz, R. A.: Ultrastructural evidence of secretion by exocytosis and of "synaptic vesicle" formation in posterior pituitary glands. Nature (Lond.) 227, 407—409 (1970).

Nishioka, R. S., Zambrano, D., Bern, H. A.: Electron microscope radioautography of amino acid incorporation by supraoptic neurons of the rat. Gen. comp. Endocr. 15, 477—483 (1970).

Norström, A.: A functional study of the hypothalamo-neurohypophyseal system of the rat with the use of a newly developed method for localized administration of labelled precursor. Brain Res. 28, 131—142 (1971a).

Norström, A.: Release in vitro of neurohypophysial proteins from neural lobe tissue slices and from isolated neurosecretory granules of the rat. Z. Zellforsch. 129, 114—139 (1972).

Norström, A.: Subcellular distribution of neurophysin in rats subjected to acute haemorrhage, salt-loading and lactation and in rats with hereditary diabetes insipidus (Brattleboro strain). Z. Zellforsch. 140, 413—424 (1973).

Norström, A., Hansson, H.-A.: Isolation and characterization of neurosecretory granules of the rat posterior pituitary gland. Z. Zellforsch. 129, 92—113 (1972).

Norström, A., Sjöstrand, J.: Axonal transport of proteins in the hypothalamo-neurohypophysial system of the rat. J. Neurochem. 18, 29—39 (1971a).

Norström, A., Sjöstrand, J.: Axonal transport and turnover of neurohypophysial proteins of the rat. J. Neurochem. 18, 2007—2016 (1971b).

Norström, A., Sjöstrand, J.: Effect of heamorrhage on the rapid axonal transport of neurohypophysial proteins in the rat. J. Neurochem. 18, 2017—2026 (1971c).

Ornstein, L.: Disc electrophoresis. I. Background and theory. Ann. N. Y. Acad. Sci. 121, 321—349 (1964).

Palay, S. L.: An electron microscope study of the neurohypophysis in normal hydrated and dehydrated rats. Anat. Rec. 121, 348 (1955).

Pickering, B. T., Jones, C. W.: The biosynthesis and intraneuronal transport of neurohypophysial proteins: preliminary studies in the rat. Mem. Soc. Endocr. 19, 327—351 (1971).

Poisner, A. M., Douglas, W. W.: A possible mechanism of release of posterior pituitary hormones involving adenosine triphosphatase in the neurosecretory granules. Molec. Pharmacol. 4, 531—540 (1968).

Sachs, H., Share, L., Osinchak, J., Carpi, A.: Capacity of the neurohypophysis to release vasopressin. Endocrinology 81, 755—770 (1967).

Sachs, H., Takabatake, Y.: Evidence for a precursor in vasopressin biosynthesis. Endocrinology 75, 943—948 (1964).

Sloper, J. C.: Hypothalamo-neurohypophysial neurosecretion. Int. Rev. Cytol. 7, 337—389 (1958).

Sloper, J. C., Arnott, D. J., King, B. C.: Sulphur metabolism in the pituitary gland and hypothalamus of the rat: a study of radioisotope uptake after injection of (^{35}S) DL-cysteine, methionine and sodium sulphate. J. Endocr. 20, 9—23 (1960).

Thorn, N. A.: Role of calcium in the release of vasopressin and oxytocin from posterior pituitary protein. Acta endocr. (Kbh.) 50, 357—364 (1965).

Thorn, N. A.: In vitro studies on the release mechanism for vasopressin in rats. Acta endocr (Kbh.) 53, 644—654 (1966).

Valtin, H.: Hereditary hypothalamic diabetes insipidus in rats (Brattleboro strain). Amer. J. Med. 42, 814—827 (1967).

Warberg, J., Thorn, N. A.: In vitro studies on the release mechanism for vasopressin in rats. III. Effect of metabolic inhibitors on the release. Acta endocr. (Kbh.) 61, 415—424 (1969).

Weiss, P.: Damming of axoplasm in constricted nerve: a sign of perpetual growth in nerve fibers. Anat. Rec. 88, 464 (1944).

Recent Functional Studies
on the Caudal Neurosecretory System of Teleost Fishes

K. Lederis, H. A. Bern, M. Medakovic, D. K. O. Chan, R. S. Nishioka, A. Letter, D. Swanson, R. Gunther, M. Tesanovic, and B. Horne

Division of Pharmacology and Therapeutics, Faculty of Medicine, University of Calgary and Department of Zoology and its Cancer Research Laboratory, University of California, Berkeley (USA)

Introduction

For many years now the caudal neurosecretory system and its neurohemal organ in teleosts, the urophysis, have been the subject of intensive morphological investigation. Although many of the more recent studies have been functionally oriented, the nature of the urophysial hormone(s) and their actual physiological role remain incompletely understood (cf. Bern, 1969, 1971, 1972; Lederis, 1970, 1971, 1972; Lederis et al., 1971; Chan, 1971; Berlind, 1973). At present, substantial data point to the existence of a number of urophysial principles or urotensins. Urotensins I and II have been extensively studied pharmacologically. Urotensin II appears to have a general smooth muscle-contracting effect including a hypertensive influence in fish, as well as bladder-contracting (Lederis, 1970a, b; Berlind, 1972a), lymph heart-stimulating (Chan, 1971) and sperm duct-contracting (Berlind, 1972b) activities. An association of the caudal system with reproduction continues to appear from time to time in the literature (Dixit, 1971).

Urotensin I is a potent hypotensive agent in mammals without significant effects on fish systems (Lederis, 1972; Medakovic and Lederis, 1972). Urotensin II activity has been found in the caudal spinal cords of all groups of fish except cyclostomes and lungfish (Bern et al., 1973); knowledge of urotensin I is so far confined to teleosts. Urotensin IV occurs only in some teleosts (Lacanilao and Bern, 1972); it has proved to date to be indistinguishable from arginine vasotocin (Lacanilao, 1972a, b). Urotensin III is a presumed osmoregulatory principle (Maetz et al., 1964), not arginine vasotocin, for the existence of which indirect suggestive indications also continue to recur (Carvajal and Vallowe, 1972).

The present survey proposes to consider three areas of "urophysiological" research which have received particular attention in our laboratories in the past year or two: (1) the nature of the neural input to the caudal neurosecretory system; (2) the evidence for the existence of unique urophysial proteins that may prove to be the carrier "urophysins" of this system, analogous to the "neurophysins" of the hypothalamo-neurohypophysial system; and (3) the chemical and pharmacological characterization of urotensin I and some comparisons with urotensin II on mammalian and piscine systems.

I. Aminergic Input to the Caudal Neurosecretory System

The caudal neurosecretory neurons are recognized as not forming an autonomous system (cf. Yagi and Bern, 1965; Baumgarten et al., 1970). It seems evident that aminergic input to these neurosecretory neurons is particularly prominent (Baumgarten et al., 1970; Wilén and Fridberg, 1973), although Baumgarten et al. feel that cholinergic fibres terminate on most if not all of the caudal neurons in *Esox lucius*, whereas aminergic input is received only by some of them.

The Falck-Hillarp histochemical technique (Falck et al., 1962) for induction of fluorescence from monoamines was utilized to investigate the relationship between the aminergic nervous system and the caudal neurosecretory system in *Gillichthys mirabilis*. It was found that the caudal neurosecretory cell bodies in the spinal cord are surrounded by small green varicosities, similar to the color and characteristics of fluorescence of noradrenaline- and dopamine-containing neurons in other systems. No fluorescence characteristic of other monoamines was observed in the system and the neurohemal organ (urophysis) was devoid of induced fluorescence. Drug treatments were applied to some fish as follows: 1.875 mg of pargyline in 0.5 ml distilled water were injected intraperitoneally into fishes weighing about 25 g 3, 24 or 48 h prior to sacrifice; 10 mg/kg reserpine in 0.5 ml distilled water were injected intraperitoneally into fishes 12 or 24 h prior to sacrifice.

Bright-green fluorescent varicosities were found surrounding the cell bodies (Fig. 1a) and axons of the caudal neurosecretory cells in the spinal cord, ventral and lateral to the central canal. Fluorescence was associated with the bilateral neurosecretory cell tracts along their entire course from the fifth or sixth preterminal vertebra to the area of the spinal cord dorsal to the urophysis; lesser amounts of fluorescence occur in the filum terminale. Animals varied with respect to intensity of fluorescence and completeness of fluorescence along the tracts.

Green fluorescent varicosities of this type have been shown to be characteristic of noradrenaline and dopamine in other tissues. Electron microscopy reveals endings of nerve fibers in association with the neurosecretory perikarya with a multivesicular ultrastructure characteristic of type "B" (aminergic) terminals, including the presence of large granular vesicles (Fig. 1b). However, although Baumgarten et al. (1970) found numerous varicosities in the caudal neurosecretory system of the pike *(Esox lucius)*, the levels of catecholamines were unexpectedly low as measured by chemical assay, raising the possibility that the endings may not contain catecholamine.

Pargyline treatment increased the apparent size and number of varicosities. Reserpine treatment reduced the green fluorescence, and in some cases completely eliminated varicosities in the entire system. These findings correlate with the presence of catecholamines. Analysis of *Tilapia mossambica* showed similar distribution of smaller varicosities which exhibited similar reactions to pharmacological treatments. No caudal cells filled with fluorescent material, as reported by Baumgarten et al. (1970) in the pike, were observed in either *Gillichthys* or *Tilapia*.

It appears that in both *Gillichthys* and *Tilapia*, the caudal neurosecretory neuron perikarya and extra-urophysial axons receive an elaborate aminergic

innervation. However, there was no evidence in either of these species for cholinergic
input. The aminergic control system here is of unknown physiological significance,
but is reminiscent of the aminergic contribution to the median eminence encountered in many vertebrates.

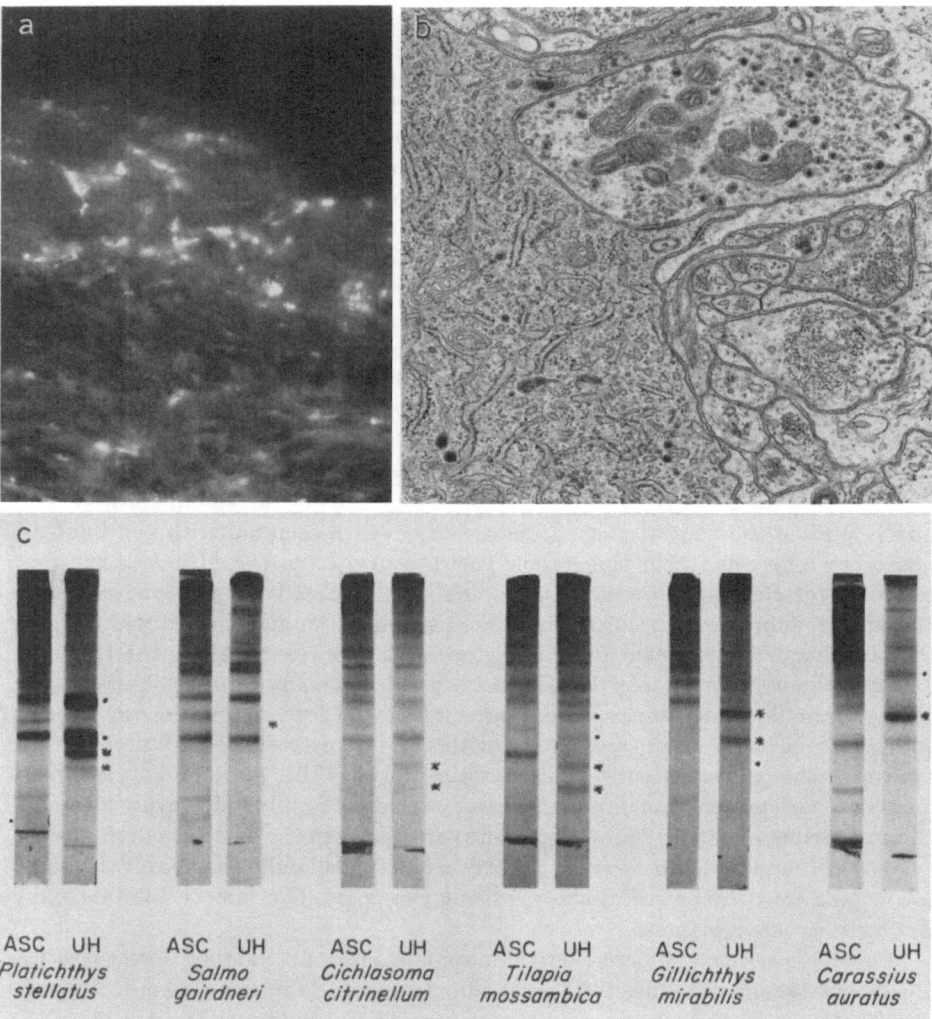

Fig. 1. a Area of spinal cord to show caudal neurosecretory perikarya of *Gillichthys mirabilis*
outlined by green fluorescent varicosities indicating the presence of aminergic nerve endings.
Falck-Hillarp method. × 320. b Electron micrograph of periphery of perikaryon of a caudal
neurosecretory neuron of *Gillichthys mirabilis* to show prominent aminergic ending. × 20000.
c Comparison of polyacrylamide gel disc electrophoretograms of anterior spinal cord (ASC)
and urophysis (UH) of 6 teleost fish species. Asterisks indicate location of prominent unique
urophysial proteins; black dots indicate location of minor components which may also be
unique

II. Unique Proteins in the Urophysis (Urophysins)

In 1972, Berlind et al. reported the existence of two unique proteins in the urophysis of *Gillichthys mirabilis*, which could serve as candidates for the putative carrier proteins of the caudal neurosecretory system. These "urophysins" would then be comparable to the "neurophysins" of the cranial (hypothalamo-neurohypophysial) system. Disc-gel electrophoresis (DE) was carried out on the urophysis (UH), anterior spinal cord (ASC), posterior spinal cord (PSC), plasma, and in some cases, the pituitary of six species of teleost fishes (Fig. 1c). Basically the method outlined by Davis (1965) was used for preparation of gel solutions, and for electrophoresis on 10% acrylamide gel.

In all cases except the flounder *(Platichthys stellatus)*, the tissues were removed from fresh fish. In the flounder, the ASC and tails were frozen over dry ice and kept several days before being used. On the day DE was performed, the tails were thawed and the UH and PSC removed. While removing the UH, the spinal cord (both anterior and posterior to it) was cut off. The PSC was taken 1—3 vertebral segments just anterior to the UH. The ASC was taken from the area of the operculum.

Several DE runs were conducted for each species, and an attempt was made to alter the amount of material to give relatively uniform staining. Therefore, because of the differences in fish sizes and inherent species differences, various numbers and different lengths of tissue were used. The pituitary and plasma showed bands totally different from the urophysis and contained none of the proteins unique to the UH. The PSC closely resembled the ASC.

Figure 1c demonstrates that, for the most part, there is little evidence of similarity in the location of the bands unique to the urophysis after DE. One or two major components are present in each species examined, with indications of minor unique components as well. However, the two major unique bands in the *Cichlasoma* and *Tilapia* species appear to have similar Rf's. Inasmuch as these two species belong to the same family (Cichlidae), it is possible that more uniformity will generally be encountered when more closely related species are compared.

The functional significance of these protein bands remains uncertain. Berlind et al. (1972) reported that urotensin II migrated closely to the slower-moving "urophysin", however, no direct identity has been established. Studies are presently being conducted to determine any association of biological activity with the bands, and also to analyze isolated urophysial neurosecretory granules for their content of unique protein(s).

III. Chemical and Pharmacological Studies on Urotensin I

A. Chemical Characterization of Urotensin I

The presence of rat blood pressure lowering activity in acidic extracts of carp urophyses was reported by Kobayashi and his coworkers (Kobayshi et al., 1968), with an indication of long- and short-acting components (cf. Lederis, 1972). These findings have been confirmed and extended by Zelnik and Lederis (1973), when it could be shown by gel-filtration in columns of Bio-Gel P2, P10, and P60 that: (a) three different substances could be isolated: a long-acting and a short-acting urotensin I both of which were active on rat blood pressure, without a demonstrable pharmacological effect in fishes, and a urotensin II having fish-smooth-muscle-contracting and eel pressor activities, (b) urotensin I activity (long-acting) as obtained by acetic acid extraction, being associated with a substance of molecular weight between 20000—60000, (c) after extraction with 0.1 N hydrochloric acid, urotensin I (long-acting) was eluted from Bio-Gel P10 columns over a broad spectrum indicating a molecular weight range from < 6000 to > 20000, (d) urotensin II was eluted, in all systems, at a rate indicating a molecular size of < 1800.

In more recent experiments (Letter et al., 1973, and unpublished observations), aimed mainly at purification of the long-acting urotensin I, gel chromatography was continued in Bio-Gel P10, P6, and P2 columns, using acetone-dried urophyses of the common sucker *(Catostomus commersoni)* extracted either in acetic acid (Bern and Lederis, 1969) or in 0.1 N hydrochloric acid. More meaningful studies became possible after the isolated hind limb of the rat was found to be a useful, sensitive and specific (under appropriate pharmacological conditions) means for quantitative estimations of the long-acting urotensin I (Medakovic and Lederis, 1972). With this assay it was found that comparable yield of the long-acting rat-hypotensive activity could be obtained after either 0.25% acetic or 0.1 N hydrochloric acid extraction (heating for 3 min and 5 min respectively).

Preliminary purification was carried out by chromatography on Bio-Gel P10 columns of HCl extracts, eluting with HCl. In contrast to the earlier experiments (Zelnik and Lederis, 1973) in which the rat-hypotensive activity was found to be associated with an undetermined number of molecular weight species from < 6000 to > 20000, in the recent experiments, urotensin I emerged in one peak at K_D 0.73—1.02 corresponding to one or more components of a molecular weight of < 6000.

The active fractions from the Bio-Gel P10 column were pooled and re-chromatographed on Bio-Gel P6. Two peaks of urotensin I activity were found: one at K_D 0—0.32, indicating a molecular weight of 4000 or greater, and another peak in the K_D 0.42—0.96 range, indicating a molecular weight of about 2000 daltons. Because a variation in the proportion of activity in the two peaks was observed in individual experiments, a series of control chromatography experiments on Bio-Gel P6 columns was devised: three batches of equal quantities (10 mg) of acetone-dried urophysis powder were homogenized in 0.1 N HCl and heated in a boiling water bath for 5, 10 or 15 min. Each batch was chromatographed under identical conditions, and eluted with 0.25% acetic acid. The amount of the "low-molecular weight" (M.wt. about 2000) urotensin I fraction increased with increasing heating, with a corresponding decrease of the "high-molecular weight" (i.e. > 4000) component(s). The percentage distribution of the "high"- and "low"-molecular weight urotensin I changed from 94 : 6 after heating for 5 min to 15 : 85 after heating of the extract for 15 min. The total amounts of urotensin I activity were comparable in all cases. A further chromatography experiment in a Bio-Gel P2 column of the "low-molecular weight" urotensin I fraction (obtained from the P6 chromatography) in which urotensin I activity was excluded from the gel confirmed the unit size of near to M.wt. 2000.

The pharmacological properties of this "low-molecular weight urotensin" have raised a question as to the existence of a short-acting component of urotensin I: routine assays of eluates from the different gel chromatography experiments have repeatedly indicated that low doses of this peptide produce only a short-lasting hypotensive effect, similar to that reported by Kobayashi (in Lederis, 1972); an increase in the dose of a given "short-acting" fraction invariably produced a typical long-lasting effect. Subject to further chemical and pharmacological investigations, it is tempting to conclude at this time that a "short-acting" urotensin I does not exist.

B. Subcellular Distribution of Urotensins I and II

Differential centrifugation experiments (Lederis et al., 1971) showed that urotensin II was located in cell particles sedimenting at a centrifugal force comparable to that required to isolate the neurohypophysial hormone containing granules under identical conditions (density of medium, temp., etc.; Barer et al., 1963).

Subcellular distribution of both urotensins (i.e., I and II) has now been studied by sucrose density gradient centrifugation (Horne and Lederis, 1973). Homogenates of 100—150 sucker urophyses were centrifuged at $178\,000 \times g$ for 90 min over layered gradients of 1.0—1.7 M sucrose. The main peak of urotensin II activity was found in 1.4 M sucrose layer. Urotensin I activity was found in the 1.4—1.55 M sucrose region of the gradient with a peak in the 1.45 M layer (Fig. 2 c), suggesting that the two urotensins may be associated with two different populations of cell particles. Electron microscopy showed that this region of the gradient, in which the urotensin I and urotensin II peaks were found, was rich in electron dense granules such as are seen in nerve terminals of the urophysis. It remains to be investigated whether the granules containing urotensin I and urotensin II, can be differentiated by electron microscopy.

C. Pharmacological Observations on Urotensins I and II

Adaptation of the isolated hind limb of the rat for assays of urotensin I has made possible studies of its pharmacological properties. Perfusion of both exsanguinated hind limbs with modified Krebs' solution containing noradrenaline $10^{-6}—10^{-7}$ g/ml at 1.2—2.5 ml/min (Medakovic and Lederis, 1972) is effected through a cannula inserted into the abdominal aorta. The cannula is connected by means of a three-way tap from a perfusion pump (LKB, Vario-Perpex) to a Statham (P23 Db) pressure transducer, water manometer and the recording instrument (Beckman RN Dynograph). The threshold dose of urotensin I varies from 0.1—1 mU and thus gives a range of sensitivity 1—2 orders of magnitude greater than that of the conscious or anaesthetized rat. Figure 2 a shows a typical response of the hind limb to urotensin I and Fig. 2 b a comparison of dose-response relationships for urotensin I, acetylcholine and bradykinin.

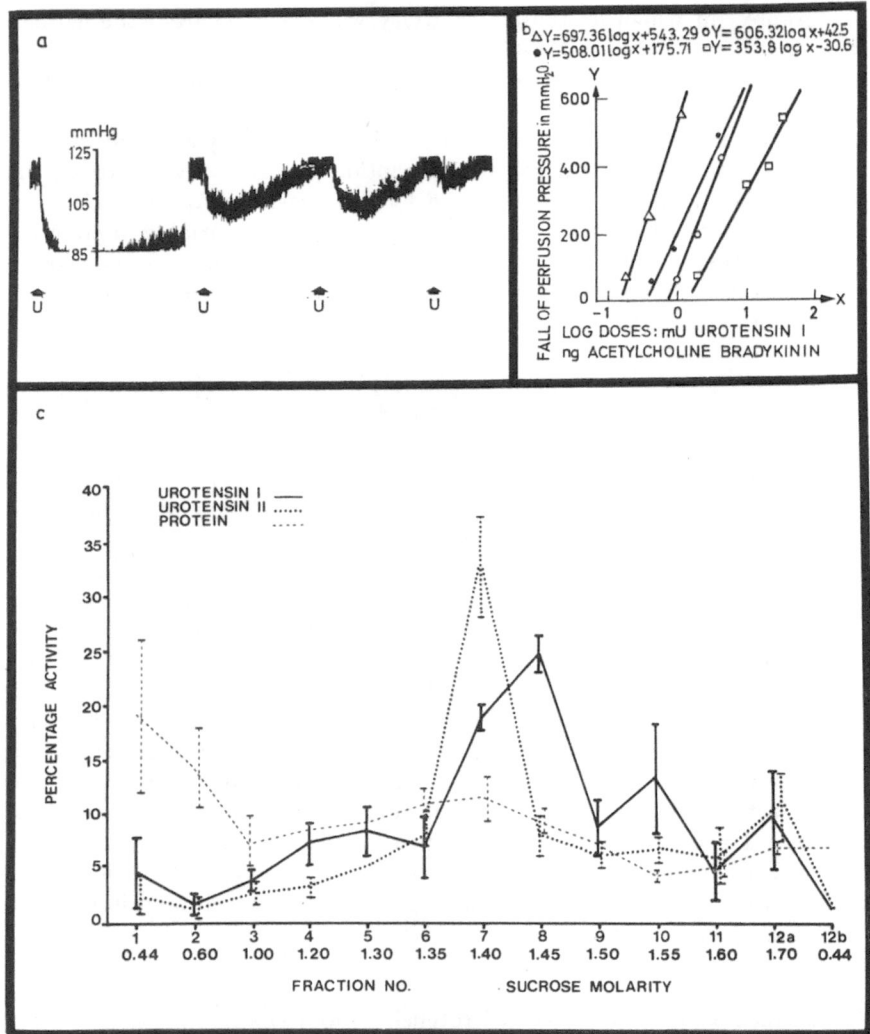

Fig. 2. a Responses of the isolated hind limb of the rat to urotensin I. From left to right (at arrow), effects of 4 mU, 2 mU, 2 mU, 1 mU. Note: decreasing extent and duration of response with decreasing doses. b Dose-response curves of two samples of urotensin I (O and ●), acetylcholine (▲) and bradykinin (■). c Density gradient centrifugation of urophysial homogenates. Percentage distribution of urotensin I, urotensin II activities, and of proteins (Folin-Lowry) in gradient fractions (Means ± S.E. from 4 experiments)

1. Mode and Site of Action of Urotensin I in the Rat

The pharmacological properties of urotensin I (the long-lasting blood pressure—lowering effect in the rat) have been found to vary considerably, depending on the experimental preparation used and on the route of administration chosen (Lederis and Medakovic, 1973):

In the conscious rat, doses of urotensin I in the range of 1—20 mU/100 g b.wt. lowered the mean blood pressure by 10—50% of pre-injection values for 10 to 120 min. Both the extent of the fall and duration of action were dose dependent. Moreover, the higher the initial (pre-injection) blood pressure, the greater were the effects of urotensin I. Rats with congenital hypertension were more sensitive to urotensin I: in female (basal pressure 144.9 ± 8.6 mm Hg) and male hypertensive rats (basal pressure 170.6 ± 2.3 mm Hg) a given dose of urotensin (e.g. 10 mU/100 g b.wt.) lowered the mean arterial blood pressure by 17.9 ± 1.5% and 28.9 ± 1.1% respectively, as compared to 12.4 ± 1.3% in normotensive controls. In all cases, the blood presure-lowering effects were accompanied by a reflex increase in heart rate which could be blocked by propranolol or by ganglion blocking drugs (e.g., hexamethonium, mecamylamine). The blood pressure effects were due to a direct vasodilator action on peripheral blood vessels and were not modified by cholinergic, α- and β-adrenergic blockers or antihistamines.

After *subcutaneous* or *intramuscular* administration to conscious rats, the duration of the hypotensive effect of urotensin I was prolonged considerably lasting for >24 h after s.c. injection of higher doses.

In rats anaesthetized with thiopental, pentobarbital, chloralose, or urethane, the duration of the hypotensive and cardiac effects of urotensin I was intermediate between that found after i.v. and s.c. administration in conscious rats.

2. Effects of Urotensin I on Renal Function in the Rat

Hypotensive doses of crude urophysial extracts or of partially purified urotensin I induced a dose-dependent antidiuresis in the ethanol-anaesthetized, water-loaded rat (Medakovic et al., 1973). The antidiuretic effects differed from those caused by vasopressin or arginine vasotocin: (a) urotensin antidiuresis lasted from 10—20 min in a dose-dependent manner, (b) there was little or no increase in urine conductivity (i.e. excretion of dilute urine), and (c) the antidiuretic potency of urotensin was not diminished after treatment with Na-thioglycollate.

Concomitant with the antidiuretic effect, decreases were observed in ^{14}C-inulin and ^{3}H-PAH clearances and lowered urinary output of Na and K.

It is likely, therefore, that the antidiuretic action of urotensin I was directly related to its hypotensive action causing a decrease in glomerular filtration and renal plasma flow rates.

3. Effects of Urotensin I on Different Vascular Beds in the Rat

An attempt to localize the vascular action of urotensin I was made by a study of changes in blood volume (measured with ^{51}Cr-labelled erythrocytes) in different vascular beds of the pentobarbital-anaesthetized rat during peak hypotension elicited by a relatively high dose of urotensin I (usually 50 mU/100 g b.wt.). An increase in blood volume, indicating vasodilatation, was found in skeletal muscle, kidney, intestine, ear (cutaneous blood flow) and adrenals. A decrease in blood volume was found in the liver and spleen, whereas no changes were observed in the heart, lungs and diaphragm. Concomitant determination of inulin space in the corresponding vascular beds showed an increase in extracellular space in the areas of the most pronounced vasodilatation (i.e., skeletal muscle, intestine, adrenals).

The tissue/plasma inulin ratio in the kidney increased considerably, suggesting a relative increase in water reabsorption.

Urotensin II did not produce measurable effects either on systemic blood pressure or on blood space in the vascular beds of the rat studied, other than in the renal cortex, outer and inner medulla (Chan, Medakovic and Lederis, unpublished observations).

4. Effects of Urotensins I and II in the Eel

Both urotensins increased blood pressure in the free swimming eel by producing vasoconstriction in the vascular beds of both the dorsal and ventral aortae (Chan et al., unpublished observations). However, urotensin II was at least ten times more effective than urotensin I (wt/wt).

The renal effects of urotensins I and II in the eel differed: whereas both urotensins increased urine flow, the GFR (^{14}C-inulin clearance) *increased* after urotensin II but *decreased* after urotensin I. Further investigation of the urotensins in the eel (and in fishes generally) appears to be indicated to establish their actions on the cardiovascular and renal systems and to determine which urotensin causes the effects on the earlier reported sodium fluxes (Maetz et al., 1964). Such studies may be expected to throw some light on the physiological role of this peptide (and of the caudal neurosecretory system) in fishes.

Acknowledgments. Aided by Medical Research Council of Canada Grant MT 3911 to K. Lederis and National Science Foundation Grant GB 35329 × to H. A. Bern. (K. Lederis is an Associate of the Medical Research Council of Canada.)

References

Barer, R., Heller, H., Lederis, K.: The isolation, identification and properties of the hormonal granules of the neurohypophysis. Proc. roy. Soc. B **158**, 388—416 (1963).

Baumgarten, H. G., Falck, B., Wartenberg, H.: Adrenergic neurons in the spinal cord of the pike *(Esox lucius)* and their relation to the caudal neurosecretory system. Z. Zellforsch. **107**, 479—498 (1970).

Berlind, A.: Teleost caudal neurosecretory system: sperm duct contraction induced by urophysial material. J. Endocr. **52**, 567—574 (1972a).

Berlind, A.: Teleost caudal neurosecretory system: release of urotensin II from isolated urophyses. Gen. comp. Endocr. **18**, 557—560 (1972b).

Berlind, A.: Caudal neurosecretory system: a physiologist's view. Amer. Zool. (1973). (In Press.)

Berlind, A., Lacanilao, F., Bern, H. A.: Teleost caudal neurosecretory system: Effects of somotic stress on urophysial proteins and active factors. Comp. Biochem. Physiol. **42 A**, 345—352 (1972).

Bern, H. A.: Urophysis and caudal neurosecretory system: In: Fish Physiology (W. S. Hoar, D. J. Randall, Eds.), Vol. 11, p. 399—418. New York: Academic Press 1969.

Bern, H. A.: The urophysis as an endocrine organ—some unanswered questions. In: Memoirs of the Society for Endocrinology. No. 19: Subcellular Organization and Function in Endocrine Tissues (H. Heller, K. Lederis, Eds.), p. 843—851. London, New York: Cambridge University Press 1971.

Bern, H. A.: Some questions on the nature and function of cranial and caudal neurosecretory systems. Progress Brain Res. **38**, 85—96 (1972).

Bern, H. A., Gunther, R., Johnson, D. W., Nishioka, R. S.: Occurrence of urotensin II (bladder-contracting activity) in the caudal spinal cord of anamniote vertebrates. Acta zool. (Stockh.) **54**, 15—19 (1973).

Bern, H. A., Lederis, K.: A reference preparation for the study of active substances in the caudal neurosecretory system of teleosts. J. Endocr. **45**, 11—12 (1969).

Carvajal, S., jr., Vallowe, H. H.: Development and osmoregulatory role of the urophysis of the teleost *Xiphophorus helleri*. Proc. Penn. Acad. Sci. **46**, 35—36 (1972).

Chan, D. K. O.: The urophysis and the caudal circulation of teleost fish. In: Memoirs of the Society for Endocrinology. No. 19: Subcellular Organization and Function in Endocrine Tissues (H. Heller, K. Lederis, Eds.), p. 391—412. London, New York: Cambridge University Press 1971.

Davis, B. J.: Disc electrophoresis—II. Clinical applications. Method and application to human serum proteins. Ann. N. Y. Acad. Sci. **121**, 404—427 (1964).

Dixit, V. P.: The karyometric response of caudal neurosecretory cells in *Clarias batrachus* to sex steroids. Gen. comp. Endocr. **17**, 561—563 (1971).

Falck, B., Hillarp, N.-Å., Thieme, G., Torp, A.: Fluorescence of catecholamines and related compounds condensed with formaldehyde. J. Histochem. Cytochem. **10**, 348—354 (1962).

Horne, B. L., Lederis, K.: Separation of urotensins I and II by density gradient centrifugation. Canad. Fed. Biol. Soc. **16** (419), 105 Abstract (1973).

Kobayashi, H., Matsui, T., Hirano, T., Iwate, T., Ishii, S.: Vasodepressor substance in the fish urophysis. Annot. Zool. Jap. **41**, 154—158 (1968).

Lacanilao, F.: The urophysial hydrosmotic factor of fishes: I. Characteristics and similarity to neurohypophysial hormones. Gen. comp. Endocr. **19** (3), 405—412 (1972a).

Lacanilao, F.: The urophysial hydrosmotic factor of fishes: II. Chromatographic and pharmacologic indications of similarity to arginine vasotocin. Gen. comp. Endocr. **19** (3), 413—420 (1972b).

Lacanilao, F., Bern, A.: The urophysial hydrosmotic factor of fishes. III. Survey of fish caudal spinal cord regions for hydrosmotic activity. Proc. Soc. exp. Biol. (N. Y.) **140** (4), 1252—1253 (1972).

Lederis, L.: Active substances in the caudal neurosecretory system of bony fishes. In: Hormones and the Environment (G. Benson, J. Phillips, Eds.). Mem. Soc. Endocr. **18**, 465—484 (1970a).

Lederis, K.: Urophysis: I. Bioassay of an active principle on the isolated urinary bladder of the rainbow trout *(Salmo gairdnerii)*. Gen. comp. Endocr. **14**, 417—426 (1970b).

Lederis, K.: Urophysis: II. Biological and pharmacological properties of a smooth muscle-contracting principle. Gen. comp. Endocr. **14**, 427—437 (1970c).

Lederis, K.: Recent progress in research on the urophysis. Gen. comp. Endocr. Suppl. **3**, 339—344 (1972).

Lederis, K., Bern, H. A., Nishioka, R. S., Geschwind, I. I.: Some Observations on Biological and Chemical Properties and Subcellular Localization of Urophysial Active Principles In: Memoirs of the Society for Endocrinology. No. 19: Subcellular Organization and Function in Endocrine Tissues (H. Heller, K. Lederis, Eds.), p. 413—433. London, New York: Cambridge University Press 1971.

Letter, A., Lederis, K.: Molecular weight estimation of the urophysial hypotensive principle be gel-filtration. Canad. Fed. Biol. Soc. **16** (420); 105 (1973).

Maetz, J., Bourguet, J., Lahlouh, B.: Urophyse et osmorégulation chez *Carassius auratus*. Gen. comp. Endocr. **4**, 401—414 (1964).

Medakovic, M., Chan, D. K. O., Lederis, K., Gosbee, J. L.: Antidiuretic effects of urotensin I. Canad. Fed. Biol. Soc. **16** (462), 116 (1973).

Medakovic, M., Lederis, K.: Rat hypotensive activity in extracts of fish urophysis. In: V. Int. Cong. Pharm. San Francisco 1972, p. 154.

Wilén, P. E., Friberg, G.: Ultrastructural studies on the ontogenesis of the caudal neurosecretory system in the roach, *Leuciscus nutilus*. Z. Anat. Entwickl.-Gesch. **139**, 207—216 (1973).

Yagi, K., Bern, H. A.: Electrophysiologic analysis of the response of the caudal neurosecretory system if *Tilapia mossambica* to osmotic manipulations. Gen. comp. Endocr. **5** (5), 509—526 (1965).

Zelnik, P., Lederis, K.: Chromatographic separation of urotensins. Gen. comp. Endocr. **20** (2), 392—400 (1973).

Bioassay and Characterization of Crustacean Limb Growth-Controlling Factors*

DOROTHY E. BLISS and PENNY M. HOPKINS**

Department of Living Invertebrates, The American Museum of Natural History, New York (USA)

For close to 70 years, biologists have known that removal of eyestalks from a decapod crustacean induces molting and precocious ecdysis (Zeleny, 1905; Megušar, 1912). For almost half that time, they have known that reimplantation of eyestalks reverses this effect (Brown and Cunningham, 1939; Scudamore, 1947). Accordingly, they have postulated the existence of a crustacean molt-inhibiting hormone (MIH). In 1953, the work of Passano (1953) implicated neurosecretory cells in the x organs of the eyestalks as a major source of MIH.

An integral part of crustacean molting—and thus presumably capable of being inhibited by MIH—is proecdysial limb regeneration, which normally is completed by ecdysis. Induced by exposure to darkness or by destalking, proecdysial limb regeneration can be inhibited by light (Bliss, 1956; Bliss and Boyer, 1964) or by implantation of the contents of two eyestalks (Altman, 1965; Bliss et al., 1966). This inhibition is assumed to be due to MIH, but there is no direct evidence to support this assumption.

The task of characterizing and isolating crustacean limb growth-controlling factors has involved (1) developing a suitable bioassay; (2) quantifying the activity of the factors; and (3) applying appropriate physical and chemical treatments to extracts and fractions of central nervous (CN) tissues, thereby to establish the characteristics of the active factors and their relationship to MIH. In our laboratory we have given this problem major attention for some years. This report is a brief summary of results to the present time. Detailed accounts are in preparation for publication elsewhere.

Part I. Bioassay of Limb Growth-Controlling Factors

A. Procedures

Groundwork for a suitable bioassay for crustacean limb growth-controlling factors was laid in 1956 when Bliss, following a suggestion by J. B. Durand, expressed the

* This work was supported by Research Grants GB-11254, GB-4380, GB-12373, and GB-31796× from the National Science Foundation.
** We thank Morris D. Altman, Jane R. Boyer, Edwin A. Martinez, and Stefanie W. Sheehan for their valuable contributions to this work.

growth of a limb bud as a series of R values, each representing length of limb bud as per cent of width of carapace. With this method it has been possible to compare regeneration in different limbs, in different individuals, and at different stages of the intermolt cycle. Furthermore, it has been possible to estimate the progress of an animal through the intermolt cycle. Within limits, a given limb reaches a certain final R value just prior to ecdysis, regardless of the size of the individual. Among investigators employing this method are Demeusy (1965, 1973); Rao (1966); Tchnernigovtzeff (1965, 1972); Rao et al. (1971); Stevenson and Henry (1971); Adiyodi (1972); Flint (1972); and Skinner and Graham (1972).

Not an absolute value of R, however, but the slope of a limb regeneration curve best signifies the proximity of an individual crustacean to ecdysis. This fact, first emphasized by Bliss and Boyer (1964), is the basis of a new method of quantifying the activity of limb growth-controlling factors. This method will be described in Section A2.

In a bioassay for growth-controlling factors, the extract to be tested must be introduced into an animal in such a way as to exert optimal — if not maximal — effect. Two possibilities are via single injection and infusion; a third is through injection of aliquots in series. All three methods were used and are evaluated later in this paper.

1. Experimental Technique

Unless otherwise indicated, extracts were prepared by grinding the contents of freshly removed eyestalks of *Gecarcinus lateralis*[1] with 0.25 ml cold *Gecarcinus* perfusion fluid (Skinner et al., 1965), centrifuging at 10000 RPM and —4° C for five minutes, and removing the supernatant by syringe (0.25 ml). A crab was injected through the arthrodial membrane at the base of the fourth walking leg (fifth pereiopod). Infusions were made through polyethylene tubing (bore = 0.6 mm), previously sealed into the crab above the heart.

During infusions the crab was immobilized in a plastic box, the syringe containing extract was mounted on an infusion pump, and extract was introduced over five, 10, or 20 h. The crab remained at room temperature (about 25° C) in all experiments; the extract was at 25° C in some experiments, at 4° C in the rest.

Eyestalk tissue was implanted into the thoracic musculature of a crab as described by Bliss et al. (1966).

All crabs used in bioassay were destalked individuals *(G. lateralis)* that had progressed halfway through proecdysis [i.e. R value for third walking leg (R_3) equals 13—15].

2. Quantification of Activity

When R_3 values of destalked *G. lateralis* are plotted, the slope of the resulting curve is determined as follows: For two consecutive R_3 values, the tangent EF/DE of the arc angle at D is calculated (Fig. 1 B). Since DE has a value of one (i.e. one

---

[1] Specimens of *G. lateralis* were made available by the Lerner Marine Laboratory, Bimini, Bahamas, and by the Bermuda Biological Station for Research, Inc. We are grateful to these institutions for providing these animals.

day), tan D equals EF. From tan D the arc angle at D is determined. This is the slope of DF, which represents rate of limb regeneration from one day (point D) to the next (point F).

When the arc angle at D is determined for each point on the R_3 value curves of destalked crabs, a standard rate curve (SRC) can be plotted (Fig. 1C, broken line). An experimental rate curve (ERC), derived from R_3 values of destalked crabs receiving eyestalk extract, can also be plotted (Fig. 1C, solid line). The area separating these curves represents the retardation (RE) or acceleration (AC) in rate of limb growth following treatment (T).

Note that SRC is refitted on ERC where experimental rate (ER) reattains its level at T (Fig. 1C, right). Refitting SRC makes possible the determination of RE and AC of the "recovery period." From T to the point of refit is the inhibitory (I) period or promotive (Pr) period; from point of refit to the beginning of terminal plateau (Bliss and Boyer, 1964) is the post-inhibitory (PI) or post-promotive (PPr) period.

To express activity of limb growth-controlling factors, the following formulas have been established:

— average experimental rate (AER): $\Sigma ER/n$,
— average standard rate (ASR): $\Sigma SR/n$,
— average relative activity (ARA): $AER/ASR \times 100$,

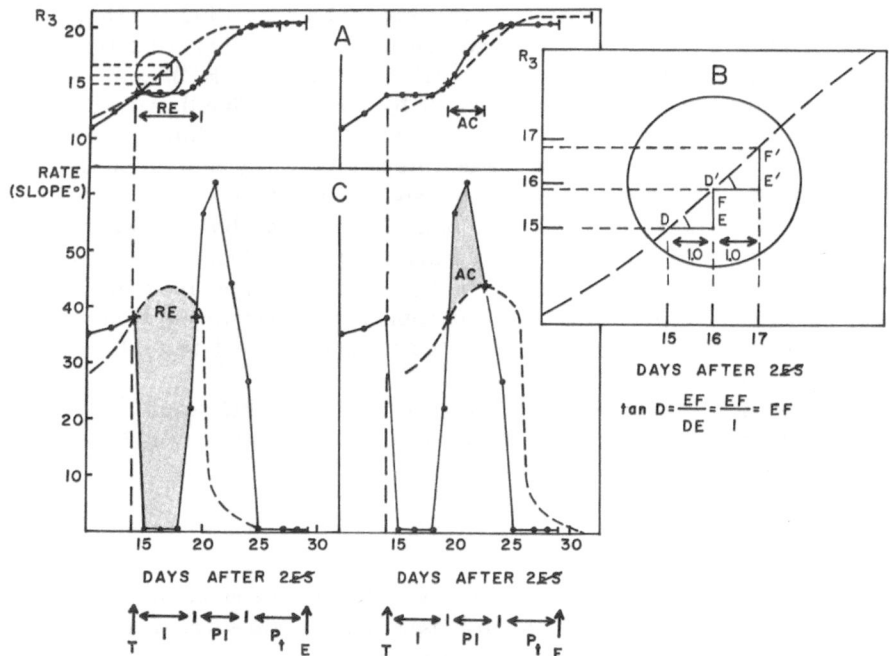

Fig. 1. (A) R_3, (B) derivation of rate, (C) rate. Destalked crabs: untreated - - -, infused (4 ESEq, 10 h, 4° C) ——. RE, retardation; AC, acceleration; I, inhibitory period; PI, post-inhibitory period; Pt, terminal plateau; T, treatment; E, ecdysis

— difference in average relative activity (ΔARA): ARA—100,
— total activity (TA): ΔARA × no. days.

Difference in average relative activity (ΔARA) measures the extent to which AER falls below (negative value; inhibition or retardation) or rises above (positive value; promotion or acceleration) ASR. Total activity (TA) reflects degree and persistence of retardation or acceleration.

B. Results

To characterize and isolate crustacean limb growth-controlling factors, it first proved necessary to establish optimal conditions of bioassay. Should bioassay be through single injection of extract, through injection of small aliquots in series, or through infusion ? If the latter, what are optimal concentration and temperature of extract and duration of infusion ?

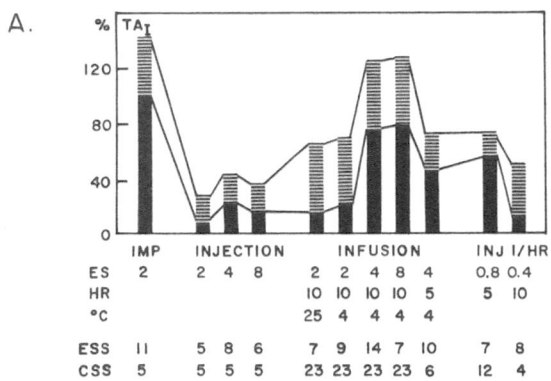

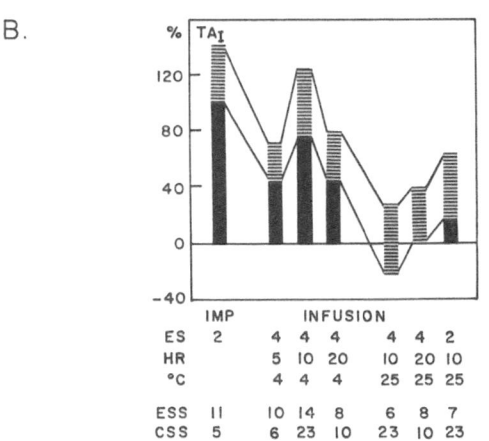

Fig. 2 A and B. Mean TA_I [in % of TA_I of 2 ES implant (IMP) minus control]. ES, eyestalks or eyestalk equivalents; INJ, injection; HR, hours. Samples: ■ net experimental (ESS, size); ≡ control (CSS, size)

In Fig. 2A the first bar shows as 100% the mean net total activity of the inhibitory period (TA_I) for an implant of two eyestalks (2 ES), after the mean TA_I of implant controls (leg muscle or leg nerve) has been substracted. All other mean TA_I's of Fig. 2A are referred, in per cent, to mean net TA_I of implants.

A single injection of extract containing two, four, or eight eyestalk equivalents (ESEq) results in low activity (27—42%). When activity of injection controls (0.25 ml perfusion fluid) is subtracted, net activity from single injections is still lower (8—22%).

Infusion of 2 ESEq for 10 h with extract at 25° C yields somewhat higher activity (66%), but TA_I following control infusion (0.25 ml perfusion fluid) for 10 h is also high; thus net activity of 2 ESEq is low (17%).

Chilling the extract (4° C) during a 10-hour infusion enhances net activity of 2 ESEq slightly (19%). Raising concentration to 4 ESEq while keeping temperature at 4° C yields much higher net activity (75%). Further rise to 8 ESEq yields approximately equal net activity (77%). When 4 ESEq are infused for 5 h at 4° C, net activity is less (45%).

Effects of infusing 4 ESEq for 5 h at 4° C could be surpassed by injecting serially the chilled extract at one injection (0.8 ESEq) per hour for five hours (total 4 ESEq); net activity (54%) was higher than after infusion (45%). But serial injection of aliquots (0.4 ESEq) hourly for 10 h (total 4 ESEq) yielded much lower net activity (11%). Reduction in net activity was due partly to activity of the corresponding control: after hourly injection of aliquots (0.025 ml) of perfusion fluid over 10 h, activity was fairly high (38%), compared with that following hourly injection of aliquots (0.05 ml) of perfusion fluid over five hours (19%).

Infusion of 4 ESEq for 10 or 20 h with the extract at room temperature (25° C) yielded zero net activity (Fig. 2B). At 4° C, however, infusion of 4 ESEq for 20 h resulted in moderately high net activity (41%), which still was low when compared with net activity (75%) following infusion of 4 ESEq at 4° C over a period of 10 h.

These data indicate infusions of 4 ESEq for 10 h at 4° C to be a method of choice. Accordingly, such infusions were used almost exclusively in experiments designed to establish characteristics of crustacean limb growth-controlling factors (see Part II).

C. Discussion

In bioassaying for crustacean limb growth-inhibiting activity, the superiority of implantation and infusion is demonstrable in results presented here. Throughout its lifetime, an implant of hormonally active tissue presumably releases small amounts of highly active material, much as does tissue in situ. Within limits, infusions may function as do implants. In work described here, 10 h appear optimal for infusion, possibly because some 10 h may be required to stop ongoing proecdysial processes.

A single injection of eyestalk extract, even in high concentration, may serve only as a transitory stimulus, providing sudden, excessive amounts of active material that cannot be used by the animal. Equivalent amounts of material are effective when injected serially over five hours, but not when injected over 10 h.

The high activity of a 10-hour control for serial injections suggests that a crab can not tolerate 10 punctures with a needle over 10 h. Stress is clearly important in a crab's responses. During infusions also, a crab undergoes stress, due no doubt to its confinement within a box and to entry of fluid into its body.

When extract is kept at room temperature during infusion, it elicits less activity than when kept at low temperature. From subsequent experimentation (see Part II) one can presume the loss of activity to be due to enzymatic breakdown of active factors at higher temperatures. Doubling concentration from 2 ESEq to 4 ESEq favors increase in limb growth-inhibiting activity but not from 4 ESEq to 8 ESEq. Possibly lower concentrations of active material fail to saturate tissues, while higher concentrations entail competitive inhibition within the active factor.

Part II. Characterization of Limb Growth-Controlling Factors

A. Methods

Extracts of eyestalks of *G. lateralis* were prepared as described earlier (Part I, Section A 1) or as indicated below. In all cases, the residue of the first extraction was re-extracted twice and supernatants combined. Following experimental treatment, the extract was lyophilized. Subsequently, lyophilized material was taken up in perfusion fluid (0.25 ml) and infused (4 ESEq, 10 h, 4° C) into *G. lateralis*. Total activity (TA$_I$) was calculated (see Part I, Section A 2).

1. Determination of Solubility Characteristics

Initially, aqueous extractions were made with perfusion fluid (Skinner et al., 1965); subsequently, with distilled demineralized (dd) water. Absolute ethanol, methanol, acetone, and acetic acid (0.1 M) were also used as solvents. In some experiments, the residue after extraction with perfusion fluid was re-extracted with absolute ethanol; in others, the residue of ethanol extraction was re-extracted with dd water.

2. Gel Filtration

Freshly removed or acetone-dried eyestalks were extracted (dd water) and combined supernatants lyophilized. Lyophilized material was re-extracted in acetic acid (0.1 M; 0.5 ml) and the mixture centrifuged. The supernatant was passed through Sephadex G-50 (fine; 1.25 cm × 40 cm; flow rate 10.0 ml/h) equilibrated with acetic acid (0.1 M). Absorbance of effluent was monitored (280 mμ; LKB Uvicord). The effluent was collected, pooled to form six fractions, lyophilized, and bioassayed. From four to eight crabs were used during bioassay of each fraction. Oxytocin and α-chymotrypsin (Sigma Chemical Co.) were passed through the G-50 column as molecular weight markers.

Pooled fractions from G-50 (fractions 3—6) containing all of the limb growth-inhibiting activity were passed through Sephadex G-25 (fine; 1.25 cm × 50 cm;

flow rate 2.5 ml/h) equilibrated with acetic acid (0.1 M). The effluent was collected, pooled to form five fractions, and bioassayed.

Residue after evaporation of solvent following ethanol extraction of fresh eyestalks was re-extracted in acetic acid (0.1 M) and passed through Sephadex G-50. The effluent was collected, lyophilized, and bioassayed.

3. Heating

Fresh eyestalks, whole or scraped from the eyestalk exoskeleton, were extracted (perfusion fluid or dd water) and centrifuged. The supernatant was heated (15 min) in a boiling water bath, with occasional stirring. After re-centrifugation, the supernatant was lyophilized and bioassayed. Active fractions from gel filtration through Sephadex G-50 were heated in a boiling water bath, treated as above, and bioassayed.

4. Enzymatic Digestion

Fresh eyestalks were extracted (dd water). Following centrifugation, the supernatant was lyophilized, re-extracted in acetic acid (0.1 M), and centrifuged. This supernatant was passed through Sephadex G-50 (fine), and active fractions were collected and lyophilized. Subsequently, these fractions were taken up in solution (pH 7.8) of the proteolytic enzyme Pronase (Sigma Chemical Co.) and incubated (2 h; 38° C). Incubated fractions were then boiled (15 min) to destroy the enzyme and centrifuged. The supernatant was lyophilized and later resuspended in perfusion fluid for bioassay.

5. Dialysis

Fresh eyestalks were extracted (dd water) and the extract placed in a dialysis bag (cellulose dialyzer tubing, diameter 6.35 mm, pore diameter 48 Å), which was suspended in a test tube (75 ml) of dd water in a refrigerator (4° C). The bathing fluid (dialysate) was stirred continuously by a magnetic stirrer. Dialysis continued for 24 h. Every hour for the first six hours and four times thereafter, the dialysate was removed. Pooled dialysates were lyophilized and bioassayed, as was fluid remaining within the bag.

B. Results

When extracts of eyestalks, or fractions thereof, were bioassayed, retardation in experimental rate below standard rate of destalked crabs was taken to indicate activity (TA_I) of limb growth-inhibiting factor (LGIF). Acceleration in experimental rate above standard rate was taken to indicate activity (TA_{Pr}) of limb growth-promoting factor (LGPF). Allowance was made for TA_I of controls.

Results of physical and chemical treatment of extracts and fractions lead us to conclude the following to be true of LGIF and LGPF:

1. Solubility: LGIF is soluble in *Gecarcinus* perfusion fluid, dd water, and acetic acid (0.1 M); it is insoluble in methanol, acetone, and absolute ethanol. LGPF is soluble in absolute ethanol.

2. Molecular Size: LGIF is a small molecule; its molecular weight is close to that of oxytocin (approximately 1000). On a column of Sephadex G-50, LGIF activity is eluted in tubes 18 through 22 and oxytocin in tubes 18 and 19. On a column of Sephadex G-25, LGIF activity is eluted in tubes 23 through 33, while oxytocin is eluted in tube 25.

Figure 3 shows the elution pattern and LGIF activity of eyestalk extract filtered through Sephadex G-50 and G-25.

LGPF is a small molecule. It is eluted from a Sephadex G-50 column in tubes 18 through 24.

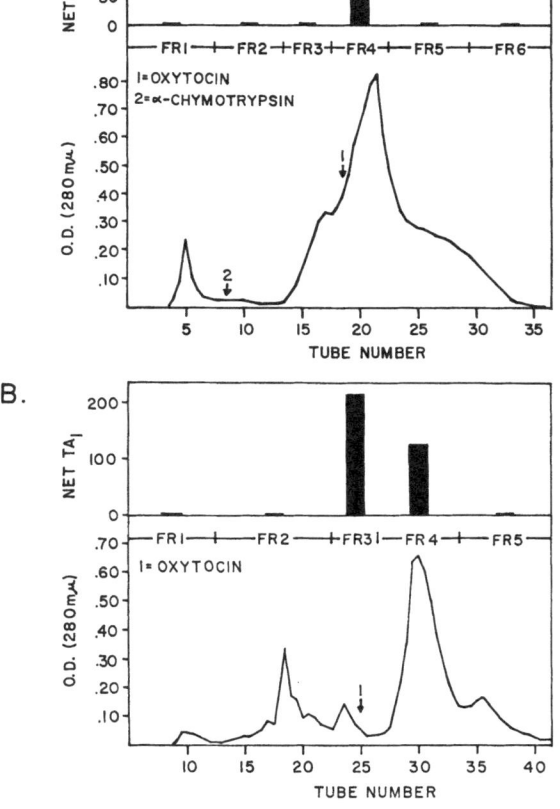

Fig. 3 A and B. Elution profile and LGIF activity of fractions (FR) from (A) Sephadex G-50, (B) Sephadex G-25 columns (see text). Collected volume/tube: 3.25 ml. Net TA_I: experimental minus control. O. D., optical density

3. Resistance to Heating: LGIF is resistant to heating (100° C, 15 min) if the crude extract, prior to heating, is lyophilized and filtered through Sephadex G-50.

4. Resistance to Enzymatic Digestion: LGIF is apparently a peptide. The proteolytic enzyme Pronase destroys LGIF activity within two hours. Denatured Pronase causes no reduction in LGIF activity.

5. Dialyzability: LGIF is a small, dialyzable molecule. After dialysis (24 h), LGIF activity is present only in the dialysate.

C. Discussion

In *Gecarcinus lateralis* LGIF is a small molecule, dialyzable and resistant to heat. Since its activity is destroyed by Pronase, LGIF must require some intact peptide linkages for activity. The preferential solubility of LGIF in more polar solvents suggests its own molecular polarity. LGPF is a small molecule, somewhat less polar than LGIF.

Little can be said of the relationship between LGIF and molt-inhibiting hormone, MIH. With concentrations of eyestalk extract employed here, LGIF does not increase significantly the period of time between removal of eyestalks and ecdysis. Yet implants of eyestalk tissue, which presumably contain LGIF, do delay ecdysis of destalked *G. lateralis.*

Results in part contradict those of Rao (1965), who reported for the crab *Ocypode macrocera* dramatic molt-inhibiting effects from a substance, MIH, isolated from the crab's eyestalks. But when eyestalk extract from *G. lateralis* was treated according to Rao's (1965) MIH-isolating protocol and the purified material infused into *G. lateralis,* there resulted no inhibition of limb regeneration and no delay in ecdysis. Possibly Rao's protocol, when used on eyestalk tissues of *G. lateralis,* does not isolate MIH (= LGIF ?).

In some respects, however, our results with crude extracts of eyestalk tissue from *G. lateralis* do not contradict those of Rao (1965). Clearly seen in limb regeneration curves of *G. lateralis,* when a crab has received eyestalk extract by infusion (2 ESEq or 4 ESEq, 10 h, 4° C), is a four- or five-day period of almost total inhibition (plateau of proecdysis; Bliss and Boyer, 1964). This period of inhibition would be expected to delay ecdysis. Yet when inhibition terminates, the limb bud displays a spurt of growth that lifts rates of regeneration above the standard rate derived from limb buds of destalked but otherwise untreated crabs. Ecdysis, therefore, is not significantly delayed.

In the hemolymph of recipient destalked crabs, there apparently is a limb growth-promoting factor, LGPF, which expresses itself visibly in an accelerated rate of regeneration when the inhibitory effect of LGIF wears off. This LGPF may be synthesized in parts of the CNS other than the eyestalks and released via the sinus glands. Some species of crabs remain in intermolt condition when sinus glands are removed (Bliss, 1953; Passano, 1953), as long as the source of MIH (x organs) is intact (Passano, 1953). In like manner, if a major source of LGPF lies outside of the eyestalks, destalking of crabs should remove the primary site of LGPF release but not of its synthesis, and the crabs should demonstrate rapid proecdysial limb regeneration.

Acceleration of proecdysial limb regeneration comparable to that following inhibition also occurs when aqueous extract of the alcohol-soluble fraction of eyestalks, which presumably contains LGPF, is infused into destalked crabs. This fraction accelerates limb growth and shortens the period of time from eyestalk removal to ecdysis.

Over the past 20 years, neurohormones that promote various proecdysial processes have been demonstrated in other decapod crustaceans (Carlisle, 1953; Carlisle and Dohrn, 1953; Scheer and Scheer, 1954; McWhinnie and Kirchenberg, 1962; McWhinnie, Cahoon and Johanneck, 1969; McWhinnie and Mohrherr, 1970). Thus the hypothesis that proecdysial processes are controlled by promoting, as well as inhibiting, factors has considerable support. Such dual control of molting may have selective advantage for a crustacean. More delicate regulation may result when it depends upon interaction between two opposing factors rather than upon a rise and fall in concentration of a single inhibiting factor acting alone.

Summary

This paper describes a new method for quantifying activity of crustacean limb-growth-controlling factors. With this method, several techniques of bioassay — implantation, injection, and infusion — have been evaluated. Infusion of 4 ESEq for 10 h with the extract at 4° C proved most effective in eliciting high activity from extracts of eyestalk tissues prepared from the crab *Gecarcinus lateralis* and assayed on that species.

With the use of such infusions and the new method of quantifying activity, effects of physical and chemical agents applied to eyestalk extract were determined and characteristics of limb growth-controlling factors defined.

There are at least two such factors, a limb growth-inhibiting factor (LGIF) and a limb growth-promoting factor (LGPF). LGIF is a small molecule, dialyzable, resistant to heat, soluble in polar solvents, and destroyed by the proteolytic enzyme Pronase. LGPF is a small molecule that is somewhat less polar than LGIF.

Relationships between LGIF and molt-inhibiting hormone, MIH, and between LGPF and molt-promoting hormones are discussed.

References

Adiyodi, R. G.: Wound healing and regeneration in the crab *Paratelphusa hydrodromus*. Int. Rev. Cytol. **32**, 257—289 (1972).

Altman, M. D.: Effects of eyestalk removal, eyestalk implantation, and eyestalk extracts on *Gecarcinus lateralis* Freminville (Crustacea, Decapoda). Thesis, New York University, New York 1965.

Bliss, D. E.: Endocrine control of metabolism in the land crab, *Gecarcinus lateralis* (Fréminville). I. Differences in the respiratory metabolism of sinusglandless and eyestalkless crabs. Biol. Bull. **104**, 275—296 (1953).

Bliss, D. E.: Neurosecretion and the control of growth in a decapod crustacean. In: Bertil Hanström, Zoological papers in honour of his sixty-fifth birthday, Nov. 20, 1956 (K. G. Wingstrand, Ed.), p. 56—75. Lund: Zoological Institute, 1956.

Bliss, D. E., Boyer, J. R.: Environmental regulation of growth in the decapod crustacean *Gecarcinus lateralis*. Gen. comp. Endocr. **4**, 15—41 (1964).

Bliss, D. E., Wang, S. M. E., Martinez, E. A.: Water balance in the land crab, *Gecarcinus lateralis*, during the intermolt cycle. Amer. Zool. **6**, 197—212 (1966).

Brown, F. A., jr., Cunningham, O.: Influence of the sinus gland of crustaceans on normal viability and ecdysis. Biol. Bull. **77**, 104—114 (1939).

Carlisle, D. B.: Studies on *Lysmata seticaudata* Risso (Crustacea, Decapoda). III. On the activity of the moult-accelerating principle when administered by the oral route. Pubbl. Staz. zool. Napoli **24**, 279—285 (1953).

Carlisle, D. B., Dohrn, P. F. R.: Studies on *Lysmata seticaudata* Risso (Crustacea, Decapoda). Experimental evidence for a growth- and molt-accelerating factor obtainable from eyestalks. Pubbl. Staz. zool. Napoli **24**, 69—83 (1953).

Demeusy, N.: Croissance somatique et fonction de reproduction chez la femelle du décapode brachyoure *Carcinus maenas* Linné. Arch. Zool. exp. gén. **106**, 625—663 (1965).

Demeusy, N.: Libération d'appendices thoraciques au cours de leur régénération chez le crabe *Carcinus maenas* L. et poursuite de leur évolution. Cahiers Biol. mar. **14**, 189—204 (1973).

Flint, R. W.: Effects of eyestalk removal and ecdysterone infusion on molting in *Homarus americanus*. J. Fish. Res. Bd. Canada **29**, 1229—1233 (1972).

McWhinnie, M. A., Cahoon, M. O., Johanneck, R.: Hormonal effects on calcium metabolism in Crustacea. Amer. Zool. **9**, 841—855 (1969).

McWhinnie, M. A., Kirchenberg, R. J.: Crayfish hepatopancreas metabolism and the intermolt cycle. Comp. Biochem. Physiol. **6**, 117—128 (1962).

McWhinnie, M. A., Mohrherr, C. J.: Influence of eyestalk factors, intermolt cycle and season upon ^{14}C-leucine incorporation into protein in the crayfish *(Orconectes virilis)*. Comp. Biochem. Physiol. **34**, 415—437 (1970).

Megušar, F.: Experimente über den Farbwechsel der Crustaceen. Arch. Entwickl.-Mech. **33**, 462—665 (1912).

Passano, L. M.: Neurosecretory control of molting in crabs by the X-organ sinus gland complex. Physiol. comp. Oecol. **3**, 155—189 (1953).

Rao, K. R.: Isolation and partial characterization of the moult-inhibiting hormone of the crustacean eyestalk. Experientia (Basel) **21**, 593—594 (1965).

Rao, K. R.: Studies on the influence of environmental factors on growth in the crab, *Ocypoda macrocera* H. Milne-Edwards. Crustaceana **11**, 257—276 (1966).

Rao, K. R., Fingerman, M., Hays, C.: Effects of α-ecdysone and 20-hydroxyecdysone on limb regeneration and molting in the fiddler crab, *Uca pugilator*. Amer. Zool. **11**, 644 (1971).

Scheer, B. T., Scheer, M. A. R.: The hormonal control of metabolism in crustaceans. VII. Moulting and colour change in the prawn *Leander serratus*. Pubbl. Staz. zool. Napoli **25**, 397—418 (1954).

Scudamore, H. H.: The influence of the sinus glands upon molting and associated changes in the crayfish. Physiol. Zool. **20**, 187—208 (1947).

Skinner, D. M., Graham, D. E.: Loss of limbs as a stimulus to ecdysis in Brachyura (True crabs). Biol. Bull. **143**, 222—233 (1972).

Skinner, D. M., Marsh, D. J., Cook, J. S.: Physiological salt solution for the land crab, *Gecarcinus lateralis*. Biol. Bull. **129**, 355—365 (1965).

Stevenson, J. R., Henry, B. A.: Correlation between the molt cycle and limb regeneration in the crayfish *Orconectes obscurus* (Hagen) (Decapoda, Astacidea). Crustaceana **20**, 301—307 (1971).

Tchernigovtzeff, C.: Multiplication cellulaire et régénération au cours du cycle d'intermue des crustacés décapodes. Arch. Zool. exp. gén. **106**, 377—497 (1965).

Tchernigovtzeff, C.: Régénération et cycle d'intermue chez le crabe *Gecarcinus lateralis*. I. — Étude de la relation entre la croissance préexuviale des bourgeons de pattes et les étapes de la morphogenèse des soies dans les épipodites branchiaux des maxillipèdes. Arch. Zool. exp. gén. **113**, 197—213 (1972).

Zeleny, C.: Compensatory regulation. J. exp. Zool. **2**, 1—102 (1905).

c) Electrophysiology

The Neurosecretory Impulse

B. A. Cross*

Department of Anatomy, University of Bristol, Bristol (Great Britain)

First Hypothalamic Recordings

This story begins twenty years ago with the publication of C. von Euler's (1953) note on hypothalamic "osmopotentials", significantly in the same year as the first symposium on neurosecretion. At that time much more was known of the role of antidiuretic hormone and its control by osmotic stimuli (Verney, 1947) than of the other neurohypophysial hormone, oxytocin, whose primary function appeared to be in the milk-ejection reflex (Cross and Harris, 1952). There followed a number of investigations with EEG electrodes oriented stereotaxically through the brain in attempts to locate the osmoreceptor mechanism postulated by Verney. Sawyer and his associates at UCLA were most active in this area and described EEG responses to acute osmotic stimuli in various forebrain structures (Sawyer and Gernandt, 1956; Holland et al., 1959a; Holland et al., 1959b). The specificity of the effects, however, was called in question by the finding that the osmotic stimuli used not only released neurohypophysial hormones but also induced a sympathetic discharge (Holland et al., 1959a, 1959b). Moreover, hypothalamic "islands", excluding the forebrain areas where the EEG changes occurred were quite capable of preserving osmotic homeostasis via secretion of ADH (Sundsten and Sawyer, 1961; Woods et al., 1966).

Microelectrode Recording

Because of the problems of interpreting records obtained by macroelectrodes, Cross and Green (1959) resorted to recording from the hypothalamus with steel microelectrodes. We were delighted at the profusion of action potential activity accessible to these electrodes. Units responding in various ways to intracarotid injections of hyperosmotic solutions were found in the thalamus, septum, preoptic areas as well as in the magnocellular nuclei. Many of these units were also influenced by nociceptive or other stimuli. Disappointingly the extracellular action potentials of supposedly neurosecretory neurones in the supraoptic nucleus were not distinguishable from those of ordinary neurones elsewhere but spontaneous firing

---

* Present address: ARC Institute of Animal Physiology, Babraham, Cambridge (Great Britain)

rates tended to be low. More information on the responses of single units in or near the magnocellular nuclei was gathered by Brooks and his collaborators (Brooks et al., 1962; Suda et al., 1963; Koizumi et al., 1964; Brooks et al., 1966) and by Joynt (1964). With the benefit of hindsight we can appreciate that conclusions from all these experiments were at best provisional since there was no sure way of knowing which units were true neurosecretory cells (i.e. with axons passing to neural lobe) and which were representatives of a diverse population of inter-neurones. In this connection the paper of Brooks et al. (1966) reporting activation by mammary and uterine stimuli of PV neurones associated with release of oxytocin was important as the first positively connecting unit activity with secretion of oxytocin, but it now seems likely that the units recorded were mostly interneurones.

Undoubtedly the most important methodological advance (outweighing even the development of conscious recording techniques) was that initiated by Kandel (1964) by intracellular recording of antidromically identified neurosecretory neurones in the goldfish. He demonstrated that following the initial spike there was a long hyperpolarising after potential, accounting no doubt for the slow firing rate generally observed in neurosecretory cells. He also presented evidence that a hyperpolarisation of the cell could result from inhibitory recurrent collateral axons. Antidromic stimulation of mammalian neurosecretory neurones was first reported by Yagi et al. (1966) and has since become a routine procedure in studies of supraoptic (Dyball and Koizumi, 1969; Dyball, 1971; Barker et al., 1971b; Dreifuss and Kelly, 1972a, 1972b; Hayward and Jennings, 1973a, 1973b; Vincent et al., 1972) or paraventricular (Sundsten et al., 1970; Novin et al., 1970; Koizumi and Yamashita, 1972; Negoro and Holland, 1972; Wakerley and Lincoln, 1973a) neurosecretory cells. Precise techniques vary in different laboratories. Recording microelectrodes may be steel, tungsten or glass micropipettes oriented stereo-taxically through the brain from above, or under visual control by a ventral approach after partial removal of the basisphenoid bone. Electrophysiological criteria for establishing true antidromic conduction also vary, but usually include a stable latency, accurate following of a brief high frequency burst of stimuli (at, say, 100/sec) and collision, i.e. the cancellation of an antidromic spike by an ortho-dromic action potential (Fig. 3A).

Electrical Properties of Neurosecretory Cells

The general properties of mammalian neurosecretory cells that have been so revealed are well exemplified by the study of Koizumi and Yamashita (1972) for the cat and dog. Conduction velocity is in the C range for unmyelinated axons, i.e. 0.3—0.9 m/sec. The typical extracellular waveform (Fig. 1B, C) is positive-negative with an inflexion in the positive wave separating the A spike (initial segment, I.S. spike) from the B spike (soma-dendritic, SD spike). The absolute refractory period of the SD spike is 5—10 msec. The A and B spikes of a unit action potential can thus be dissociated by high frequency stimuli (Fig. 1E, F) and may also fire separately in spontaneous activity. This latter seems a primitive characteristic of the neurosecretory cell for it occurs often in Aplysia ganglion cells (Tauc, 1962) but not in mammalian spinal motor neurones. It would be unwise however to suppose too hard and fast a set of characters for all mammalian neurosecretory cells for there is plenty of evidence that these various parameters may vary both between species and between cells in the same animal.

Since Kandel's (1964) original observation in the goldfish it has now become quite clear that recurrent inhibitory collateral axons to neurosecretory cells are

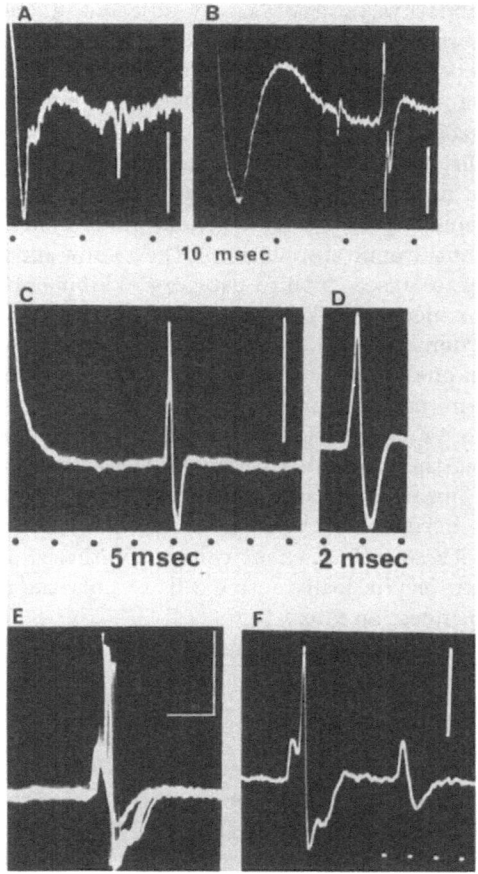

Fig. 1 A—F. Oscilloscope photographs showing unit waveforms of neurosecretory cells in the PV nucleus of rabbits produced by antidromic stimulation from the neural lobe (from Novin et al., 1970; Sundsten et al., 1970). Positive deflection of trace is upward. A Negative spike occurring 15 msec after antidromic shock (artefact on left of trace). Often this is the first sign that microelectrode is approaching cell. Voltage calibration 0.2 mV. B Another small negative going spike at 18 msec preceding a typical antidromic action potential at 26 msec. Voltage calibration 0.2 mV. C and D Two characteristic action potentials. In A artefact at left shows latency to be 20 msec. Note the inflexions in the positive going traces. Voltage calibration 1 mV. E Superimposed oscilloscope sweeps to show fractionation of action potential into A spike by a rapid volley of antidromic shocks. Calibrations 2 msec and 1 mV. F Fractionation of action potential by paired antidromic shocks 5 msec apart. The waveform on the left shows a pronounced inflexion demarcating the A and B spikes and the waveform on the right shows the A spike only. Voltage calibration 1 mV

also present in mammals (Kelly and Dreifuss, 1970; Dreifuss and Kelly, 1972a; Barker et al., 1971a; Negoro and Holland, 1972; Koizumi and Yamashita, 1972; Hayward and Jennings, 1973b). A single antidromic shock may inhibit spontaneous discharges in a neurosecretory cell for about 100 msec and intracellular recordings show a hyperpolarisation (IPSP) during this period. The inhibition can result even if the stimulus intensity is inadequate to propagate an antidromic action potential in the axon of the cell actually being recorded. This implies that convergence occurs from recurrent pathways activated by adjacent axons and excludes the possibility that membrane changes induced by an antidromic impulse are the cause of the inhibitory period. Koizumi and Yamashita (1972) described "Renshaw-like" units in the SO and PV nuclei that discharge 5—7 spikes at high frequency (500—800/sec) following a single antidromic shock, and these are obvious candidates for inhibitory interneurones. As yet however no adequate morphological basis for recurrent inhibition of neurosecretory cells has been supplied.

A proportion of neurosecretory cells are silent and would easily escape detection in the absence of antidromic stimulation. Others show spontaneous discharges at variable rates of up to 10/sec. A third category exhibit bursts of activity with intervening lapses into silence (Wakerley and Lincoln, 1971; Dreifuss and Kelly, 1972b; Dyball and Pountney, 1973; Hayward and Jennings, 1973a). Whether units can change from one category to another is not certain but it is of interest that the three patterns are seen in several different species and in conscious animals as well as those anaesthetised with several different anaesthetic agents. Hayward (1974) raises the possibility that the three firing patterns might be related to the type of hormonal product released, viz. oxytocin, vasopressin, and the newly postulated hormone "coherin". Alternatively, he suggests they correspond to the secretory state, e.g. silent cells to synthesis, active cells to tonic release and intermittent or phasically active cells to pulsatile release of hormone. We shall return to this question later.

Osmoreceptors and ADH Secretion

With the availability of the antidromic method for positive identification of true neurosecretory neurons, several investigators turned again to the problem of osmoreceptor function and secretion of ADH. Dyball (1971) found that a significant increase in action potential activity in identified supraoptic neurosecretory neurones was induced in rats under urethane by intracarotid injection of 0.25 ml/M NaCl. The electrical response was completed in 1 min though peak concentrations of plasma ADH occurred at 3 min. In conscious monkeys Vincent et al. (1972) reported that cells in the supraoptic region fell into two classes of specific osmosensitive cells (using the nomenclature of Vincent and Hayward, 1970), i.e. one responding monophasically to intracarotid injections (1 ml 2.7% NaCl in 5 sec) and the other responding biphasically to the same stimuli—usually by excitation followed by inhibition. The former were not invaded antidromically when the neural lobe was stimulated and these were taken to be osmoreceptor cells. On the other hand, most of the biphasic units were antidromically activated, defining them as true neurosecretory cells. This neat solution to the problem, which accords with evidence from pharmacological blockade (Bridges and Thorn, 1970) that at least one synapse intervenes between the osmoreceptor and neurosecretory cell, deserves confirmatory work in other species. Because of the great variability in spontaneous unit activity and in the response to rapid osmotic stimuli it is difficult to attach great precision to the terms "specific", "monophasic", and "biphasic" (cf. Hayward and Jennings, 1973b; Dyball and Pountney, 1973). For example, how could a biphasic response be detected in a "silent" cell where there was no spontaneous activity to reveal an inhibitory rebound?

Further it is highly questionable how far intracarotid injections may substitute for normally occurring osmotic changes. For that reason Dyball and Pountney (1973) have studied firing rates in neurosecretory cells, identified by antidromic stimulation in rats given 2% NaCl instead of drinking water for 3 days. The dehydration thus caused depleted the neural lobes of vasopressin and oxytocin and significantly increased the firing rate of neurosecretory PV and SO neurones but not that of a control population of neurones elsewhere in the hypothalamus. Unfortunately these results tell us little about the identity of osmoreceptors and leave in doubt which of the recorded neurones were secreting vasopressin-ADH and which were secreting oxytocin. We may fairly assume that the two hormones are secreted by distinct cells and it is a matter of some importance to devise methods to distinguish them *in vivo*.

Oxytocin Cells

The best progress on this score is undoubtedly the work of Wakerley and Lincoln (1973a, 1973b). They have shown that about half the antidromically identified neurosecretory cells in both magnocellular nuclei exhibit a very distinctive pattern of accelerated firing at a fixed interval before each milk-ejection response in suckled anaesthetised animals. The recurrent milk ejections correspond in magnitude to the response evoked by intravenous injection of 1 mU oxytocin. They are abolished in glands receiving an intra-arterial injection of the specific antagonist N-carbamyl-O-methyl-oxytocin and occur in the absence of measurable releases of ADH (Wakerley et al., 1973). It would seem therefore that the neurones that reveal themselves in this highly characteristic style are indeed oxytocin cells. Possibly some of the unresponsive units are also oxytocin cells, temporarily in abeyance, but the greater likelihood is that many of them are vasopressin neurones. Unfortunately, since there are no known stimuli that reliably release vasopressin-ADH without some concomitant release of oxytocin this inference will be difficult to check. Some of the implications of the discovery of the oxytocin neurone have been discussed elsewhere (Cross, 1974) but one aspect should detain us here, and that is the fundamental question of the relationship between the neurosecretory impulse and the release of hormone.

Action Potentials and Hormone Release

In most of the work on neurohypophysial hormone secretion it has been tacitly assumed that increased action potential traffic in neurosecretory cells means more

hormone released—so that for example a general speeding up of discharge rate
from, say, 1/sec to 3/sec betokens a similar increase in hormone output. This
assumption would explain the results of Koizumi et al. (1966), and Dyball (1971),
on the acute release of oxytocin and vasopressin respectively; also the chronic
experimental results of Dyball and Pountney (1973) in saltloaded rats and Dyball
and Dyer (1971) in rats with hypothalamic islands. However, the notable fact
about the oxytocin neurones of Wakerley and Lincoln (1973a, 1973b) is that
preceding each measurable release of oxytocin they increased their firing rate
not twofold but twenty to fortyfold (Fig. 2B). Peak discharge rates were 40—80/sec,
but the bursts were usually maintained for only a very few seconds to be followed by an inhibitory rebound before recovery to the spontaneous low level of

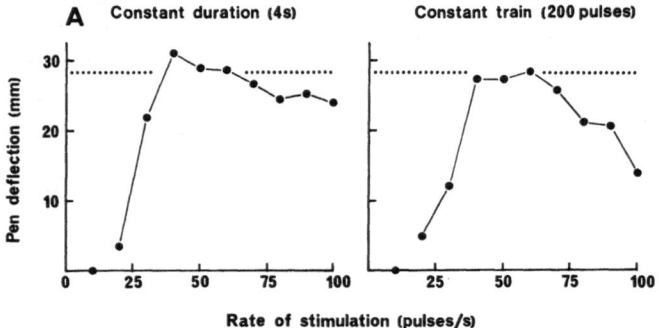

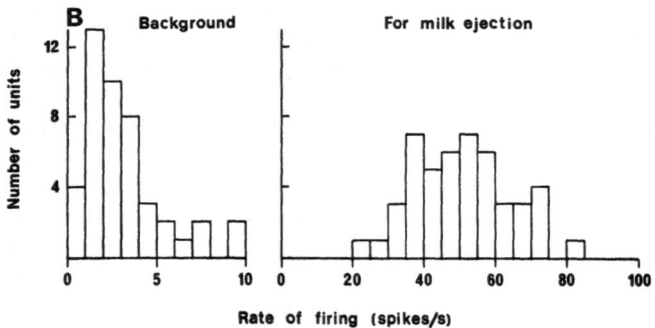

Fig. 2A and B. Relationship of discharge rate in neurosecretory axons to release of hormone
from neural lobe (Lincoln, D.W., and Wakerley, J.B., unpublished). A Graphs showing effect
of frequency of electrical stimulation (biphasic 2 mS pulses at <1 mA) on size of milk-
ejection response (measured in mm of polygraph pen deflection). The horizontal dotted line
gives the mean response to 1 mU oxytocin i.v. which corresponds to the release in natural milk
ejection. Note that whether the stimulus is of constant duration or constant number of pulses,
there is little response at frequencies below 25/sec and a decline in response at frequencies above
75/sec. B Histograms showing distribution of firing rates of antidromically identified neurosecretory (oxytocin) cells in the PV and SO nuclei. Left, low spontaneous firing rates
between milk ejection responses. Right, peak firing rates of bursts preceding a reflex release of
oxytocin. Note that most excited oxytocin cells had peak discharge rates of 40—60/sec i.e.
corresponding to the optimum stimulation frequency as seen above in A

firing. We have therefore a picture of many thousands of unmyelinated axons synchronously discharging a rapid volley of impulses lasting 2—3 sec in order to release 1 mU oxytocin.

The question arises, why such prodigality of impulses ? Almost certainly there is a connection with the observations of Harris et al., (1969), Sundsten et al. (1970) and Wakerley and Lincoln (1973a) that electrical stimulation of the pituitary stalk *in vivo* fails to evoke milk-ejection in lactating rabbits or rats if the pulse frequency of the stimulation drops below 20—30/sec, and frequencies of 50/sec are about optimal (Fig. 2A). Further insight can be gained from the experiments of Dreifuss and his co-workers (Dreifuss et al., 1971; Nordmann and Dreifuss, 1972) with rat neurohypophyses incubated *in vitro*. Release of hormone into the medium was much more effective with high frequency stimulation, i.e. the amount of oxytocin released by identical numbers of pulses increased if the pulses were delivered at high frequency. Exclusion of calcium from the medium blocked the release of hormone as was previously demonstrated for vasopressin by Mikiten and Douglas (1965). Evidently a depolarisation of the terminal membrane of the neurosecretory axon discharges the hormone stored in neurosecretory granules by a calcium-dependent mechanism. The details of this release mechanism are still the subject of speculation (see Poisner, 1973). However, there is impressive evidence that neurosecretory granules are discharged by a process of exocytosis (Douglas et al., 1971; Dreifuss, 1973; see also Douglas this volume, p. 302) in which vasopressin or oxytocin are extruded along with their respective neurophysins.

Douglas and Sorimachi (1971, for vasopressin) and Nordmann and Dreifuss (1972, for oxytocin) have shown that stimulation of the neural stalk fibres in sodium free media liberates hormone in the absence of recordable action potentials. Nevertheless we may be reasonably certain that in the intact animal the requisite depolarisation effect is brought about only by a rapid succession of action potentials arriving at the axon terminal. This must surely be the primary role of the neuro-secretory impulse—to release intragranular hormone stores from the axon terminals. There is no evidence to suggest that neurosecretory impulses have a significant part to play in the synthesis of secretory products and very little indicating a role in axonal transport. In hypothalamic islands action potential activity in the paraventricular nucleus is drastically reduced while oxytocin disappears from the blood plasma (Dyball and Dyer, 1971) and accumulates in the perikarya of the neurosecretory cells (Dyer et al., 1973).

There is another important implication of this recent work which might be called the principle of inequality of impulses. An action potential contributes to hormone discharge if it is one of a rapid train of impulses (Fig. 2B). To put it another way, we could say that a million neurosecretory axons firing at 1/sec would release significantly less hormone than 10000 axons firing at 100/sec. It is the distribution of impulses in time and space, not their number, that determines the end result in the neural lobe. We have here a good example of neural coding in the light of which the high frequency bursts of the oxytocin cell in lactating rats and the phasically active neurosecretory cells seen in rats (Wakerly and Lincoln, 1971; Dreifuss and Kelly, 1972b) and monkeys (Hayward and Jennings, 1973a) assume a clear functional significance. If our interpretation is correct this code of neuro-secretory impulses ensures that with a relatively fixed number of spikes the release of hormone is determined by their distribution in time. Thus the synchronous bursts of the oxytocin cells in suckled rats are balanced by the subsequent inhibitory pause (recurrent inhibition?) giving an overall discharge frequency not much different from that in the unsuckled animal.

Afferent Synaptic Mechanisms

Since the neurosecretory impulses are generated in the hypothalamus it is there we must look for the synaptic mechanisms that ultimately govern discharge of neurohypophysial hormones.

Concerning the source and distribution of afferent terminations on neurosecretory cells in the magnocellular nuclei our morphological information is regrettably sparse. The Golgi technique, though adequate for depicting terminal boutons in other nuclei of the hypothalamus, unfortunately fails to impregnate neurosecretory cells. Electron microscopy reveals synaptic endings very adequately but does not always permit reliable differentiation of neurosecretory axons and dendrites, as the latter lack typical dendritic spines and may contain neurosecretory granules. Nevertheless, in a preliminary study on the PV nucleus of the rat, J. F. Morris (1974) found 70% of the synaptic bags on the membrane of neurosecretory cell bodies possess dense-cored vesicles, usually thought of as containing catecholamines. Synaptic bags on dendritic shafts, however, have significantly fewer dense-cored vesicles and mostly contain synaptic vesicles of the classical cholinergic type. These findings are consistent with the presence of a cholinergic excitatory input and a monoaminergic inhibitory input, and for this idea there is a fair amount of experimental support.

Use of the Koelle technique for choline esterase has shown that cholinergic fibres are undoubtedly present in the magnocellular nuclei (Shute and Lewis, 1966), while the Falck technique for the detection of catecholamines has established the presence also of noradrenergic endings (Fuxe and Hökfelt, 1967; see also Fuxe et al. this volume, p. 223). Dopamine and serotonin were apparently absent from the nuclei, and there is little evidence for the occurrence of other possible neurotransmitter substances therein, e.g. GABA (Robinson and Wells, 1973).

A presumption that acetylcholine may be excitatory to neurosecretory cells and noradrenaline (or adrenaline) inhibitory stems from the work of Verney (1947) and Pickford and her associates (Abrahams and Pickford, 1954; Duke and Pickford, 1951; Pickford, 1960) who found that suitable injections of acetylcholine (e.g. intracarotid) released oxytocin and vasopressin while a preceding injection of adrenaline could prevent the release of these hormones from the neurohypophysis.

As it is now fairly certain that release of oxytocin or vasopressin under physiological conditions requires the despatch of volleys of action potentials from the appropriate neurosecretory cells an important source of evidence is the effect of iontophoretic application of transmitter agents to antidromically identified units in the PV or SO nuclei. In our laboratory a study in the rabbit paraventricular nucleus (Moss et al., 1972) revealed that 91% of the neurosecretory cells were excited by iontophoretic injection of acetylcholine and 81% were inhibited by noradrenaline. Tests on 12 cells with the nicotinic blocker dihydro-β-erythroidine

Table 1. Effects of iontophoretic injection of neurotransmitter agents on units in rabbit PV nucleus (data from Moss et al., 1972b)

Agent	Neurosecretory cell responses				Non-neurosecretory cell responses			
	No. tested	% excited	% inhibited	% unaf-fected	No. tested	% excited	% inhibited	% unaffected
Acetylcholine	127	91	4	5	98	16	76	8
Noradrenaline	60	5	83	12	57	81	12	7
L-glutamic acid	95	100	0	0	46	100	0	0
GABA	14	0	100	0	12	0	100	0
Serotonin	30	37	30	33	15	33	66	0
Dopamine	19	47	53	0	16	35	65	0
Nicotine	33	51	28	21	11	64	9	27

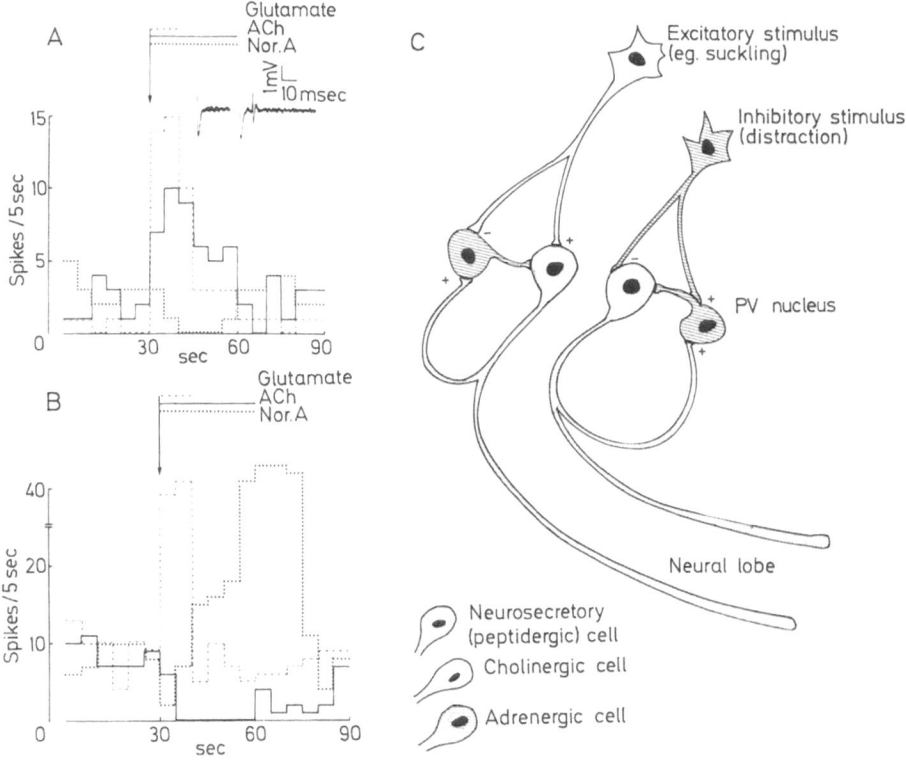

Fig. 3 A—C. Neurochemical transmission at PV neurosecretory cell in the rabbit (Moss et al., 1972b). A Superimposed graphs of responses of PV neurosecretory cell to iontophoretic application at 6 nanoamps of acetylcholine, noradrenaline and glutamate. Inset at top right shows the collision test for this cell whereby a double antidromic shock triggered by an orthodromic spike failed to elicit an antidromic spike to the first shock. B Superimposed graphs of responses of non-neurosecretory PV cell (not antidromically excited) to same doses of transmitter substances as in A. Note that in this cell noradrenaline excites and acetylcholine inhibits, i.e. opposite effect to that in A, while glutamate excites both cells. C Diagram of a possible arrangement of synaptic connexions of the oxytocin cell. The interneuronal cells (adrenergic) are depicted as playing a part both in reflex stimulation or inhibition of oxytocin release and in recurrent inhibition via peptidergic collateral axons from the neurosecretory cells

indicated that 8 were excited via nicotinic receptors, and tests in 13 cells with atropine suggested that acetylcholine may have been exciting via muscarinic receptors in 6 cases. Non-neurosecretory cells in the nucleus were chiefly distinguished by their response to acetylcholine and noradrenaline which were the reverse of the neurosecretory cells (Table 1). In other experiments in rats, Moss, Dyball and Cross (1971) found that neurosecretory cells in both PV and SO nuclei were predominantly excited by acetylcholine and depressed by noradrenaline. Dreifuss and Kelly (1972b) found that 70% of neurosecretory cells in the SO nucleus of the rat were excited by acetylcholine and they also obtained evidence for the existence of both nicotinic and muscarinic receptors. However, Barker et al., (1971b) in the cat reported that the majority of supraoptic neurosecretory cells were inhibited by acetylcholine and the responses were atropine sensitive, while the minority of excitatory responses to acetylcholine were blocked by dihydro-β-erythroidine. But in agreement with the other workers Barker et al. (1971b) found that noradrenaline inhibited most of the supraoptic cells, and that some at least of these responses were mediated by β-adrenergic receptors.

It would certainly be an oversimplication to say that the neurosecretory cells possess excitatory nicotinic receptors and inhibitory β-adrenergic receptors but that is the trend of the evidence so far. Much more neuropharmacological analysis with intracellular recordings, together with orthodromic stimulation and inhibition will be required to settle this issue.

The Problem of Recurrent Inhibition

We have already noted the absence of a morphological basis for recurrent inhibition of neurosecretory cells other than the occurrence of synaptic endings on their perikarya. Yet the neurophysiological evidence for the existence of such inhibitory connexions is overwhelming.

One idea that was quick to germinate suggested that collateral axons from neurosecretory cells might release vasopressin or oxytocin directly on to the membrane of the cell body and suppress discharge without the help of an interneurone (Nicoll and Barker, 1971). I think this view can be discounted. It is based on Dale's Law which states that a given nerve cell must release the same chemical at any of its endings. In the case of oxytocin Moss et al. (1972a) found that iontophoretic injection of the hormone on to neurosecretory cells in rabbits and rats produced a pronounced excitation though non-neurosecretory cells were unaffected. This result was surprising but it could hardly provide a mechanism for recurrent inhibition. Moreover, we have seen that for release of oxytocin from neural lobe terminals a rapid volley of impulses is required, but a single antidromic shock can produce a prolonged inhibitory pause in neurosecretory cell discharge. Vasopressin might appear a safer candidate as inhibitory transmitter for Nicoll and Barker (1971) have shown that in contrast to oxytocin iontophoretic injection of this hormone reduces the discharge of many neurosecretory cells in the supraoptic nucleus. But this idea is difficult to reconcile with the fact that recurrent inhibition can be readily demonstrated in Brattleboro rats which have a congenital inability to synthesise vasopressin (Dyball, 1974). Finally, if recurrent neurosecretory terminals should be regarded as a normal occurrence on or near the perikarya of PV or SO cells, why has the electron microscope not revealed such contacts with neurosecretory vesicles like those in the neural lobe terminations ?

Reference to Table 1 suggests that GABA might be a highly effective inhibitory transmitter for PV neurosecretory cells. GABA has also been shown to have powerful inhibitory effects on supraoptic neurosecretory cells in cats (Nicoll and Barker, 1971) but the indications are that neither this nor the less effective dopamine are present in the magnocellular nuclei in significant amounts. We are left then with noradrenaline which is both effective as an inhibitor and assuredly present in the nucleus.

Table 1 shows that many cells that do not send axons to the neural lobe are excited by iontophoretic injection of noradrenaline. It is attractive to think that some of these might be interneurones, perhaps of the Renshaw type described by Koizumi and Yamashita (1972) which relay back to the neurosecretory cells. Figure 3C shows in a schematic form how these cells might be concerned both with recurrent inhibition and with the afferent inputs to the magnocellular nucleus. It makes the assumptions that the internuncial cells are adrenergic and inhibitory to PV cells and that they are excited by an unknown mediator from collateral branches of neurosecretory axons. While this model serves adequately to explain much of what is known about the generation and suppression of neurosecretory impulses in the rat and rabbit there is discordant evidence for the cat, in which Nicoll and Barker (1971) failed to block recurrent inhibition in the SO nucleus by pretreatment with 5-OH dopamine though most of the noradrenaline endings in the nucleus had degenerated. To accommodate known facts about the synchronous discharge of oxytocin cells in the rat (Wakerley and Lincoln, 1973a) and reciprocal interactions between neurosecretory cells in the PV and SO nuclei (Yamashita et al., 1970), additional synaptic connexions would be needed. In the present state of knowledge this would enter too far into the realm of speculation.

Summary and Conclusions

The observations of "osmopotentials" in the anterior hypothalamus twenty years ago initiated an era of electrical recording in the hypothalamus. This was directed towards two problems: where and what are Verney's osmoreceptors, and how is the electrical activity of neurosecretory cells in the supraoptic and paraventricular nuclei related to the secretion of neurohypophysial hormones ?

Microelectrode recordings in mammals quickly established that single cells in the magnocellular nuclei exhibit typical action potentials whose discharge frequency could be influenced by osmotic and other physiological stimuli. The solution of the main questions, however, required the development of antidromic techniques for distinguishing neurosecretory cells from other neurones. This done, a profile of the electrical characteristics of the neurosecretory cells was soon mapped out. Verney's osmoreceptors are still not unequivocally identified but are probably interneurones rather than neurosecretory cells. The second question now seems to be virtually settled. There are oxytocin cells and vasopressin cells and release of hormone from their endings is determined in a fairly precise way by volleys of action potentials. These initiate the depolarisation change in the terminals that is the prerequisite for discharge of intragranular stores of hormone. Generation of the neurosecretory action potentials in the hypothalamus is facilitated by cholinergic (nicotinic receptors) mechanisms and inhibited by adrenergic (β receptors) mechanisms but the morphological and neurotransmitter basis for the recurrent inhibition of neurosecretory cell discharges remains obscure.

Acknowledgments. I wish to thank my colleagues, R. E. J. Dyball, R. G. Dyer, D. W. Lincoln, J. F. Morris and J. B. Wakerley for helpful suggestions and permission to quote their unpublished observations.

References

Abrahams, V. C., Pickford, M.: Simultaneous observations on the rate of urine flow and spontaneous uterine movements in the dog and their relationship to posterior lobe activity. J. Physiol. (Lond.) **126**, 239 (1954).

Barker, J. L., Crayton, J. W., Nicoll, R. A.: Antidromic and orthodromic responses of paraventricular and supraoptic neurosecretory cells. Brain Res. **33**, 353 (1971a).

Barker, J. L., Crayton, J. W., Nicoll, R. A.: Supraoptic neurosecretory cells: adrenergic and cholinergic sensitivity. Science **171**, 208 (1971b).

Bridges, T. E., Thorn, N. A.: The effect of autonomic blocking agents on vasopressin release *in vivo* induced by osmoreceptor stimulation. J. Endocr. **48**, 265 (1970).

Brooks, C. McC., Ishikawa, T., Koizumi, K., Lu, H. H.: Activity of neurones in the paraventricular nucleus of the hypothalamus and its control. J. Physiol. (Lond.) **182**, 217 (1966).

Brooks, C. McC., Ushiyama, J., Lange, G.: Reactions of neurons in or near the supraoptic nuclei. Amer. J. Physiol. **202**, 487 (1962).

Cross, B. A.: Functional identification of hypothalamic neurones. In press (1974).

Cross, B. A., Green, J. D.: Activity of single neurones in the hypothalamus: effect of osmotic and other stimuli. J. Physiol. (Lond.) **148**, 554 (1959).

Cross, B. A., Harris, G. W.: The role of the neurohypophysis in the milk-ejection reflex. J. Endocr. **8**, 148 (1952).

Douglas, W. W., Nagasawa, J., Schulz, R.: Electron microscopic studies on the mechanism of secretion of posterior pituitary hormones and significance of microvesicles ("synaptic vesicles"): evidence of secretion by exocytosis and formation of microvesicles as a by-product of this process. Mem. Soc. Endocr. **19**, 353 (1971).

Douglas, W. W., Sorimachi, M.: Electrically evoked release of vasopressin from isolated neurohypophyses in sodium-free media. Brit. J. Pharmacol. **42**, 647 (1971).

Dreifuss, J. J.: Mécanismes de sécrétion des hormones neurohypophysaires. Aspects cellulaires et sub-cellulaire. J. Physiol. (Paris) **67**, 5 (1973).

Dreifuss, J. J., Kalnins, I., Kelly, J. S., Ruf, K. B.: Action potentials and release of neurohypophysial hormones *in vitro*. J. Physiol. (Lond.) **215**, 805 (1971).

Dreifuss, J. J., Kelly, J. S.: Recurrent inhibition of antidromically identified rat supraoptic neurones. J. Physiol. (Lond.) **220**, 87 (1972a).

Dreifuss, J. J., Kelly, J. S.: The activity of identified supraoptic neurones and their response to acetylcholine applied by iontophoresis. J. Physiol. (Lond.) **220**, 105 (1972b).

Duke, H., Pickford, M.: Observations on the action of acetylcholine and adrenaline on the hypothalamus. J. Physiol. (Lond.) **114**, 325 (1951).

Dyball, R. E. J.: Oxytocin and ADH secretion in relation to electrical activity in antidromically identified supraoptic and paraventricular units. J. Physiol. (Lond.) **214**, 245 (1971).

Dyball, R. E. J.: Single unit activity in the hypothalamo-neurohypophysial system of Brattleboro rats. J. Endocr. In Press (1974).

Dyball, R. E. J., Dyer, R. G.: Plasma oxytocin concentration and paraventricular neurone activity in rats with diencephalic islands and intact brains. J. Physiol. (Lond.) **216**, 227 (1971).

Dyball, R. E. J., Koizumi, K.: Electrical activity in the supraoptic and paraventricular nuclei associated with neurohypophysial hormone release. J. Physiol. (Lond.) **201**, 711 (1969).

Dyball, R. E. J., Pountney, P. S.: Discharge patterns of supraoptic and paraventricular neurones in rats given a 2% NaCl solution instead of drinking water. J. Endocr. **56**, 91 (1973).

Dyer, R. G., Dyball, R. E. J., Morris, J. F.: The effect of hypothalamic deafferentation upon the ultrastructure and hormone content of the paraventricular nucleus. J. Endocr. **57**, 509 (1973).

von Euler, C.: A preliminary note on slow hypothalamic "osmopotentials". Acta physiol. scand. **29**, 133 (1953).

Fuxe, K., Hökfelt, T.: The influence of central catecholamine neurons on the hormone secretion from the anterior and posterior pituitary. In: Neurosecretion (F. Stutinsky, Ed.), p. 165. Berlin-Heidelberg-New York: Springer 1967.

Harris, G. W., Manabe, Y., Ruf, K. B.: A study of the parameters of electrical stimulation of unmyelinated fibres in the pituitary stalk. J. Physiol. (Lond.) **203**, 67 (1969).

Hayward, J. N.: Neurohormonal regulation of neuroendocrine cells in the hypothalamus. In press (1974).

Hayward, J. N., Jennings, D. P.: Activity of magnocellular neuroendocrine cells in the hypothalamus of unanaesthetised monkeys. I. Functional cell types and their anatomical distribution in the supraoptic nucleus and internuclear zone. J. Physiol. (Lond.) **232**, 515 (1973a).

Hayward, J. N., Jennings, D. P.: Activity of magnocellular neuroendocrine cells in the hypothalamus of unanaesthetised monkeys. II. Osmosensitivity of functional cell types in the supraoptic nucleus and internuclear zone. J. Physiol. (Lond.) **232**, 545 (1973b).

Hayward, J. N., Vincent, J. D.: Activity of single cells in the osmoreceptor-supraoptic complex in the hypothalamus of the waking rhesus monkey. Brain Res. **23**, 105 (1970).

Holland, R. C., Cross, B. A., Sawyer, C. H.: EEG correlates of osmotic activation of the neurohypophyseal milk-ejection mechanism. Amer. J. Physiol. (Lond.) **196**, 796 (1959a).

Holland, R. C., Sundsten, J. W., Sawyer, C. H.: Effects of intracarotid injections of hypertonic solutions on arterial pressure in the rabbit. Circulat. Res. **7**, 712 (1959b).

Joynt, R. J.: Functional significance of osmosensitive units in the anterior hypothalamus. Neurology **14**, 584 (1964).

Kandel, E. R.: Electrical properties of hypothalamic neuroendocrine cells. J. gen. Physiol. **47**, 691 (1964).

Kelly, J. S., Dreifuss, J. J.: Antidromic inhibition of identified rat supraoptic neurones. Brain Res. **22**, 406 (1970).

Koizumi, K., Ishikawa, T., Brooks, C. McC.: Control of activity of neurons in the supraoptic nucleus. J. Neurophysiol. **27**, 878 (1964).

Koizumi, K., Yamashita, H.: Studies of antidromically identified neurosecretory cells of the hypothalamus by intracellular and extracellular recordings. J. Physiol. (Lond.) **221**, 683 (1972).

Mikiten, T. M., Douglas, W. W.: Effect of Ca^{++} and other ions on vasopressin release from rat neurohypophysis stimulated electrically *in vitro*. Nature (Lond.) **207**, 302 (1965).

Morris, J. F.: A quantitative analysis of synaptic terminals in the paraventricular nucleus of the rat hypothalamus. J. Anat. In press (1974).

Moss, R. L., Dyball, R. E. J., Cross, B. A.: Responses of antidromically identified supraoptic and paraventricular units to acetycholine, noradrenaline and glutamate applied iontophoretically. Brain Res. **35**, 573 (1971).

Moss, R. L., Dyball, R. E. J., Cross, B. A.: Excitation of antidromically identified neurosecretory cells of the paraventricular nucleus by oxytocin applied iontophoretically. Exp. Neurol. **34**, 95 (1972a).

Moss, R. L., Urban, I., Cross, B. A.: Microelectrophoresis of cholinergic and aminergic drugs on paraventricular neurons. Amer. J. Physiol. **223**, 310 (1972b).

Negoro, H., Holland, R. C.: Inhibition of unit activity in the hypothalamic paraventricular nucleus following antidromic activation. Brain Res. **42**, 385 (1972).

Nicoll, R. A., Barker, J. L.: The pharmacology of recurrent inhibition on the supraoptic neurosecretory system. Brain Res. **35**, 501 (1971).

Nordmann, J. J., Dreifuss, J. J.: Hormone release evoked by electrical stimulation of rat neurohypophyses in the absence of action potentials. Brain Res. **45**, 604 (1972).

Novin, D., Sundsten, J. W., Cross, B. A.: Some properties of antidromically activated units in the paraventricular nucleus of the hypothalamus. Exp. Neurol. **26**, 330 (1970).

Pickford, M.: Factors affecting milk release in the dog and the quantity of oxytocin liberated by suckling. J. Physiol. (Lond.) **152**, 515 (1960).

Poisner, A. M.: Stimulus-secretion coupling in the adrenal medulla and posterior pituitary gland. In: Frontiers in Neuroendocrinology (Ganong, W. F., Martini, L., Eds.), p. 33. New York: Oxford University Press 1973.

Robinson, N., Wells, F.: Distribution and localisation of sites of gamma aminobutyric acid metabolism in the adult rat brain. J. Anat. (Lond.) **114**, 365 (1973).

Sawyer, C. H., Gernandt, B. E.: Effects of intracarotid and intraventricular injections of hypertonic solutions on electrical activity of the rabbit brain. Amer. J. Physiol. **185**, 209 (1956).

Shute, C. C. D., Lewis, P. R.: Cholinergic and monoaminergic pathways in the hypothalamus. Brit. med. Bull. **22**, 221 (1966).

Suda, I., Koizumi, K., Brooks, C.McC.: Study of unitary activity in the supraoptic nucleus of the hypothalamus. Jap. J. Physiol. **13**, 374 (1963).

Sundsten, J. W., Sawyer, C. H.: Osmotic activation of neurohypophysial hormone release in rabbits with hypothalamic islands. Exp. Neurol. **4**, 548 (1961).

Tauc, L.: Site of origin and propagation of spike in the giant neurone of Aplysia. J. gen. Physiol. **45**, 1077 (1962).

Verney, E. B.: The antidiuretic hormone and the factors which determine its release. Proc. roy, Soc. B. **135**, 25 (1947).

Vincent, J. D., Arnauld, E., Nicolescu-Catargi, A.: Osmoreceptors and neurosecretory cells in the supraoptic complex of the unanaesthetised monkey. Brain Res. **45**, 278 (1972).

Vincent, J. D., Hayward, J. N.: Activity of single cells in the osmoreceptor-supraoptic complex in the hypothalamus of the waking rhesus monkey. Brain Res. **23**, 105 (1970).

Wakerley, J. B., Dyball, R. E. J., Lincoln, D. W.: Milk ejection in the rat: the result of a selective release of oxytocin. J. Endocr. **57**, 557 (1973).

Wakerley, J. B., Lincoln, D. W.: Phasic discharge of antidromically identified units in the paraventricular nucleus of the hypothalamus. Brain Res. **25**, 192 (1971).

Wakerley, J. B., Lincoln, D. W.: The milk-ejection reflex of the rat: a 20—40-fold acceleration in the firing of paraventricular neurones during oxytocin release. J. Endocr. **57**, 477 (1973a).

Wakerley, J. B., Lincoln, D. W.: Unit activity in the supraoptic nucleus during reflex milk ejection. J. Endocr. In press (1973b).

Woods, J. W., Bard, P., Bleier, R.: Functional capacity of the deafferented hypothalamus: water balance and responses to osmotic stimuli in the decerebrate cat and rat. J. Neurophysiol. **29**, 751 (1966).

Yagi, K., Asuma, T., Matsuda, K.: Neurosecretory cell: capable of conducting impulses in rats. Science **154**, 778 (1966).

Yamashita, H., Koizumi, K., Brooks, C.McC.: Electrophysiological studies of neurophysiological studies of neurosecretory cells in the cat hypothalamus. Brain Res. **20**, 462 (1970).

Dynamics of Oxytocin Secretion

D. W. Lincoln

Department of Anatomy, University of Bristol, Bristol (Great Britain)

There are many technical approaches to the study of neurosecretion but so diverse are the techniques that in the past biochemists, electrophysiologists and electron-microscopists have tended to pursue their own goals in comparative isolation. The situation is changing and in some areas a measure of agreement seems to be emerging, as the results are complementary and the figures tally. With the study of the milk-ejection reflex of the rat, for example, we can identify the oxytocic-neurones, record their electrical activity and measure "on-line" the release of the hormone.

The adult lactating rat (280—320 g) nurses her young for 12—14 h each day, in periods of about 20—60 min. Milk ejection (RME) occurs at regular intervals of 5—15 min, though the pups suckle continuously. Each RME lasts 8—12 sec and is associated with (but not caused by) an abrupt increase in the suckling activity of the pups as the intramammary pressure rises (Lincoln, Hill and Wakerley, 1973). The individual RME is the result of an abrupt release of 0.5—1.5 mU oxytocin (Wakerley and Lincoln, 1971), without a measurable release of vasopressin (Wakerley et al., 1973). Estimates of total neurohypophysial oxytocin tend to vary; the Porton strain of Wistar rats on which the above studies were conducted have 175 mU oxytocin/100 g body weight (i.e. about 500 mU/rat) (Jones and Pickering, 1969). Thus, the 1 mU pulse of each RME represents only 0.2% of the neurohypophysial store. On a daily basis, however, the lactating rat has a requirement for up to 100 mU oxytocin, i.e. 60—80 RME's at 1 mU and an allowance for basal turnover. Such a daily requirement is 4—5 times the basal turnover (18 mU) of oxytocin in a male rat in water balance, a nonstimulated situation (Jones and Pickering, 1972; Pickering et al., 1974).

This pattern of oxytocin release, with the discharge of a uniform pulse of hormone every 5—15 min, represents a principle which appears to be new to endocrinology. The system is frequency modulated: it depends not on the magnitude of a prolonged release of hormone but on the number of pulses released per unit of time. A similar pattern of release is found during suckling in mice, gerbils and hamsters (Somerset et al., unpublished observations). In all these species, and in no others known to date, a "normal" pattern of RME continues during the surgical anaesthesia of the mother, and with the rat we have employed such diverse anaesthetics as ethyl carbamate (urethane), tribromoethanol ("Avertin"), sodium pentobarbitone ("Nembutal") (Lincoln et al., 1973) and ethyl alcohol (Lincoln, 1973). Whilst this pulsatile pattern of release helps some causes it hinders others. For example, the release of neurosecretory granules from the neurohypophysis is mathematically an infrequent event. A 1 mU pulse of oxytocin involves the "exocytosis" of about 1 neurosecretory granule in 1000 if one assumes that the readily releasable hormone is in a granular form — in 2 sec or less, and this is a stimulated situation. Secondly, it restricts the value of measurements of neurohypophysial and plasma oxytocin. There should be no observable depletion of neurohypophysial oxytocin, for the oxytocin released as a result of one hour of suckling will only equal 1—2% of the gland content and that assumes rather naively that there has been no replacement.

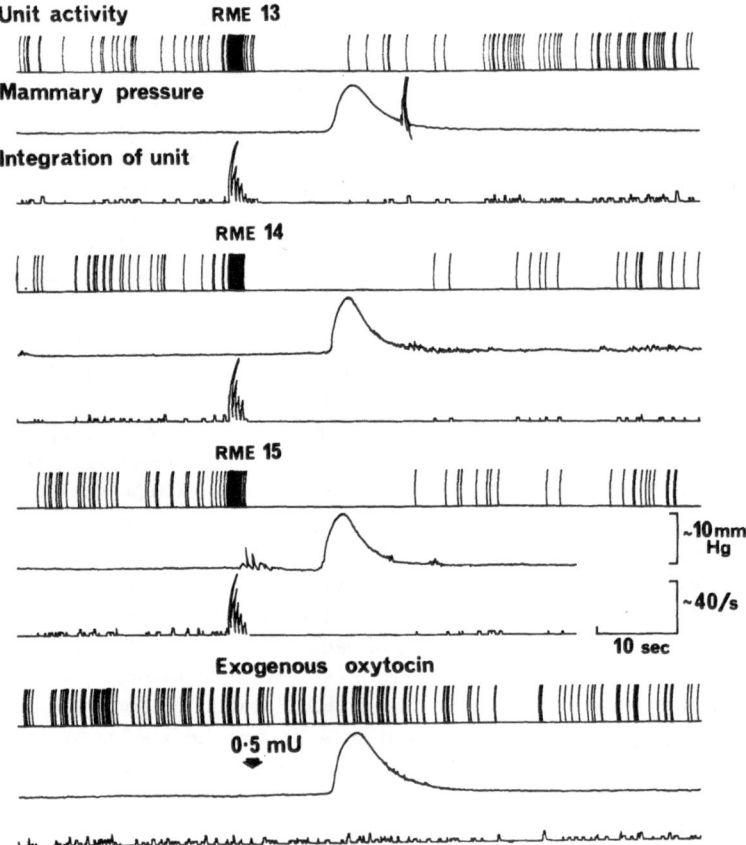

Fig. 1. A polygraph recording of a supraoptic neurone to show the accelerated spike activity that precipitates the release of oxytocin during suckling in rats. The rat (weight 320 g) was anaesthetized with urethane (1.1 g/Kg, i.p.), stereotaxically restrained and suckled by a litter of 8—10 pups. The supraoptic unit was antidromically identified by stimulation of the neurohypophysis; antidromic invasion occurred at a latency of 11 ms (S/N, 100/1). Intramammary pressure was recorded from a cannulated teat duct; oxytocin was injected into the great saphenous vein. Milk ejections (RME) are numbered from the onset of suckling. Note: (i) the magnitude and uniformity of the acceleration in activity, (ii) the period of inhibition following the response, (iii) the 12—13 sec latency from the acceleration in spike activity to the rise in intramammary pressure, and (iv) the failure of exogenous oxytocin and the induced milk ejection to influence the spike activity of the neurone

Each pulse of oxytocin is precipitated by a stereotyped acceleration, of 2—4 sec duration, in the spike activity of about 50% of the neurosecretory cells in the supraoptic and paraventricular nuclei (Fig. 1) (Lincoln and Wakerley, 1972; Wakerley and Lincoln, 1973a, b). This synchronous discharge of the "oxytocic-neurones" precedes RME by 12—18 sec and involves the generation of 40 to 80 spikes/unit. The latency of 12—18 sec is the time it takes for hormone release, circulation in the blood and action on the myoepithelial cells of the mammary gland. The acceleration in spike activity is not a "square-wave" function, it is rapid in onset and exponential in decay. Thus the peak frequency of 40—80 spikes/sec is only obtained for about 0.5 sec (see Fig. 2, Cross, 1973). Note: this peak frequency exceeds the critical frequency of stimulation that is necessary to elicit oxytocin release both *in vivo* (Cross and Harris, 1952; Harris et al., 1969) and *in vitro* (Ishida, 1970; Dreifuss et al., 1971).

These electrophysiological studies and recent immunohistochemical (Burlet et al., 1974) and biochemical work (Burford et al., 1973) all support the view that the supraoptic and paraventricular nuclei are both involved in the biosynthesis and control of oxytocin (and vasopressin). If any dichotomy of function does exist between these nuclei then it is small, but at the same time the nuclei should not be considered equal. Observations must be weighted according to the size of the nuclei. The supraoptic nuclei with 13000—15000 neurosecretory cells are 3—4 times the size of the paraventricular nuclei: at 3500—4500 cells (Bodian and Maren, 1951; Bandaranayake, 1971).

Now, if all the neurones of the supraoptic and paraventricular nuclei are anti-dromically invaded, during both the generation of the orthodromic spike and when antidromically driven from the neurohypophysis—and the current evidence suggests that they are (Novin et al., 1970; Dyball and Koizumi, 1969; Wakerley and

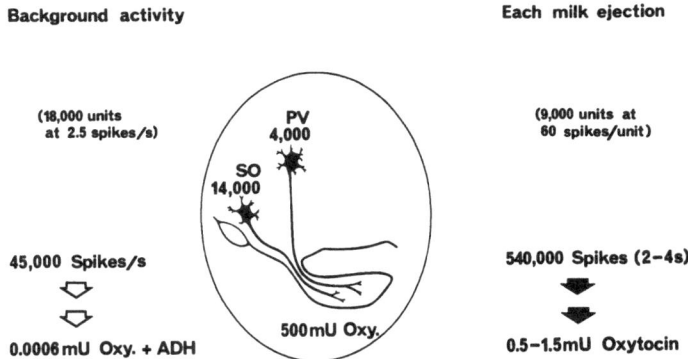

Fig. 2. A summary of the relationship between electrical activity of neurosecretory cells and the release of oxytocin in rats. The number of supraoptic (SO) and paraventricular (PV) neurones and the oxytocin content of the neurohypophysis are given in the centre of the figure. The total spike traffic in the hypothalamo-neurohypophysial tract is compared to the "basal" release of oxytocin (on the left) and the pulsatile release of oxytocin during suckling (on the right). In the latter calculation the contribution to spike activity of the 9000 unresponsive SO and PV cells has been ignored. Note the 100-fold facilitation in the amount of hormone released per spike in the burst of activity that causes milk ejection

Lincoln, 1973a), — then some 540000 spikes must pass along the hypothalamo-neurohypophysial tract within a space of 2—4 sec to precipitate the release of each 1 mU pulse of oxytocin for RME. Thus one spike equates to a release of 3—4 fg (10^{-15} g) of hormone. This burst of activity must involve considerable enhancement in the amount of hormone released per spike, for there are some 45000 spikes/sec passing along the tract when the animals are not being suckled. If this background activity caused a release of 3—4 fg/spike the neurohypophysis would be emptied of all hormone within 2 h. From biochemical studies we know that the nonstimulated gland only turns over about 5% of its content/day (Pickering et al., 1974).

A summary of the dynamics of oxytocin release is given in Fig. 2. Undoubtedly with time these calculations will improve.

References

Bandaranayake, R. C.: Morphology of the accessory neurosecretory nuclei and of the retrochiasmatic part of the supraoptic nucleus of the rat. Acta anat. (Basel) **80**, 14—22 (1971).

Bodian, D., Maren, T. H.: The effect of neuro- and adenohypophysectomy on retrograde degeneration in hypothalamic nuclei of the rat. J. comp. Neurol. **94**, 485—511 (1951).

Burford, G. D., Dyball, R. E. J., Moss, R. L., Pickering, B. T.: Are oxytocin and vasopressin synthetized in different hypothalamic nuclei? J. Anat. (Lond.) **114**, 306 (1973).

Burlet, A., Marchetti, J., Duheille, J.: Immunohistochemistry of vasopressin: study of the hypothalamo-hypophysial system of normal dehydrated and hypophysectomized rat. Proc. VI. Int. Symp. Neurosecretion. In press (1974).

Cross, B. A.: The neurosecretory impulse. In: Proc. VI. Int. Symp. Neurosecretion. In press (1974).

Cross, B. A., Harris, G. W.: The role of the neurohypophysis in the milkejection reflex. J. Endocr. **8**, 148—161 (1952).

Dreifuss, J. J., Kalnins, I., Kelly, J. S., Ruf, K. B.: Action potentials and release of neurohypophysial hormones in vitro. J. Physiol. (Lond.) **215**, 805—817 (1971).

Dyball, R. E. J., Koizumi, K.: Electrical activity in the supraoptic and paraventricular nuclei associated with neurohypophyseal hormone release. J. Physiol. (Lond.) **210**, 711—722 (1969).

Harris, G. W., Manabe, Y., Ruf, K. B.: A study of the parameters of electrical stimulation of unmyelinated fibres in the pituitary stalk. J. Physiol. (Lond.) **203**, 67—81 (1969).

Ishida, A.: The oxytocin release and the compound action potential evoked by electrical stimulation of the isolated neurohypophysis of the rat. Jap. J. Physiol. **20**, 84—96 (1970).

Jones, C. W., Pickering, B. T.: Comparison of the effects of water deprivation and sodium chloride inhibition on the hormone content of the neurohypophysis of the rat. J. Physiol. (Lond.) **203**, 449—458 (1969).

Jones, C. W., Pickering, B. T.: Intra-axonal transport and turnover of neurohypophysial hormones in the rat. J. Physiol. (Lond.) **227**, 553—564 (1972).

Lincoln, D. W.: Milk ejection during alcohol anaesthesia in the rat. Nature (Lond.) **243**, 227—229 (1973).

Lincoln, D. W., Hill, A., Wakerley, J. B.: The milk-ejection reflex of the rat: an intermittent function not abolished by surgical levels of anaesthesia. J. Endocr. **57**, 459—476 (1973).

Lincoln, D. W., Wakerley, J. B.: Accelerated discharge of paraventricular neurosecretory cells correlated with reflex release of oxytocin during suckling. J. Physiol. (Lond.) **222**, 23—24P (1972).

Pickering, B. T., Jones, C. W., Burford, G. D.: Biochemical aspects of the hypothalamo-neurohypophysial neurone. In: Proc. VI. Int. Symp. Neurosecretion. (F. Knowles, L. Vollrath, Eds.). Berlin-Heidelberg-New York: Springer 1974.

Wakerley, J. B., Dyball, R. E. J., Lincoln, D. W.: Milk ejection in the rat: the result of a selective release of oxytocin. J. Endocr. **57**, 557—558 (1973).

Wakerley, J. B., Lincoln, D. W.: Intermittent release of oxytocin during suckling in the rat. Nature New Biology **233**, 180—181.

Wakerley, J. B., Lincoln, D. W.: The milk-ejection reflex of the rat: a 20- to 40-fold acceleration in the firing of paraventricular neurones during oxytocin release. J. Endocr. **57**, 477—493 (1973a).

Wakerley, J. B., Lincoln, D. W.: Unit activity in the supraoptic nucleus during reflex milk ejection. J. Endocr. **57**, 46—47 (1973b).

B. Hypophysiotropic Neurosecretion

Recent Advances in the Study of the Hypothalamic Releasing Factors

L. MARTINI

Department of Endocrinology, University of Milano, Milano (Italy)

Several hypothalamic releasing and inhibiting factors have recently been obtained in a pure form. This has permitted the elucidation of their structure and their synthesis. Table 1 provides an up to date summary (September 1973) of the releasing and inhibiting factors already prepared by total synthesis.

Table 1. Synthetic hypothalamic releasing and inhibiting factors

TSH-RF	(Burgus et al., 1969)	
	pyroGlu-His-Pro-NH$_2$	
LH-RF	(Matsuo et al., 1971)	
	pyroGlu-His-Trp-Ser-Tyr-Gly-Leu-Arg-Pro-Gly-NH$_2$	
GH-RF	(Schally et al., 1971a)	
	Val-His-Leu-Ser-Ala-Glu-Glu-Lys-Glu-Ala	
GH-IF	(Somatostatin) (Brazeau et al., 1973)	
	Ala-Gly-Cys-Lys-Asn-Phe-Phe-Trp-Lys-Thr-Phe-Thr-Ser-Cys-OH	
MIF	(Celis et al., 1971a)	
	Pro-Leu-Gly-NH$_2$	
MIF	(Nair et al., 1972)	
	Pro-His-Phe-Arg-Gly-NH$_2$	
MIF	(Bower et al., 1971)	
	Cys-Tyr-Ile-Gln-Asn-Cys-OH	
MRF	(Celis et al., 1971b)	
	Cys-Tyr-Ile-Gln-Asn-Cys-OH	

It is now a generally accepted view that these factors are synthesized in specialized hypothalamic neurons and are subsequently transported by nerve fibers to the median eminence, which is the region of the hypothalamus specifically responsible for their storage. From this area, the hypothalamic releasing and inhibiting factors are secreted into the pituitary portal vessels and transported down to the anterior pituitary where they exert their biological effects (Harris, 1955; Porter et al., 1971; Vale et al., 1973). More than one aspect of the complex physiology of the releasing and inhibiting factors had not been clarified so far. This paper represents the author's contribution toward the elucidation of some of these unsolved problems. The following topics will be selected for discussion:

I) The localization of the nuclei which synthesize the gonadotropin releasing factors.

II) The participation of cholinergic mediators in the process of release of the gonadotropin releasing factors.

III) The effect of the intracarotid administration of synthetic LH-RF on the release of LH and FSH.

I. Localization of the Nuclei which Synthesize Gonadotropin Releasing Factors

Three groups of experiments have been performed in order to clarify which regions of the hypothalamus synthesize the releasing factors which control the secretion of pituitary gonadotropins.

A. Hypothalamic Lesions

The first technique was that of placing separate electrolytic lesions in each of the hypothalamic areas which are believed to play a role in the control of gonadotropin secretion (Szentágothai et al., 1968), and of studying whether such lesions modify the concentrations of the FSH-Releasing Factor (FSH-RF) and of the LH-Releasing Factor (LH—RF) at the level of the median eminence. It was assumed

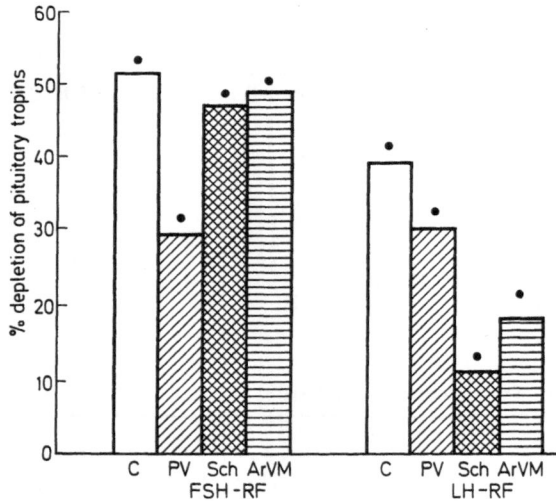

Fig. 1. Effect of lesions localized in the paraventricular (PV), suprachiasmatic (Sch) and arcuate-ventromedial (ArVM) regions on FSH-RF and LH-RF activities of the median eminence of male rats. Columns represent the depletion of pituitary gonadotropins induced in normal male rats by the intracarotid injection of hypothalamic extracts prepared from non-lesioned controls (C) or from animals with the different hypothalamic lesions

that a lesion placed exactly in an area in which a releasing factor is produced would prevent its synthesis and consequently reduce its accumulation in the median eminence. Three independent areas of the brain were bilaterally lesioned. They will be referred to as: a) paraventricular area; b) suprachiasmatic area; and c) arcuate-ventromedial area. Five days following placement of the lesions, the rats were killed and their median eminences were collected in order to evaluate their content in FSH-RF and in LH-RF. For the assays of these principles the "pituitary depletion methods" described by Motta et al. (1970a) were employed. Using this approach it has been possible to localize, within the hypothalamus, a circumscribed region in which FSH-RF is synthesized; it has actually been shown that lesions in, or around, the paraventricular nuclei are the only ones which reduce the concentration of this releasing factor at median eminence level (Fig. 1). The synthesis of LH-RF takes place apparently in two different regions, since the content of this releasing factor in the median eminence is reduced when lesions are placed either in the suprachiasmatic area or in the arcuate-ventromedial nuclei (Fig. 1) (Mess et al., 1967; Martini et al., 1968).

B. Hypothalamic Deafferentation

The second approach devised to study the localization of the nuclei synthesizing the releasing factors which control the secretion of pituitary gonadotropins was that of evaluating the concentrations of FSH-RF and LH-RF in the hypothalamic islands of rats submitted to a complete hypothalamic deafferentation (Halász, 1969). This operation permits a total separation of the paraventricular region from the rest of the hypothalamus. Consequently, if it is true that FSH-RF originates in the paraventricular area, the complete disappearance of FSH-RF from the

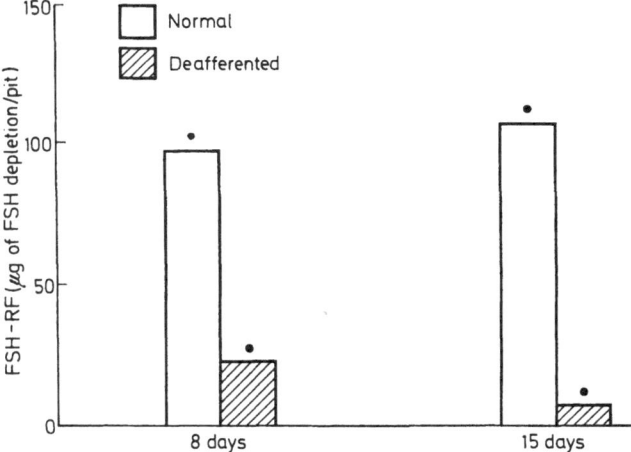

Fig. 2. Effect of hypothalamic deafferentation on the FSH-RF content of the hypothalamic island of adult male rats (eight and fifteen days after the operation). Columns represent the depletion of pituitary FSH induced in normal male rats by the intracarotid injection of hypothalamic extracts prepared from normal or from deafferented animals

island a few days after the operation would be expected. On the other hand, the suprachiasmatic and the arcuate-ventromedial regions are still included within the hypothalamic island. Consequently, if LH-RF is really produced by these two zones, its concentrations in the island should not be reduced following the operation. The content of FSH-RF and of LH-RF in the deafferented islands was measured eight and fifteen days following the operation, using the techniques described by Motta et al. (1970a). The results shown in Fig. 2 indicate that FSH-RF stores are significantly reduced in the hypothalamic island eight days after a complete deafferentation; FSH-RF disappears completely from the isolated hypothalamus fifteen days after the operation. Eight and fifteen days after deafferentation LH-RF is still present in the isolated island (Fig. 3). Surprisingly

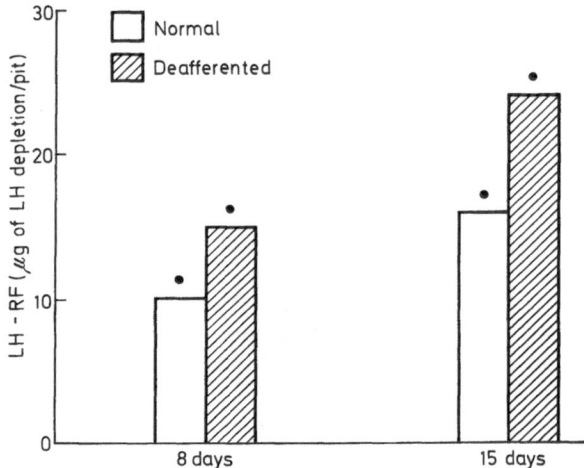

Fig. 3. Effect of hypothalamic deafferentation on the LH-RF content of the hypothalamic island of adult male rats (eight and fifteen days after the operation). Columns represent the depletion of pituitary LH induced in normal male rats by the intracarotid injection of hypothalamic extracts prepared from normal or from deafferented animals

the concentration of this releasing factor in deafferented animals is even higher than usual (Tima et al., 1969; Motta et al., 1970b). These data confirm with a new technique that FSH-RF is synthesized in the paraventricular region, and that LH-RF is probably manufactured in the suprachiasmatic and in the arcuate-ventromedial regions. The fact that the stores of LH-RF are increased following deafferentation suggests that, after the operation, all the LH-RF which is synthesized is accumulated in the island, because the extrahypothalamic neural stimuli necessary for its release are no longer transmitted to the hypothalamus (see below) (Tima et al., 1969; Motta et al., 1970b).

C. Hypothalamic Implants of Inhibitors of Protein Synthesis

In the third group of experiments, the hypothesis that FSH-RF might be synthesized in the paraventricular nuclei was tested by implanting cycloheximide

(Actidione), an inhibitor of protein synthesis, into the paraventricular region, and by evaluating the effects of such implants on FSH-RF stores in the median eminence. Cycloheximide was implanted either unilaterally or bilaterally. When unilateral implants were performed, at the time of autopsy median eminence tissue was collected in a way which permitted the separation of the half median eminence corresponding to the implanted side from the half corresponding to the non-implanted one. The two halves of the median eminence were then tested separately for their content of FSH-RF and of LH-RF according to the usual "pituitary depletion method" (Motta et al., 1970a). The data shown in Fig. 4 indicate that, five days after unilateral implant of cycloheximide into one paraventricular nucleus, FSH-RF disappears only from the ipsilateral half of the median eminence; complete disappearance of FSH-RF from the median eminence is induced by bilateral implants. It may be concluded from these results that inhibition of protein synthesis in the cells of the paraventricular nuclei interferes with some biochemical process which is essential for the synthesis of FSH-RF in this region. It is also clear from the results that fibers originating in one paraventricular nucleus do not cross, and carry FSH-RF only to the ipsilateral half of the median eminence (Motta et al., 1971). Figure 5 shows once more that the paraventricular region is not strictly involved in the synthesis of LH-RF. Rats implanted with cycloheximide either unilaterally or bilaterally in this region of the brain have normal amounts of LH-RF in the median eminence (Motta et al., 1971).

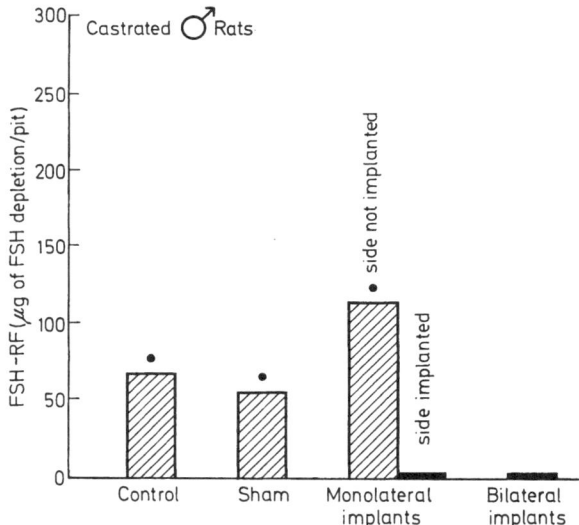

Fig. 4. Effect of implants of cycloheximide (Actidione) in the paraventricular region on the FSH-RF content of the median eminence of adult castrated male rats. See text for more details. Columns represent the depletion of pituitary FSH induced in normal male rats by the intracarotid injection of hypothalamic extracts prepared from controls or from implanted animals. Control: unimplanted animals; Sham: animals implanted with empty cannulae; Monolateral implants: animals implanted with cycloheximide in one paraventricular nucleus; Bilateral implants: animals implanted with cycloheximide in both paraventricular nuclei

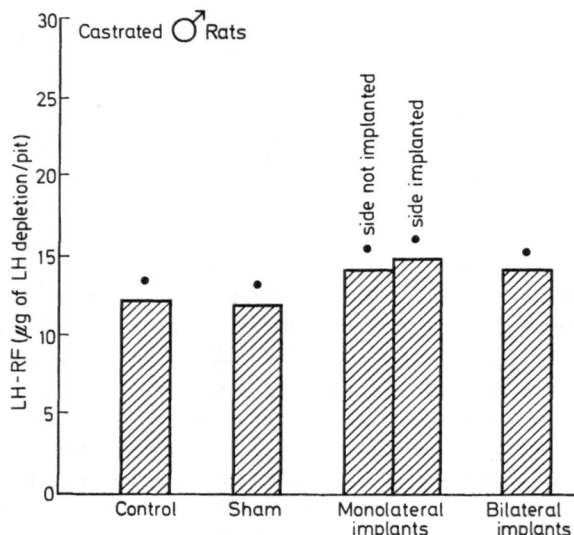

Fig. 5. Effect of implants of cycloheximide (Actidione) in the paraventricular region on the LH-RF content of the median eminence of adult castrated male rats. See text for more details. Columns represent the depletion of pituitary LH induced in normal male rats by the intra-carotid injection of hypothalamic extracts prepared from controls or from implanted animals. Control: unimplanted animals; Sham: animals implanted with empty cannulae; Monolateral implants: animals implanted with cycloheximide in one paraventricular nucleus; Bilateral implants: animals implanted with cycloheximide in both paraventricular nuclei

D. Conclusions

The following conclusions may be derived from these three sets of experiments: 1. the median eminence region is not directly responsible for the synthesis of the gonadotropin releasing factors; 2. the paraventricular region is specifically involved in the synthesis of FSH-RF, while the suprachiasmatic and the arcuate-ventro-medial zones are specifically devoted to the synthesis of LH-RF; 3. it is possible to modify intrahypothalamic stores of one gonadotropin releasing factor without changing those of the other. This finding does not seem compatible with the hypo-thesis that one single hypothalamic factor might control the release of both LH and FSH as recently suggested (Matsuo et al., 1971; Schally et al., 1971b).

II. Participation of Cholinergic Mediators in the Process of Release of the Gonadotropin Releasing Factors

It is a generally accepted concept that extrahypothalamic nervous structures (e.g. amygdala, hippocampus, midbrain, cerebral cortex, etc.) may influence the neurons which secrete the gonadotropin releasing factors (Mess and Martini, 1968; Szentá-gothai et al., 1968; Halász, 1969). The validity of this concept is proved once more by the observation, reported in a previous section of this paper, that LH-RF is

Table 2. Effect of acetylcholine (ACh) and atropine (Atr) on the release of FSH by anterior pituitaries (AP) incubated *in vitro* alone or with basal hypothalamus-median eminence tissue (ME)[a]

Groups[b]		FSH release in the medium (µg/ml/4 h)	Significance (P)
A. AP	(9)	4.64 ± 0.57	
B. AP + ACh 10 µg/ml	(6)	4.36 ± 0.73	NS *vs* A
C. AP + 2 ME	(9)	7.16 ± 0.84	<0.0125 *vs* A
D. AP + 2 ME + ACh 10 µg/ml	(9)	16.68 ± 1.88	<0.0005 *vs* C
E. AP + Atr 20 µg/ml	(3)	3.41 ± 0.52	NS *vs* A
F. AP + 2 ME + Atr 20 µg/ml	(3)	3.73 ± 0.87	<0.025 *vs* C
G. AP + 2 ME + ACh 10 µg/ml + Atr 20 µg/ml	(3)	9.70 ± 3.55	<0.01 *vs* D

[a] Values are means ± SE.
[b] Number of assays in parentheses.

accumulated in the deafferented hypothalamic island when all inputs from extra-hypothalamic structures are eliminated. The chemical nature of the humoral mediator(s) involved in transferring the information from extrahypothalamic centers to the hypothalamic nuclei has not been fully clarified so far. A lot of data seem to suggest that traditional central nervous system mediators (e.g., epinephrine, norepinephrine, serotonin, dopamine, acetylcholine, etc.) may be involved in such a process (Ganong and Lorenzen, 1967; Fuxe and Hökfelt, 1969; Kobayashi and Matsui, 1969; Piva et al., 1969). The possibility that cholinergic mediators might intervene in the control of the secretion of the gonadotropin releasing factors has recently been tested in the author's laboratory using an *in vitro* procedure similar to that described by Kamberi et al. (1970). Anterior pituitaries of normal rats were incubated for 4 h either alone or in the presence of hypothalamic tissue. In some experiments, acetylcholine (ACh), or drugs inhibiting its effects, were added to the incubation media. At the end of the incubation period FSH was evaluated in the media by the method of Steelman and Pohley (1953). Table 2 indicates that the anterior pituitary, when incubated alone, secretes very low amounts of FSH. The release of FSH from the incubated pituitaries is increased by the addition of fragments of rat hypothalamus. ACh, added to incubation flasks containing only anterior pituitary tissue, does not increase FSH output. On the contrary, the drug does enhance FSH secretion in flasks containing simultaneously hypothalamic fragments and anterior pituitary tissue (Simonovic et al., 1971; Motta and Martini, 1972). Since ACh added to the anterior pituitary alone does not have any effect on FSH output, it is obvious that the effect of the cholinergic agent must be mediated through some hypothalamic mechanism. It may be suggested that ACh stimulates the release of FSH-RF from the incubated hypothalami. FSH-RF released under the influence of ACh in turn enhances the secretion of FSH from the incubated pituitaries. These preliminary results indicate then that cholinergic mechanisms may be involved in liberating the releasing factors from the neurons in which they are manufactured. This interpretation is supported by the experiments in which atropine, a typical blocker of cholinergic impulses, was used. When atropine is added to the media containing only anterior pituitary tissue, it does not greatly change the secretion of FSH (Table 2). However, atropine inhibits the small increase in the release of FSH, which is observed when hypothalamic tissue is added to the anterior pituitary. Atropine also reduces the effect ACh exerts on FSH secretion when added to the media containing simultaneously anterior pituitary tissue and hypothalamic fragments (Simonovic et al., 1971; Motta and Martini, 1972). In a similar set of experiments it was shown that ACh may play a role also in the release of LH-RF (Fiorindo and Martini, unpublished observations). It is interesting to note that the stimulating effect ACh exerts on the liberation of the releasing factors seems to be specific for those principles controlling the secretion of pituitary gonadotropins. In an *in vitro* study ACh was shown to be completely unable to affect the secretion of growth hormone releasing factor (Collu and Martini, unpublished observations).

III. Effect of an Intracarotid Administration of Synthetic LH-RF on the Release of LH and FSH

As previously mentioned, it has been recently proposed that one single hypothalamic factor might control the release of both LH and FSH (Matsuo et al., 1971; Schally et al., 1971 b). This suggestion was mainly based on the observation that the synthetic LH-RF decapeptide prepared by Matsuo et al. (1971) is able to release FSH as well as LH in several types of experimental preparations. According to this hypothesis, the direction of the response of the anterior pituitary gland, when stimulated by the endogenous or by the exogenous LH-FSH-RF, would be modulated by the levels of circulating sex steroids. However, there are several physiological observations which are not easily explained on the basis of the existence of only one single hypothalamic gonadotropin releasing factor (Faiman and Ryan, 1967; Swerdloff et al., 1971).

It was believed that a careful study of the endocrinological effects exerted by the synthetic decapeptide in animals submitted to different experimental manipulations might help in solving the problem of the unity or of the plurality of the gonadotropin releasing factor(s).

Figure 6 shows the effects of the intracarotid injection of graded amounts of synthetic LH-RF into castrated female rats pretreated with estradiol benzoate (50 µg/rat/day/2 days). In this experiment the rats were killed for blood collection 15 min following the intracarotid injection of the decapeptide. It appears that, under the conditions of this experiment, synthetic LH-RF liberates very significant amounts of LH and operates in a dose-related fashion. On the other hand, the effect of LH-RF on FSH is of lower magnitude and does not show any dose-response relationship. In this and in the subsequent experiments LH and FSH have been evaluated using specific radioimmunological procedures (Daane and Parlow, 1971; Niswender et al., 1968).

At this point, it was felt appropriate to evaluate the relationship of the release of LH and FSH after the intracarotid injection of a standard dose of synthetic

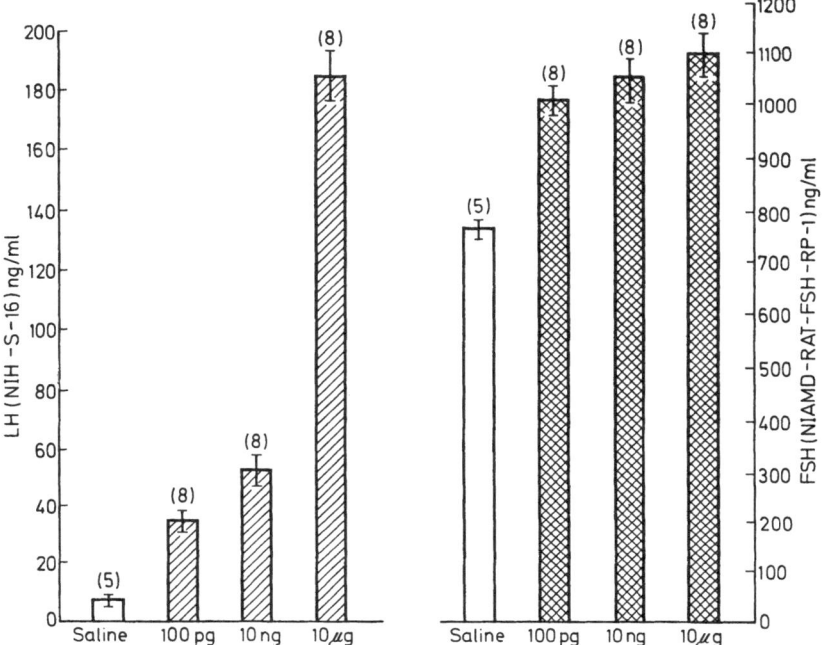

Fig. 6. Effect of intracarotid injection of graded doses of synthetic LH-RF on serum levels of LH and FSH of adult female rats castrated for three weeks and pretreated with estradiol benzoate (50 μg/rat/day/2 days)

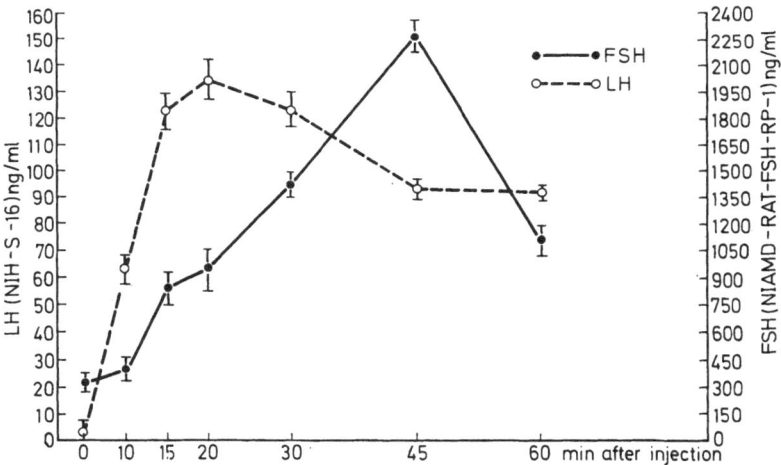

Fig. 7. Effect of intracarotid injection of synthetic LH-RF on serum levels of LH and FSH of adult female rats castrated for three weeks and pretreated with estradiol benzoate (50 μg/rat/day/2 days)

LH-RF (10 μg/rat). Figure 7 indicates that in castrated estrogen-pretreated female rats, the release of LH and that of FSH follow a completely different pattern. The maximal secretion of LH is obtained 15—20 min following intracarotid injection of synthetic LH-RF, while that of FSH occurs only 45 min following injection.

In another set of experiments, synthetic LH-RF was injected in increasing doses into adult castrated male rats pretreated either with estradiol benzoate (50 μg/day/2 days) or with testosterone propionate (2 mg/rat/day/6 days). The data

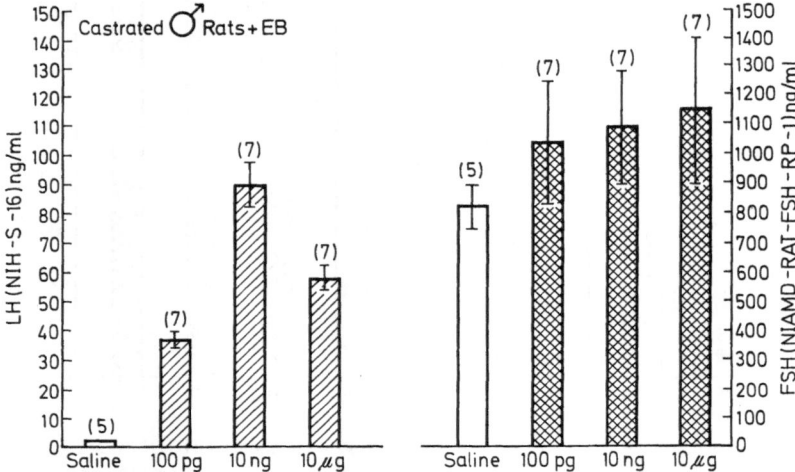

Fig. 8. Effect of intracarotid injection of graded doses of synthetic LH-RF on serum levels of LH and FSH of adult male rats castrated for three weeks and pretreated with estradiol benzoate (EB, 50 μg/rat/day/2 days)

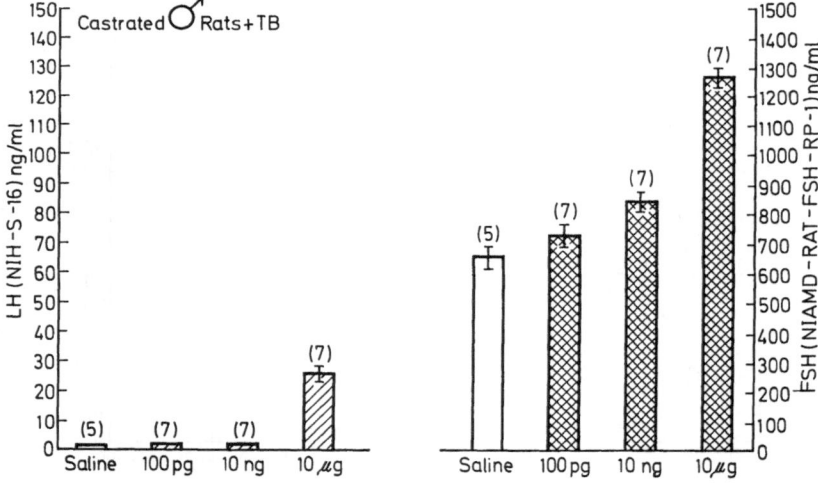

Fig. 9. Effect of intracarotid injection of graded doses of synthetic LH-RF on serum levels of LH and FSH of adult male rats castrated for three weeks and pretreated with testosterone propionate (TP, 2 mg/rat/day/6 days)

shown in Fig. 8 clearly indicate that the administration of synthetic LH-RF to castrated male rats pretreated with estrogens results in the liberation of high amounts of LH, but does not influence FSH release. This result is exactly similar to that previously obtained in castrated females pretreated with estradiol (Fig. 6). Figure 9 shows that pretreatment with testosterone markedly reduces the ability of the anterior pituitary to release LH under the influence of exogenous LH-RF. On the contrary, the release of FSH seems to be augmented.

The fact that the synthetic decapeptide has a clear-cut effect on the release of LH but only a minor one on that of FSH when tested at an interval of 15 min in castrated estrogen-treated rats might suggest that this peptide is specifically related to the release of LH. There is no doubt however that the synthetic decapeptide does release FSH in the same animal preparation when tested at a different interval. This result might be interpreted in several ways. The first possibility is obviously that suggested by Matsuo et al. (1971) and by Schally et al. (1971 b) that LH-RF and FSH-RF are just one and the same substance. A second possibility is that synthetic LH-RF might have some intrinsic FSH-RF activity without being the real FSH-RF. Examples of overlapping of activities in peptide hormones are very numerous. One may recall for instance that vasopressin has intrinsic oxytocic activities (Martini, 1966). A third possibility is that the release of FSH following the administration of synthetic LH-RF might be due entirely to indirect mechanisms (e.g. via the stimulation of estrogen secretion induced by the peptide). Such a possibility cannot be disregarded at the moment, mainly because of the large lag between the release of LH and that of FSH reported in this paper.

The data obtained in castrated male rats pretreated with estrogen or testosterone are the only ones which, in the author's opinion, would support the hypothesis that there is only one gonadotropin releasing factor and that its activity on the pituitary gland is directed or modulated by the levels of circulating sex steroids. In the present experiment it has indeed been possible to augment the release of LH by the administration of estrogens and that of FSH by the administration of testosterone. However, one must keep in mind that these observations have been made using supraphysiological levels of sex steroids. It is urgently needed to establish whether this phenomenon also occurs with physiological amounts of estrogens and androgens.

Acknowledgement. The work described in this paper has been supported by a Grant of the Ford Foundation, New York. Synthetic LH-RF has been kindly supplied by Hoffmann-La Roche, Basel.

References

Bower, S.A., Hadley, M.E., Hruby, V.J.: Comparative MSH release-inhibiting activities of tocinoic acid and L-Pro-L-Leu-Gly-NH$_2$. Biochem. Biophys. Res. Commun. **45**, 1185—1191 (1971).
Brazeau, P., Vale, W., Burgus, R., Ling, N., Butcher, M., Rivier, J., Guillemin, R.: Hypothalamic polypeptide that inhibits the secretion of immunoreactive pituitary growth hormone. Science **179**, 77—79 (1973).

Burgus, R., Dunn, T. F., Desiderio, D., Guillemin, R.: Structure moléculaire du facteur hypothalamique hypophysiotrope TRF d'origine ovine: évidence par spectométrie du masse de
la séquence PCA-His-Pro-NH₂. C. R. Acad. Sci. (Paris) **269**, 1870—1893 (1969).

Celis, M. E., Taleisnik, S., Walter, R.: Regulation of formation and proposed structure of the
factor inhibiting the release of melanocyte-stimulating hormone. Proc. nat. Acad. Sci. **68**,
1428—1433 (1971a).

Celis, M. E., Taleisnik, S., Walter, R.: Release of pituitary melanocyte-stimulating hormone by
the oxytocin fragment, H-Cys-Tyr-Ile-Gln-Asn-OH. Biochem. Biophys. Res. Commun. **45**,
564—569 (1971b).

Daane, T. A., Parlow, A. F.: Periovulatory patterns of rat serum follicle stimulating hormone
and luteinizing hormone during the normal estrous cycle: effect of pentobarbital. Endocrinology **88**, 653—663 (1971).

Faiman, C., Ryan, R. J.: Serum follicle-stimulating hormone and luteinizing hormone concentrations during the menstrual cycle as determined by radioimmunoassay. J. clin. Endocr.
27, 1711—1716 (1967).

Fuxe, K., Hökfelt, T.: Catecholamines in the hypothalamus and the pituitary gland. In:
Frontiers in Neuroendocrinology (W. F. Ganong, L. Martini, Eds.), p. 47—96. New York:
Oxford University Press 1969.

Ganong, W. F., Lorenzen, L.: Brain neurohumors and endocrine function. In: Neuroendocrinology (W. F. Ganong, L. Martini, Eds.), Vol. II, p. 583—640. New York: Academic
Press 1967.

Halász, B.: The endocrine effect of isolation of the hypothalamus from the rest of the brain.
In: Frontiers in Neuroendocrinology (W. F. Ganong, L. Martini, Eds.), p. 307—342.
New York: Oxford University Press 1969.

Harris, G. W.: Neural control of the pituitary gland. London: Edward Arnold 1955.

Kamberi, I. A., Schneider, H. P. G., McCann, S. M.: Action of dopamine to induce release of FSH-
releasing factor (FRF) from hypothalamic tissue in vitro. Endocrinology **86**, 278—284
(1970).

Kobayashi, H., Matsui, T.: Fine structure of the median eminence and its functional significance. In: Frontiers in Neuroendocrinology (W. F. Ganong, L. Martini, Eds.), p. 3—46.
New York: Oxford University Press 1969.

Martini, L.: Neurohypophysis and anterior pituitary activity. In: The Pituitary Gland (G. W.
Harris, B. T. Donovan, Eds.), Vol. III. London: Butterworths 1966.

Martini, L., Fraschini, F., Motta, M.: Neural control of anterior pituitary functions. Recent
Progr. Hormone Res. **24**, 439—496 (1968).

Matsuo, H., Baba, Y., Nair, R. M. G., Arimura, A., Schally, A. V.: Structure of the porcine LH-
and FSH-releasing hormone. I. Proposed amino acid sequence. Biochem. Biophys. Res.
Commun. **43**, 1334—1339 (1971).

Mess, B., Fraschini, F., Motta, M., Martini, L.: The topography of the neurons synthesizing the
hypothalamic releasing factors. In: Hormonal Steroids (L. Martini, F. Fraschini, M. Motta,
Eds.), p. 1004—1013. Amsterdam: Excerpta Medica 1967.

Mess, B., Martini, L.: The central nervous system and the secretion of anterior pituitary trophic
hormones. In: Recent Advances in Endocrinology (V. H. T. James, Ed.), p. 1—49. London:
Churchill 1968.

Motta, M., Martini, L.: Hypothalamic releasing factors: a new class of "neurotransmitters".
Arch. int. Pharmacodyn. **196**, (Suppl.), 191—204 (1972).

Motta, M., Piva, F., Fraschini, F., Martini, L.: "Pituitary depletion methods" for the bioassay
of hypothalamic releasing factors. In: Hypophysiotropic hormones of the hypothalamus:
assay and chemistry (J. Meites, Ed.), p. 44—57. Baltimore: Williams and Wilkins 1970a.

Motta, M., Piva, F., Tima, L., Zanisi, M., Martini, L.: Feedback mechanisms and the control of
the secretion of the hypothalamic releasing factors. Mem. Soc. Endocr. **18**, 407—422 (1970b).

Motta, M., Piva, F., Tima, L., Zanisi, M., Martini, L.: Intrahypothalamic localization of the
nuclei synthesizing the gonadotropin releasing factors. J. Neuro-Visc. Relat. **10** (Suppl.),
32—40 (1971).

Nair, R. M. G., Kastin, A. J., Schally, A. V.: Isolation and structure of another hypothalamic
peptide possessing MSH-release-inhibiting activity. Biochem. Biophys. Res. Commun. **47**,
1420—1425 (1972).

Niswender, G. D., Midgley, A. R., Jr., Monroe, S. E., Reichert, L. E., Jr.: Radioimmunoassay for rat luteinizing hormone with antiovine LH serum and ovine LH-[131] I. Proc. Soc. exp. Biol. (N.Y.) **128**, 807—811 (1968).

Piva, F., Sterescu, N., Zanisi, M., Martini, L.: Non steroidal antifertility agents affecting brain mechanisms. Bull. Wld Hlth Org. **41**, 275—288 (1969).

Porter, J. C., Kamberi, I. A., Grazia, Y. R.: Pituitary blood flow and portal vessels. In: Frontiers in Neuroendocrinology (L. Martini, W. F. Ganong, Eds.), p. 145—175. New York: Oxford University Press 1971.

Schally, A. V., Arimura, A., Baba, Y., Nair, R. M. G., Matsuo, H., Redding, T. W., Debeljuk, L., White, W. F.: Isolation and properties of the FSH and LH releasing hormone. Biochem. Biophys. Res. Commun. **43**, 393—399 (1971 b).

Schally, A. V., Baba, Y., Nair, R. M. G., Bennett, C. D.: The amino acid sequence of a peptide with growth hormone-releasing activity isolated from porcine hypothalamus. J. biol. Chem. **246**, 6647—6650 (1971 a).

Simonovic, I., Motta, M., Martini, L.: Acetylcholine (ACh) and the release of follicle stimulating hormone-releasing factor (FSH-RF). Program 53rd Meeting Endocrine Soc., p. 255 (1971).

Steelman, S. L., Pohley, F. M.: Assay of the follicle stimulating hormone based on the augmentation with human chorionic gonadotropin. Endocrinology **53**, 604—616 (1953).

Swerdloff, R. S., Walsh, P. C., Jacobs, H. S., Odell, W. D.: Serum LH and FSH during sexual maturation in the male rat: effect of castration and cryptorchidism. Endocrinology **88**, 120—128 (1971).

Szentágothai, J., Flerkó, B., Mess, B., Halász, B.: Hypothalamic control of the anterior pituitary. Budapest: Akademiai Kiado 1968.

Tima, L., Motta, M., Martini, L.: Effect of "hypothalamic deafferentation" on hypothalamic follicle stimulating hormone releasing factor (FSH-RF) and on pituitary FSH. Program 51st Meeting Endocrine Soc., p. 194 (1969).

Vale, W., Grant, G., Guillemin, R.: Chemistry of the hypothalamic releasing factors—Studies on structure-function relationships. In: Frontiers in Neuroendocrinology (W. F. Ganong, L. Martini, Eds.), p. 375—413. New York: Oxford University Press 1973.

Study of the Preoptico-Infundibular
LH-RH Neurosecretory Pathway in Female Guinea-Pigs
during Gestation and the Oestrous Cycle

J. Barry and M. P. Dubois

Laboratory of Histology of the Faculty of Medicine and E. R. A. No. 175 of the CNRS, Lille (France)
Laboratory of the Physiology of Reproduction INRA-CNRZ, Nouzilly (France)

Introduction

Using antisera to synthetic LH-RH (luteinizing hormone-releasing hormone) in castrated adult male guinea-pigs, the perikarya of specifically immunoreactive neurones were demonstrated (Barry et al., 1973).

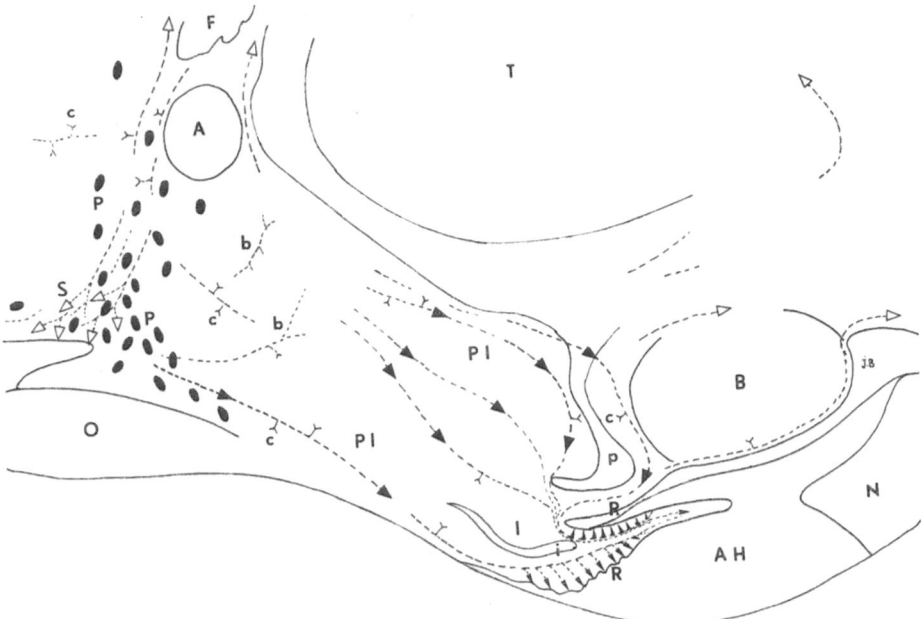

Fig. 1. General pattern of LH-RH producing cells of guinea-pig's hypothalamus. *A* anterior commissure, *AH* adenohypophysis, *B* mamillary body, *F* fornix, *I* infundibular nucleus, *O* optic chiasm, *P* perikarya of LH-RH producing cells; *PI* preoptico-infundibular pathway (black arrows) with pericapillary endings (R), *N* neural lobe, *S* supraoptic crest, *T* thalamus, white arrows: extrahypophysial LH-RH pathways, *i* infundibular recess, *p* premamillary recess. Note the branching (b) and short collaterals (c) of LH-RH axons

These perikarya are distributed throughout a very large region of the hypothalamus, mainly from the septo-preoptic region to the anterior hypothalamic and suprachiasmatic nuclei (Fig. 1).

Similar results were obtained by the use of antisera in castrated adult male guinea-pigs following intraventricular injection of methanol (50 μl of a solution methanol + distilled water, in equal parts) or of melatonin (200 μg dissolved in 50μl of the previous solution), (Barry et al., unpublished results, Figs. 5—7).

Subsequently, immunoreactive perikarya, of the same topography but much less numerous, were observed in various physiological conditions, i.e. male and female foetuses at the end of gestation; normal males; pregnant females (Figs. 2—4). Most of the axons of these cells form a "preoptico-infundibular LH-RH neurosecretory pathway" (Barry and Dubois, 1973) ending at different levels of the median eminence, by means of numerous radiating collaterals. These collaterals recall the pictures recently described with the Golgi triple impregnation technique in the same area (Barry, 1972). The region which contains the greater part of these pericapillary nerve endings is adjacent to the two adenohypophysial regions that are the richest in gonadotrophic cells detectable by immunofluorescence. Stereotaxic experiments suggest the existence of proximodistal axoplasmic transport of specifically immunoreactive material along the "preoptico-infundibular" pathway (Barry et al., 1973).

The present studies are intended to extend the above observations by an examination of the distal part of the LH-RH pathway with particular attention to the possibility of detectable variations in relation to the sexual cycle and pregnancy.

Material and Techniques

Our observations were made on 43 female guinea-pigs (26 cyclic females and 17 females, aged 5—7 months, during gestation or in the first post partum cycle).

The animals were killed by decapitation; the brains and genital tracts were removed and fixed for 48 h in Bouin-Hollande fixative without acetic acid; dehydrated; embedded in paraffin; cut in serial sections of 10 microns and mounted on slides in 0.75% gelatinized water. The brain sections were treated by the indirect fluorescent antibody technique, using a 1/40 dilution of the specific antiserum (prepared by M. P. Dubois in the rabbit) and sheep gamma globulin anti-rabbit immunoglobulin serum, conjugated with fluoresceine isothiocyanate (Pasteur Institute, Paris). All the solutions and washings were carried out with isotonic veronal buffer, pH 8.6. The reactions were studied with the Universal Zeiss fluorescence microscope, fitted for reflection (mercury vapour lamp HBO 200 W, type L_2 or L_1; excitation filter BG 12, 4 mm; barrier filter No. 530). The photomicrographs were made on Rayoscope Kodak RY 135—50 films, and printed on Brovira BN 1 No. 4 paper, with Dektol developer. Exposure time, lighting, enlargement and printing time of films and papers were kept constant.

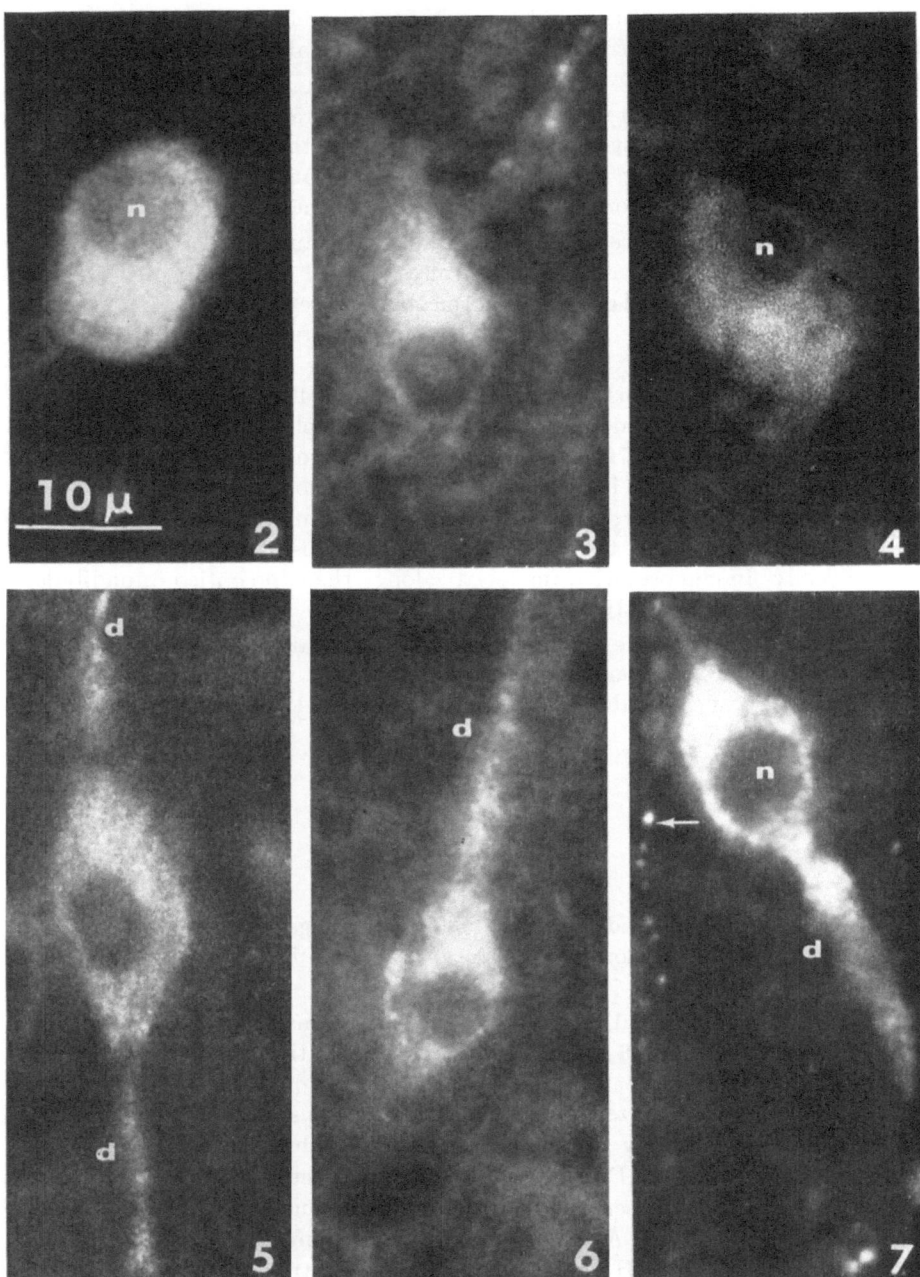

Figs. 2, 3 and 4. "Physiologically" immunoreactive perikarya. Pregnant females

Figs. 5, 6 and 7. Immunoreactive perikarya in experimental conditions (castrated male guinea-pigs, intraventricular injection of melatonin dissolved in methanol 50%). Note the immunoreactivity of the dendrites (d), n: nucleus. The arrow points to a beaded axon, coming from another perikaryon

Results

During gestation distinct variations were observed in the quantity of specifically immunoreactive infundibular material, particularly in the ventral labium of the median eminence. However these variations are generally not so conspicuous as those observed during the oestrous cycle. Toward the end of gestation there is a gradual increase in the quantity of this material (Fig. 8).

After birth of the young, and before the next ovulation, considerable depletion of the fluorescent material can be seen.

During the first post partum cycle and in normal cyclic females, significant modifications can be observed in the quantity of specifically immunoreactive material, along the distal part of the "preoptico-infundibular LH-RH neurosecretory pathway". A sudden fall to minimum concentration occurs during pro-oestrus-preovulatory oestrus (Fig. 9), followed by a progressive increase during post-ovulatory oestrus and post oestrus (Fig. 10). A maximum concentration occurs toward the end of dioestrus (Fig. 11) with some individual variations.

Discussion

The antisera used are highly specific. No significant competition between LH-RH and either hypothalamic peptides (oxytocin, vasopressin, thyroid stimulating hormone- releasing hormone) or a brain lipid-free protein extract could be demonstrated, using the indirect fluorescent antibody tests on slides, a radio-immunoassay or indirect passive hemolysis (see Barry et al., 1974, for details on the preparation of antisera, the immunization techniques, the serological study of the antisera and the criteria of specificity). The reacting neurons contain therefore a substance antigenically related to LH-RH. Topographically they coincide with the "hypophysiotropic" (Halasz et al., 1962) and "septo-arcuate" (Barraclough, 1966) areas. Moreover, the rostral position of their perikarya agrees perfectly with the localization of LH-RH in the hypothalamus, according to Crighton et al. (1970).

Finally, the specifically immunoreactive material shows characteristic modifications under various physiological conditions (neonatal period, prepuberty, oestrous cycle, gestation) and experimental conditions (castration, hypophysectomy, hormones or drug injections) linked with specific variations of the gonadotropic secretion of the pituitary pars anterior.

Therefore we consider that the neurons in question are the hypothalamic neurosecretory cells producing LH-RH.

In conclusion we would point out that certain axons (or collaterals of axons) of LH-RH producing cells form "extrahypophysial neurosecretory pathways" with preoptic, telencephalic, epithalamic or mesencephalic terminations. The existence of these pathways seems to us likely to provide a direct interpretation of certain recent experiments. Particularly, the presence of specifically immuno-reactive axon terminations in the area of the supraoptic crest and the vascular organ of the terminal lamina (Barry and Dubois, 1973) might be connected with the intervention of the median preoptic area in copulatory behavior (Hart et al.,

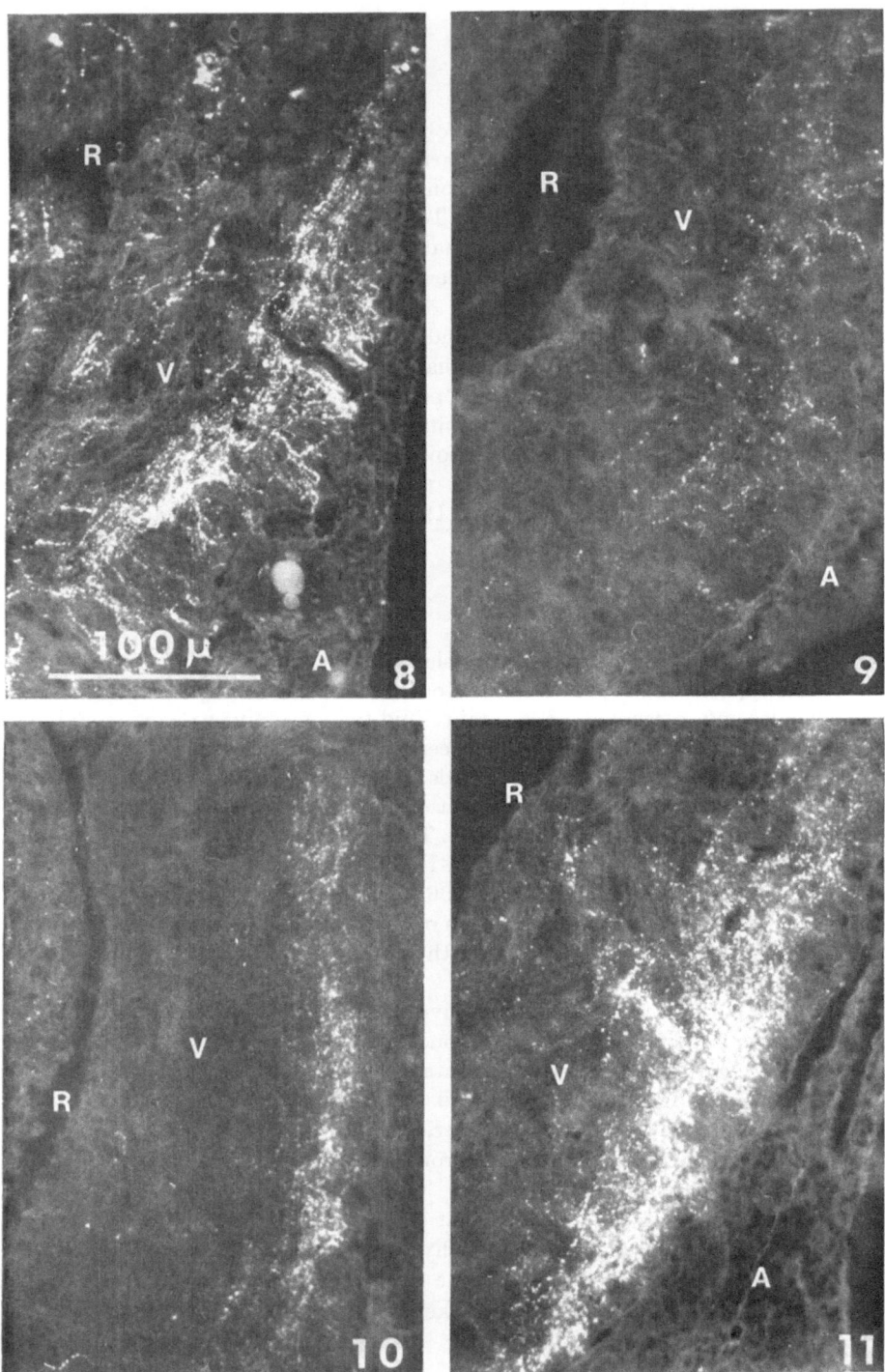

Figs. 8, 9, 10 and 11. Sagittal sections of the ventral labium (v) of the infundibular region. *R* infundibular recess, *A* adenohypophysis. Fig. 8. Female guinea-pig at the end of gestation. Fig. 9. Preovulatory oestrus. Fig. 10. Postovulatory oestrus. Fig. 11. Second half of dioestrus

1973), the inductive role of LH-RH in this behavior (Moss and McCann, 1973) or with eventual action of this hormone by the intermediary of the cerebrospinal fluid, as LH-RH is seen to be active in intraventricular administration (Weiner et al., 1973).

This work was financed by the DGRST (France) Contract n° 72-7-0375 (Pr Barry).

References

Barraclough, C. A.: Modification of the CNS regulation of reproduction after exposure of prepubertal rats to steroid hormones. Recent Progr. Hormone Res. 22, 503—536 (1966).

Barry, J.: Etude en technique de Golgi du mode de division et des terminaison des fibres du tractus hypothalamo-infundibulaire des Mammifères. C. R. Soc. Biol. (Paris) 166, 1313—1315 (1972).

Barry, J., Dubois, M. P.: Etude en immunofluorescence de la différenciation prénatale des cellules hypothalamiques élaboratrices de LH-RH et de la maturation de la voie neurosécrétrice préoptico-infundibulaire chez le cobaye. Brain Res. 67, 103—113 (1974).

Barry, J., Dubois, M. P., Poulain, P.: LRF producing cells of the mammalian hypothalamus. Z. Zellforsch. 146, 351—366 (1973).

Crighton, D. B., Schneider, H. P. G., McCann, S. M.: Localization of LH-releasing factor in the hypothalamus and neurohypophysis as determined by an in vitro method. Endocrinology 87, 323—329 (1970).

Halasz, B., Pupp, L., Uhlarik, S.: Hypophysiotrophic area in the hypothalamus. J. Endocr. 25, 147—154 (1973).

Hart, B. L., Haugen, C. M., Peterson, D. M.: Effects of medial preoptic anterior hypothalamic lesions on mating behavior of male rat. Brain Res. 54, 177—191 (1973).

Moss, R. L., McCann, S. M.: Induction of mating behavior in rats by luteinizing hormone releasing factor. Science 181, 177—179 (1973).

Weiner, R. I., Terkel, J., Blake, C. A., Schally, A. V., Sawyer, C. H.: Changes in serum luteinizing hormone following intraventricular and intravenous injections of luteinizing hormone-releasing hormone in the rat. Neuroendocrinology 10, 261—272 (1972).

A Concept of Neuroendocrine Cell Complexes

A. OKSCHE, H. J. OEHMKE, and H. G. HARTWIG

Department of Anatomy and Cytobiology, Justus Liebig University, Giessen (Federal Republic of Germany), and Department of Zoology, University of Washington, Seattle (USA)

Experimental endocrinologists criticise the concept of a mosaic-like representation of hypothalamic functions (see Szentágothai et al., 1968). In contrast to a rigid cytoarchitectonic scheme Szentágothai et al. (1968) distinguish between a "hypophysiotropic, releasing factors system" and a "release regulating system". Substances responsible for basic gonadotropin release are available in all parts of the hypophysiotropic area including the arcuate nucleus. Under these circumstances the classical cytoarchitectonic divisions of the hypothalamus appear to be only of limited value. However, a more general type of hypothalamic action does not exclude a clear-cut wiring diagram between single anatomical units. According to Cross (1973): "It may be that many hypothalamic interneurons are programmed in highly specific ways . . .". "Each cell may indeed be unique in its connectivities and sensitivities".

There is a considerable body of evidence that tuberal monoamines (dopamine) and releasing factors (e.g., LH-RF, FSH-RF) are not stored in the same neuron (Fig. 1). Hökfelt and Fuxe (1972) suggest that the dopamine neurons of the tuber influence the LH-RF systems at the level of the median eminence through axo-axonal mechanisms. Synaptoid axo-axonal contacts between aminergic and other preterminals and endings of the median eminence have been described by Kobayashi et al. (1970). The nerve endings in the external (palisade) layer of the median eminence contain different types of granular or vesicular inclusions (Kobayashi et al., 1970; Dierickx et al., 1973).

We suggest (Fig. 1): (1) that the tuberal nuclei are formed by cell clusters consisting of neurons of differing characteristics, and (2) that within individual clusters, specialized secretory elements may form functional units (see Oksche et al., 1972; Oksche and Farner, 1974). This hypothesis is supported further by the fact that distinct systems of collaterals occur within the tuberal nuclei (Szentágothai et al., 1968; Millhouse, 1973) and may function in integration and modulation at the nuclear level.

We have investigated the interrelationships of anatomical units in the arcuate nucleus of the mouse and in the tuberal complex of passerine birds. Our studies have been focussed on gonadotropic functions (cf. Dierickx et al., 1972). Investigations of avian material have the following advantages: (1) The gonadal function in many avian species of higher latitudes is controlled by photoperiod which can be easily manipulated in experiments (see Farner, 1973; Follett, 1973).

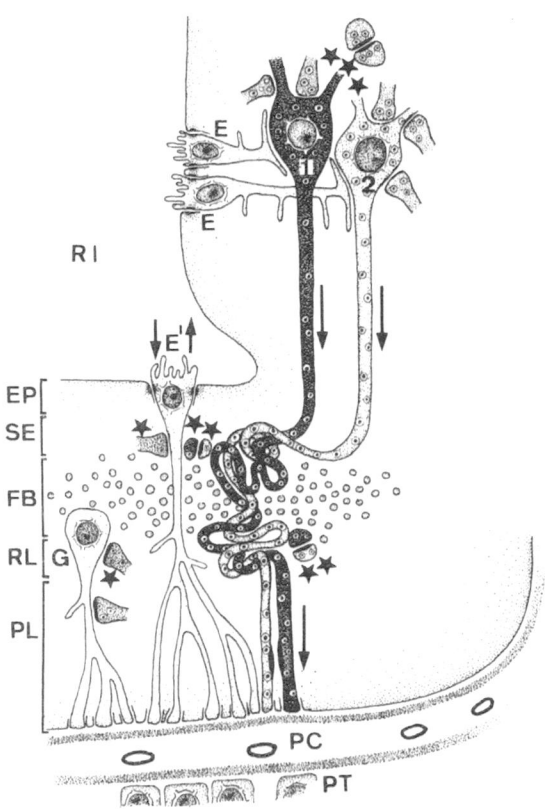

Fig. 1. Basic arrangement of neurons and ependymal cells in the region of the arcuate nucleus and in the median eminence. This diagram has been simplified, and some details are still hypothetical. The neurons of the arcuate nucleus have intimate contacts with two different populations of ependymal cells: (1) at the *central* level of the perikarya within the nuclear area, (2) at the *peripheral* level of the terminals within the median eminence. *1* aminergic and *2* peptidergic (releasing-factor producing) neurons of the arcuate nucleus. Axo-somatic and axo-dendritic synapses (***). Numerous presynaptic endings belong to ascending noradrenergic tracts. *E* ependymal tanycytes form a link between the CSF and the somata of tuberal neurons. *Arrows* indicate the direction of transport of secretory materials within the axons. A number of tuberal axons run directly into the subependymal (*SE*) and reticular (*RL*) layers of the median eminence. Some fibers traverse the fiber layer (*FB*, with the cross-sectioned supra-optico-hypophysial tract) where they may have increased contact area (exaggerated in the diagram). In the median eminence long and branched ependymal tanycytes (*E'*) extend from the ependymal layer (*EP*) covering the infundibular recess (*RI*) to the outer surface of the median eminence (*PL*, palisade layer) that is covered by the primary capillaries of the portal circulation. *PT*, pars tuberalis. *G*, glial cell with ependyma-like processes and end-feet. Synaptoid contacts (*) have been described between nerve endings of unknown origin (aminergic elements?) and ependymal or glial cells (see Kobayashi et al., 1970); further, axo-axonal contacts (**) occur in the median eminence. At the surface of the infundibular recess (*RI*) *arrows* indicate the possible direction of uptake or release of substances in the ependymal cells (*E'*)

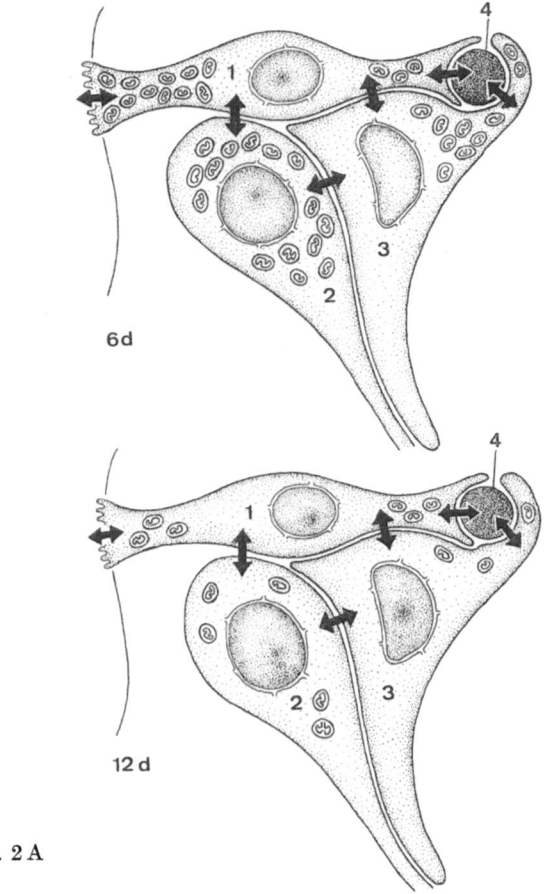

6d

12 d

Fig. 2 A

Fig. 2. (A) Diagram indicating functionally-linked subunits in the arcuate nucleus of female albino mouse. Data based on cytometric studies. *1* Ependymal cell (tanycyte), *2* neuron, *3* glial cell, *4* capillary. *Arrows* indicate probable sites of interaction. Six days (*6d*) after ovariectomy the size of arcuate neuron and adjacent ependymal nuclei is increased significantly if compared with control animals. Twelve days (*12d*) after ovariectomy these nuclei remain in an enlarged state. Between 6 and 12 days after ovariectomy there is—between other changes— a decrease of the volume density and the surface area of the mitochondria in the apical zone of the ependymal cells. At the same time there is a decrease in the volume density and the mitochondrial surface area in the arcuate neurons. It is accompanied by a decrease in volume density and surface area of mitochondria in the pericapillary terminations of glial cells. A cautious interpretation of these results (Zimmermann) speaks in favor of a functional inter- action between arcuate neurons, adjacent ependymal and glial cells, and capillaries of the arcuate nucleus. On the other hand, cytometric analyses indicate a considerable degree of functional dissociation between the tuberal (arcuate) and eminential ependyma. (B) Circumscribed groups of neurons with significantly different nuclear sizes in the arcuate nucleus of female albino mouse. The nuclear area (A_N) was estimated by the aid of a point- counting microscope (Wild). The arcuate nucleus was subdivided in arbitrary horizontal and vertical zones. Only two of the horizontal (A, D) and vertical (A, F) zones have been shown in the diagrams. Cross sections were examined along the rostro-caudal axis at distances of $30\,\mu m$, and all nerve-cell nuclei lying within a zone (dark bar) were measured. ● Nuclear area in control animals, ○ nuclear area 2 h after administering of estrogen. Note the increase in nuclear area (size) in the experimental animals. The smaller classes of neurons display a very distinct increase in their nuclear size. (Courtesy Mr. A. Schneider and Dr. P. Zimmermann, unpublished results)

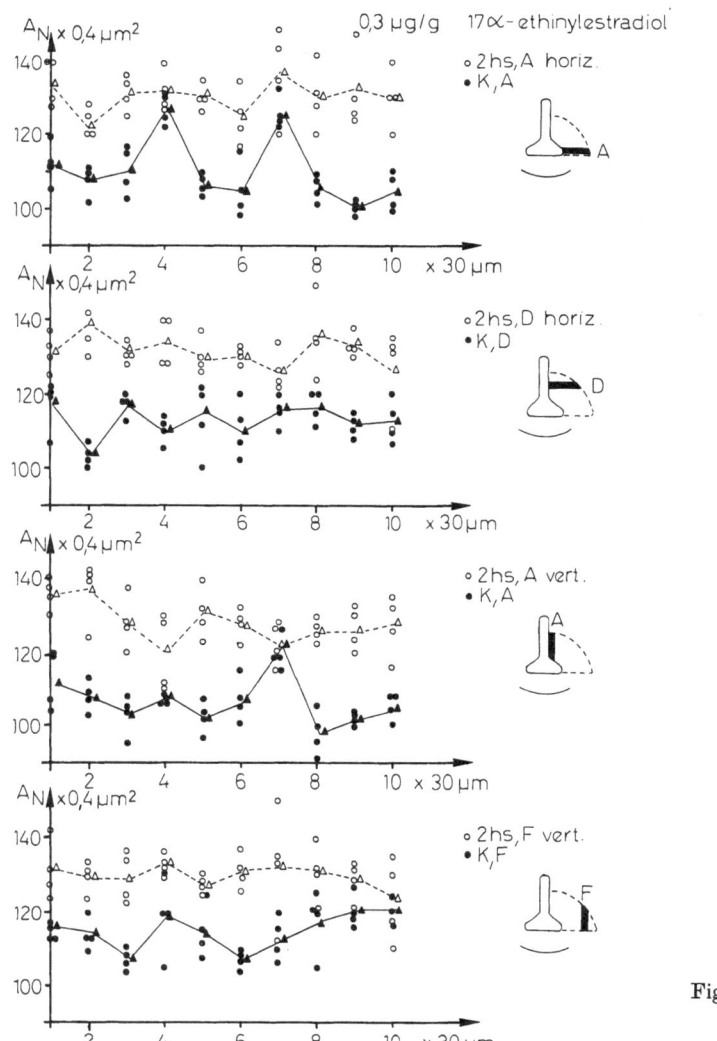

Fig. 2 B

(2) Testicular and ovarial functions of birds are completely under hypothalamic control, in contrast to thyroid and adrenal functions (see Nalbandov and Graber, 1969). (3) The gonadotropic release area of the avian hypothalamus is well outlined on the basis of stereotaxic lesions and implants (see Review by Oksche and Farner, 1974). Stereotaxic lesions placed within this area abolish the light-dependent testicular increase in weight.

It is an open question whether axons from the ventromedial nucleus of the mouse penetrate into the arcuate nucleus (Millhouse, 1973). In contrast to the ventromedial nucleus the Golgi picture of the arcuate neurons is still incomplete. Therefore, in order to study the subunits of the arcuate nucleus, a cytometric approach was chosen (see Oksche et al., 1972; in recent work the technique used previously has been improved). One of the parameters investigated was size of cell nuclei. The functional significance of the nuclear size as an indicator in functional activity of neuroendocrine cells has been reviewed critically by Szentágothai et al. (1968). We, too, are aware of the disadvantages of this method, and, therefore, our analysis has been augmented by quantitative methods at the electron-microscopic level. The latter include, e.g., estimations of the volume density and the surface area of the mitochondria. These studies can be extended to other cell organelles.

From a critical reconsideration of our pilot studies with female albino mice (see Oksche et al., 1972) the following conclusions can be drawn: (1) The arcuate nucleus consists of nerve-cell bodies that — during diestrus — fall into three different nuclear-size ranges. The neurons with the smallest nuclei are periventricular in position. They may represent the relatively small population of dopamine cells (see Hökfelt and Fuxe, 1972). (2) The nuclear size of the above mentioned three groups of neurons shows distinct changes during estrus and also 6 and 12 days after ovariectomy. (3) The arcuate neurons have intimate contacts with two different groups of ependymal cells at two different levels (Figs. 1, 2A): a) central (nuclear area), b) peripheral (median eminence). Six days after ovariectomy nuclear size increases not only in the arcuate neurons and in the adjacent ependymal cells, but also in the ependyma of the median eminence. Twelve days after ovariectomy only the ependyma of the arcuate nucleus region remains in an activated state.

Fig. 3A—D. Some hypothetical relationships of avian tuberal neurons (slightly modified after Oksche and Farner, 1974) which have to be proven definitely by anatomical and/or physiological methods. Several other arrangements of the neuroendocrine elements—including *collaterals* and *interneurons*—are open to discussion. Ependymal (*I*), subependymal (*II*), fiber (*III*), reticular (*IV*), and palisade (*V*) layers of the median eminence. Ependymal (*E*) and glial (*G*) cells. The neuroglial elements have been shown only in A. (A) Two neurons (*2*) producing the same type of releasing factor are innervated by an aminergic (possibly NA) fiber system *(asterisk)*. This system may ascend from lower portions of the brainstem. Aminergic projection into the subependymal *(arrow)* and reticular *(two arrows)* layers. o, synaptoid contacts of unknown origin with ependymal and glial cells. (B) Two neurons (*2, 3*) producing two different types of releasing factors are innervated by separate aminergic neurons *(asterisks)* of the NA type. *Arrow* and *two arrows*, see A. (C) Two neurons (*2,3*) producing different types of releasing factors are innervated not only by projecting aminergic fibers *(asterisks)* but also by a non-aminergic neuron (*4*) of a more dorsal region supposed to be a center of integration (homologue of the ventromedial nucleus?). The perikarya of these neurons are crowded with aminergic boutons *(asterisk)*. Hypothetical interneuron (*5*) with collaterals (*6*). *7*, subependymal secretory (non-aminergic) neuron (cf. Calas, 1973). (D) As fluorescent perikarya have not been demonstrated with certainty in the avian basal tuberal nucleus, there is a strong objection to a scheme showing aminergic (*1*) and releasing-factors (*2*) producing neurons in juxtaposition in one tuberal area. Principally the axons of these cells may be intertwined within the subependymal and/or reticular layers where collateral or *en passant* synapses are formed. Aminergic afferents are indicated by *asterisks*. Neurons in a more dorsal portion of the tuber (*4*) may play an integrating role. We have positive evidence that also this level of the avian tuber contains secretory perikarya. However, their connections with the median eminence and/or the basal tuberal neurons are an open question. Summarizing our hypotheses based on neuroanatomical evidence we suggest that an interaction of neuroendocrine elements of different types may occur not only within the median eminence (palisade layer) but highly probably also at the level of the nuclei of the tuberal complex

(4) At the electron-microscopic level cytometric estimations of mitochondria indicate a functional interaction between a) arcuate neurons, b) adjacent ependymal and glial cells, and c) capillaries of the arcuate nucleus (Fig. 2 A).

New karyometric investigations conducted with adult female albino mice during the first 24 h of the diestrus show that in a system of coordinates, along the rostro-caudal axis, the arcuate nucleus consists of circumscribed groups of neurons

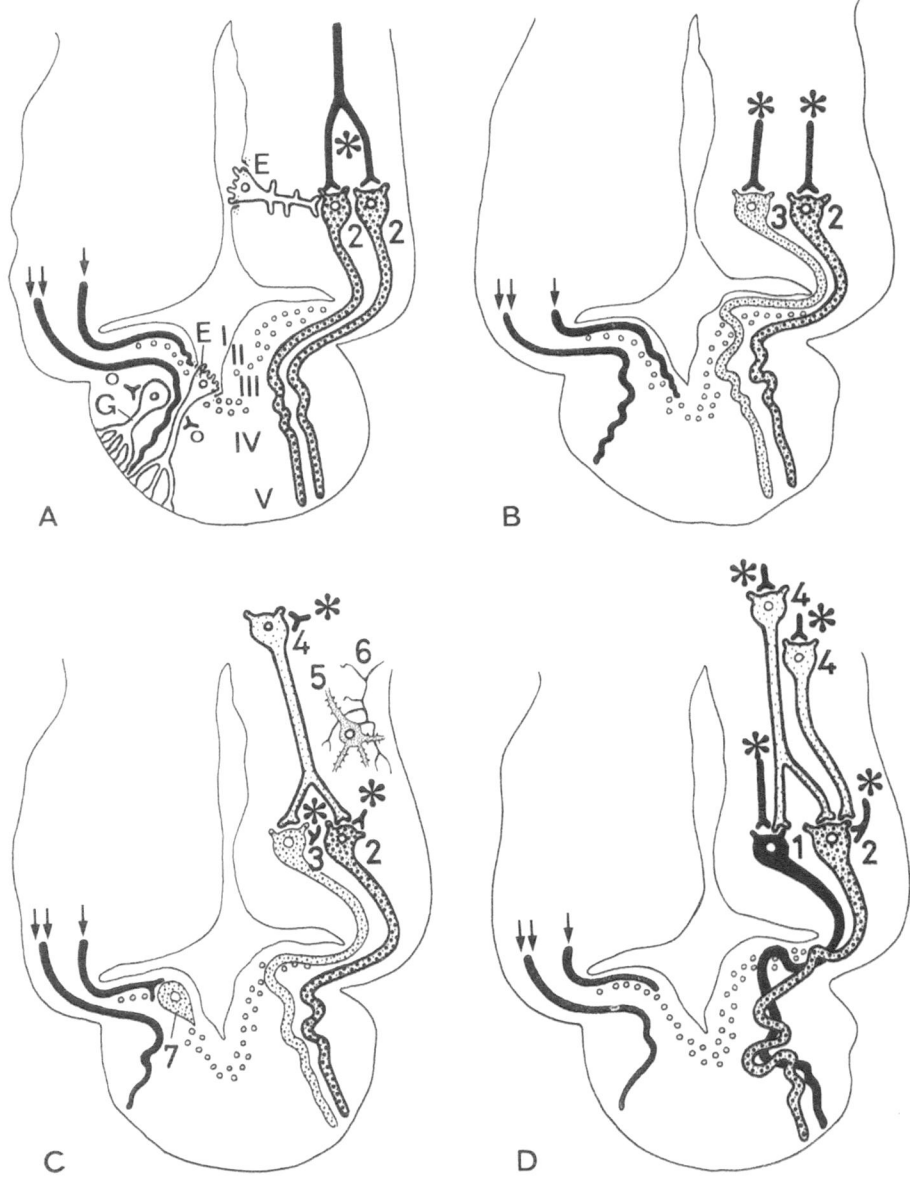

Fig. 3 A—D (Legend see p. 158)

with significantly different nuclear sizes (Fig. 2B). After administering 10 µg of
17 α-ethinyl estradiol only the smaller classes of periventricular arcuate neurons
respond with a distinct increase in their nuclear size (Schneider and Zimmermann,
unpublished). Also in female mice examined 6 and 12 days after ovariectomy by
quantitative ultrastructural analysis, only a number of arcuate neurons exhibit
a distinct response (Santolaya, unpublished results). It would be premature to
propose here a functional interpretation, but these data furnish new evidence that
the arcuate nucleus has anatomical subunits that display phasic changes in the
activity.

Cytometric procedures can also be adapted for studies of avian material. This
work is in progress, and definite data are not yet available. The avian hypothalamo-hypophysial system has attained morphological differentiation and
specialization as extensive as that of mammals (Fig. 3). In the tuberal complex of
passerine birds circumscribed clusters of neurons are even more distinct than the
arcuate nucleus of the mouse. There is a considerable body of neuroanatomical
evidence – at least in the White-crowned Sparrow, *Zonotrichia leucophrys gambelii*,
– that the serially arranged tubero-infundibular tracts establish point-to-point
relationships between circumscribed areas of the tuberal nuclei and the median
eminence (cf. Oksche and Farner, 1974).

There is, however, one point to be emphasized: Dopamine neurons have not
been demonstrated with certainty in the basal tuberal nucleus of birds. This
negative evidence is based on work with fluorescent microscopic, microspectro-
graphic and autoradiographic methods (Follett, 1973; Warren Soest et al., 1973;
Calas, 1973). The elementary granules of the range of 1000 Å which were observed
in the tuberal neurons of the House Sparrow (Oksche, 1967) probably characterize
some kind of releasing-factors-producing cells. The subependymal fiber systems in
the median eminence of the mallard (Calas et al., 1974)[1] and in the
House Sparrow (Hartwig and Oehmke, unpublished) contain noradrenaline and
apparently originate outside of the basal tuberal nucleus. Further, the tuberal
neurons are embedded in a rich terminal network formed by noradrenergic fibers.
According to Graber and Nalbandov (1972) in the domestic fowl increased hypothalamic noradrenaline concentrations occur concomitantly with increased gonadotropin activity. The anatomical situation observed in birds resembles that in frogs
in which monoamine fluorescence was completely absent in the isolated ventral
infundibular region (Dierickx et al., 1972). If technical errors can be completely
excluded, one must assume that the dopamine neurons of the mammalian arcuate
nucleus represent a specialization. This point should be considered in all working
hypotheses dealing with functional interrelationships between dopaminergic fibers
and the elements that produce releasing factors.

Even if aminergic neurons do not occur within the basal tuberal nuclei of birds
the problem of a central integration of neuroendocrine elements should be discussed. The perikarya of these neurons are embedded in a very dense neuropil rich
in axo-dendritic and axo-somatic synapses (Priedkalns and Oksche, 1969). A
number of these synapses are formed by ascending noradrenergic fibers. However,
other synapses resembling the inhibitory type have been observed in the same

---

[1] See also Calas (1974).

material. It should be kept in mind that in mammals inhibitory interneurons apparently occur in the ventromedial nucleus and in the lateral hypothalamic region (see Millhouse, 1973). In our opinion it is difficult to assume that the huge gonadotropic area of the avian hypothalamus with its serial arrangements of tubero-infundibular tracts is controlled and synchronized only by the manifold afferents. Golgi studies are in progress in our laboratory.

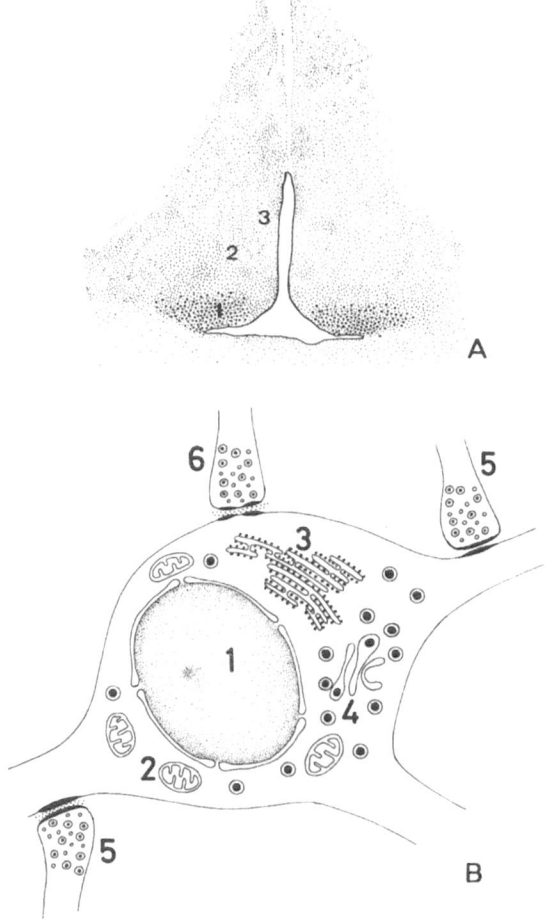

Fig. 4. (A) Transverse section through the preoptic area of a passerine bird (see Crosby and Showers, 1969; Oksche and Farner, 1974). *1 n. suprachiasmaticus, 2 n. praeopticus medialis* (continuous with the *area hypothalamica anterior*), *3 n. praeopticus periventricularis* (continuous with the *n. hypothalamicus periventricularis*). (B) Diagrammatic representation of secretory neurons observed in the *n. suprachiasmaticus, n. praeopticus medialis, n. periventricularis* and *area hypothalamica anterior* of *Passer domesticus*. The elementary granules (dense-core vesicles) of these neurons belong either to the 1300—1500 Å range or to the 1000 Å class. In addition to these types of nerve cells (which in many cases are found in juxtaposition within one cluster) other neurons show dense-core vesicles approximately 1800—2000 Å in diameter. *1* nucleus, *2* mitochondria, *3* granular endoplasmic reticulum (Nissl substance), *4* Golgi zone. *5* axo-dendritic, and *6* axo-somatic synapses containing clear and dense-core vesicles 500—800 Å in diameter

Recently, our studies on neuroendocrine cell complexes have been extended to the suprachiasmatic and preoptic regions of the avian hypothalamus (Fig. 4 A). In mammals (e.g. rat) the suprachiasmatic and anterior hypothalamic regions belong to the "release regulating system" of the gonadotropic axis (Szentágothai et al., 1968). The anterior hypothalamus is concerned with the estrogen-feedback control system. In birds the suprachiasmatic and retrochiasmatic regions are still a *terra incognita*, although Wingstrand (1951) and Oksche and Farner (1974) have shown that a conspicuous anterior hypothalamic tract to the median eminence can be traced back to this point. Moreover, Ralph (1959) found that electrolytic lesions in the rostral hypothalamus interrupt the laying cycle of hens. These effective lesions involve the region dorsal to the optic chiasma and a part of the preoptic area. In the anterior hypothalamus of the House Sparrow, Crosby and Showers (1969) distinguish between a suprachiasmatic nucleus and an anterior hypo-thalamic region (continuous with the medial preoptic nucleus). In both nuclear regions numerous secretory neurons, which do not belong to the classical supraoptic and paraventricular systems, have been observed with the electron microscope (Fig. 4B; Oksche and Kirschstein, unpublished results).[2] Both nuclei contain perikarya with three different types of granules: (1) approximately 1000 Å in diameter, (2) 1300—1500 Å in diameter, (3) 1800—2000 Å in diameter. All three types of granules are elaborated within the Golgi zone of individual neurons that display the principal characteristics of secretory elements (see Scharrer, 1969). Some of the scattered periventricular neurons containing granules of the 1500 to 2000 Å-range may belong to the "Gomori-positive" fiber system of the avian anterior median eminence. Other neurons with the larger types of elementary granules, however, are located in areas that are devoid of "Gomori-positive" elements. The secretory neurons of the suprachiasmatic nucleus and the anterior hypothalamic area are embedded in a neuropil very rich in synapses. Numerous fluorescent presynaptic endings bear dense-core vesicles 500—800 Å in diameter. So far we do not know whether the secretory suprachiasmatic and/or anterior hypothalamic neurons project into the median eminence or into some caudal hypo-thalamic area. We feel that the outstanding secretory activity of the anterior hypothalamic nuclei deserves further investigation with special reference to the connections of the different cell types. If these perikarya contribute to the very conspicuous anterior hypothalamic tract to the median eminence, the classification of the types of granulated nerve endings (see Oksche et al., 1970, 1974) should be reviewed on the basis of the new findings. Finally immunofluorescent techniques will lead to a precise identification and mapping of neurons that elaborate releasing factors.

For comparative reasons the neuroendocrine system of the earthworm, *Lumbricus terrestris*, has been included in our investigation (see Zimmermann, 1971). On the first look the close arrangement of peptidergic ("Gomori-positive") and aminergic neurons in the supraesophageal ganglion may suggest some kind of anatomical coupling. According to Myhrberg (1967) serotonin- and noradrenaline-containing neurons are found in the supraesophageal ganglion.[3] Myhrberg could not observe synaptic contacts between aminergic fibers and nonfluorescent perikarya. This finding has been confirmed by Zimmermann (personal communication). On

---

[2] See also Oksche et al. (1974).
[3] See also Koritsánszky and Hartwig (1974).

the other hand, synaptic connections between receptor afferents and neurosecretory axons have been described in the pericapillary fiber layer of the circumpharyngeal ring of Lumbricidae (see Aros, 1974, this volume). The problem of axon collaterals and interneurons requires further investigations.

Acknowledgments. The investigations reported herein were supported by research grants from the Deutsche Forschungsgemeinschaft to the authors. The authors are greatly indebted to Professor D. S. Farner, Seattle, and Dr. P. Zimmermann, Giessen, for their help in preparing this manuscript. We are also grateful to Miss D. Vaihinger for the drawings, and to Mrs. H. Dühring and Miss I. Lyncker for secretarial aid. The generous supply of test compounds provided by Dr. K.-H. Kolb, Schering AG, Berlin, is gratefully acknowledged.

References

Aros,B.: Synapses in the neurosecretory system of the earthworm. VI. International Symposium on Neurosecretion, London 1973 (this volume, 1974).

Calas,A.: L'innervation monoaminergique de l'éminence médiane — Etude radioautographique et pharmacologique chez le Canard, *Anas platyrhynchos*. I. L'innervation catécholaminergique. Z. Zellforsch. **138**, 503—522 (1973).

Calas,A., Hartwig,H.-G., Collin,J.P.: Noradrenergic innervation of the median eminence. Microspectrofluorimetric and pharmacological study in the duck, *Anas platyrhynchos*. Z. Zellforsch. **147**, 491—504 (1974).

Crosby,E.C., Showers,M.J.: Comparative anatomy of the preoptic and hypothalamic areas. In: Haymaker,W., Anderson,E., Nauta,W.I.H. (Eds.): The hypothalamus, pp. 61—135. Springfield Ill.: Ch. C. Thomas 1969.

Cross,B.A.: Unit responses in the hypothalamus. In: Martini,L., Ganong,W.F. (Eds.): Frontiers in neuroendocrinology. New York: Oxford University Press 1973.

Dierickx,K., Druyts,A., Vandenberghe,M.P., Goossens,N.: Identification of adenohypophysiotropic neurohormone producing neurosecretory cells in *Rana temporaria*. I. Ultrastructural evidence for the presence of neurosecretory cells in the tuber cinereum. Z. Zellforsch. **134**, 459—504 (1972).

Dierickx,K., Vandenberghe,M.P., Goossens,N.: Identification of adenohypophysiotropic neurohormone producing neurosecretory cells in *Rana temporaria*. II. Identification, in the median eminence, of the terminal arborizations of axons of the tubero-hypophysial neurosecretory system. Z. Zellforsch. **142**, 479—513 (1973).

Farner,D.S. (Ed.): Breeding biology of birds. Washington: National Academy of Sciences 1973.

Follett,B.K.: The neuroendocrine regulation of gonadotropin secretion in avian reproduction. In: Farner,D.S. (Ed.): Breeding biology of birds, pp. 209—243. Washington: National Academy of Sciences 1973.

Graber,J.W., Nalbandov,A.V.: Relationship of hypothalamic catecholamines and gonadotrophin levels in the chicken. Neuroendocrinology **10**, 325—337 (1972).

Hartwig,H.-G., Oehmke,H.J.: Unpublished results.

Hökfelt,T., Fuxe,K.: On the morphology and the neuroendocrine role of the hypothalamic catecholamines. In: Knigge,K.M., Scott,D.E., Weindl,A. (Eds.): Brain-endocrine interaction. Median eminence: Structure and function, pp. 181—223. Basel: Karger 1972.

Kobayashi,H., Matsui,T., Ishii,S.: Functional electron microscopy of the hypothalamic median eminence. Int. Rev. Cytol. **29**, 281—381 (1970).

Millhouse,O.E.: The organization of the ventromedial hypothalamic nucleus. Brain Res. **55**, 71—87 (1973).

Myhrberg,H.E.: Monoaminergic mechanisms in the nervous system of *Lumbricus terrestris* (L.). Z. Zellforsch. **81**, 311—343 (1967).

Nalbandov,A.V., Graber,I.W.: Neural control of the anterior and the posterior pituitary gland in birds. In: Haymaker,W., Anderson,E., Nauta,W.I.H. (Eds.): The hypothalamus, pp. 311—325. Springfield/Ill.: Ch. C. Thomas 1969.

Oksche, A.: Unpublished results.

Oksche, A.: Eine licht- und elektronenmikroskopische Analyse des neuroendokrinen Zwischen-hirn-Vorderlappen-Komplexes der Vögel. In: Stutinsky, F. (Ed.): Neurosecretion, pp. 77—88. Berlin-Heidelberg-New York: Springer 1967.

Oksche, A., Farner, D. S.: Neurohistological studies of the hypothalamo-hypophysial system of *Zonotrichia leucophrys gambelii*. With special attention to its role in the control of reproduction. Erg. Anat. Entwickl.-Gesch. 48, Fasc. 4, pp. 1—136 (1974).

Oksche, A., Kirschstein, H.: Unpublished results.

Oksche, A., Oehmke, H.-J., Farner, D. S.: Weitere Befunde zur Struktur und Funktion des Zwischenhirn-Hypophysensystems der Vögel. In: Bargmann, W., Scharrer, B. (Eds.): Aspects of neuroendocrinology, pp. 262—273. Berlin-Heidelberg-New York: Springer 1970.

Oksche, A., Zimmermann, P., Oehmke, H.-J.: Morphometric studies of tubero-eminential systems controlling reproductive functions. In: Knigge, K. M., Scott, D. E., Weindl, A. (Eds.): Brain-endocrine interaction. Median eminence: Structure and function, pp. 142—153. Basel: Karger 1972.

Priedkalns, J., Oksche, A.: Ultrastructure of synaptic terminals in nucleus infundibularis and nucleus supraopticus of *Passer domesticus*. Z. Zellforsch. 98, 135—147 (1969).

Ralph, C. L.: Some effects of hypothalamic lesions on gonadotropic release in the hen. Anat. Rec. 134, 411—431 (1959).

Santolaya, R.: Unpublished results.

Scharrer, B.: Neurohumors and neurohormones. Definitions and terminology. J. Neuro.-Visc. Relat. (Suppl.) 9, 1—20 (1969).

Schneider, A., Zimmermann, P.: Unpublished results.

Szentágothai, J., Flerkó, B., Mess, B., Halász, B.: Hypothalamic control of the anterior pituitary. Budapest: Akadémiai Kiadó 1968.

Warren Soest, S., Farner, D. S., Oksche, A.: Fluorescence microscopy of neurons containing primary catecholamines in the ventral hypothalamus of the White-crowned Sparrow, *Zonotrichia leucophrys gambelii*. Z. Zellforsch. 141, 1—17 (1973).

Wingstrand, K. G.: The structure and development of the avian pituitary from a comparative and functional viewpoint. Lund: Gleerup 1951.

Zimmermann, P.: Personal communication.

Zimmermann, P.: Die zentralnervöse Kontrolle der Dehydration bei *Lumbricus terrestris* L. Z. Zellforsch. 112, 551—571 (1971).

Added in proof:

Calas, A.: L'innervation peptidergique et monoaminergique de l'éminence médiane. Etude cytophysiologique chez les Oiseaux. Thèse, pp. 1—140. Académie de Montpellier, Université des Sciences et Techniques du Languedoc, 1974.

Koritsánszky, S., Hartwig, H. G.: The regeneration of the monoaminergic system in the cerebral ganglion of the earthworm, *Allolobophora caliginosa*. A morphological and micro-spectrofluorimetrical analysis. Cell Tiss. Res. 151, 171—186 (1974).

Oksche, A., Kirschstein, H., Hartwig, H. G., Oehmke, H. J., Farner, D. S.: Secretory parvo-cellular neurons in the rostral hypothalamus and in the tuberal complex of *Passer domesticus*. Cell Tiss. Res. 149, 363—370 (1974).

Cellular Localization of Thyrotropic Releasing Factor (TRF) after Intraventricular Administration*

David E. Scott**, Willis K. Paull, Gerald P. Kozlowski, Gerda Krobisch Dudley, and Karl M. Knigge

Department of Anatomy, University of Rochester, School of Medicine, Rochester (USA)
University of Vermont, College of Medicine and the Colorado State University, Colorado (USA)

Introduction

The historic hypotheses postulated by Green and Harris (1947) over a quarter of a century ago have stood the test of time and have clearly established parvicellular neurosecretory neurons and the hypophyseal portal vasculature as the vital linkage in the transduction of bioelectric energy into blood-borne signals, the releasing factors. Recent evidence has suggested, in addition, the presence of parallel mechanisms which may serve as an alternative way in which biologically active molecules reach the portal bed. The purpose of this investigation was to test the distribution of radio-labelled releasing factors in the mammalian hypothalamus with autoradiography.

Material and Methods

Sprague Dawley rats were anesthesized with sodium pentobarbital (5 mg/kg) and placed in a stereotaxic apparatus. Tritium labelled thyrotropic releasing factor (TRF) 40 c/mmol was infused with a 28° cannula into the lateral ventricle following the techniques of Knigge et al. (1973). Rats were killed 5, 10, 15, and 30 min following infusion and prepared for light and electron microscopic autoradiography after the techniques of Scott et al. (1973).

Observations

The light microscopic autoradiograms of rats killed 10 and 15 min following intraventricular infusion of ^{3}H-TRF demonstrated heavy labelling of the palisade contact zone of the median eminence (Fig. 1). Tanycyte terminals as well as perivascular glia demonstrated distinct and selective sequestration of silver grains over their cytoplasm. In addition some neurons of the arcuate nucleus also exhibited selective uptake of ^{3}H-TRF (Figs. 2 and 3).

* Supported by U.S.P.H.S. Grants NS 08171 and AM 10002.
** U.S.P.H.S. Career Development Awardee RO4 GM 70001.

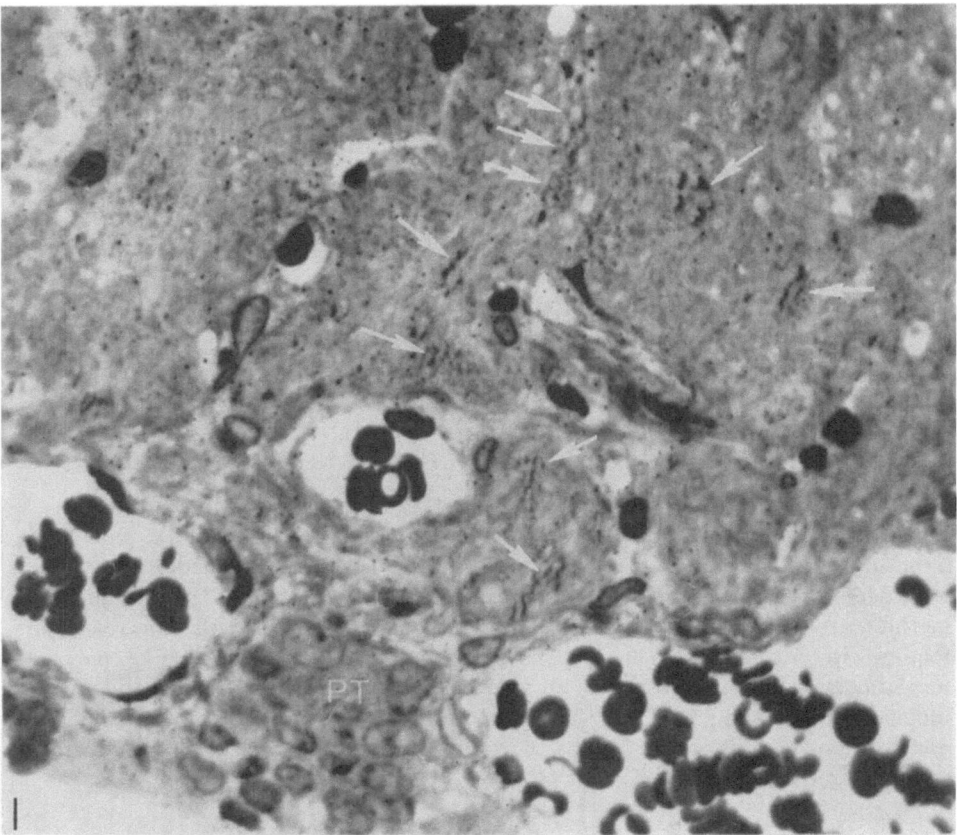

Fig. 1. Palisade contact zone of median eminence of rat killed 10 min following intraventricular infusion of ³H-TRF. Cell processes (arrows) are laden with silver grains near portal vessels PT, Pars Tuberalis × 640

Discussion

The original observations of Löfgren (1959–1961) drew attention to the tanycyte of the median eminence as a potential link for active communication between the cerebrospinal fluid (CSF) of the third ventricle and the pituitary portal vasculature. A wealth of morphologic data has described the ultrastructural complexity of this region of the brain (Mazzuca, 1966; Matsui, 1966; Monroe, 1967; Knowles and Kumar, 1969; Scott and Knigge, 1970; Raisman and Field, 1971). The tanycyte (Horstmann, 1954) draws the attention of morphologists because of its steric orientation and structural imposition between the CSF and the portal bed. This anatomical configuration has led a number of investigators to postulate that tanycytes possess a transport capacity for certain substances from the CSF to the portal bed and may serve as a parallel, alternative mechanism that influences

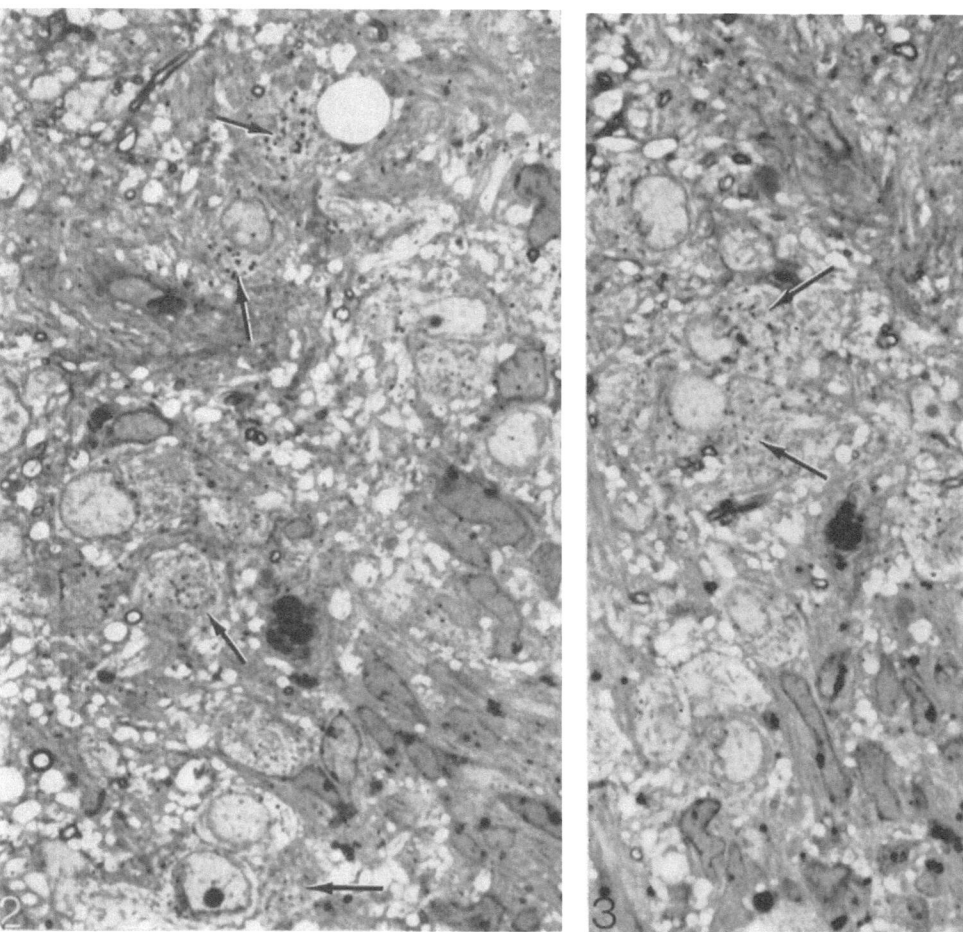

Fig. 2. Arcuate nucleus in proximity to the wall of the third ventricle. Certain arcuate neurons (arrows) are labelled selectively with ³H-TRF 10 min following intraventricular infusion. × 640

Fig. 3. Arcuate neurons (arrows) located deep within the nuclear group at its lateral edge. Despite the distance from the ventricular lumen selective uptake is observed in the form of silver grains over neuronal cytoplasm. × 640

adenohypophysial metabolism (Scott and Knigge, 1970; Kobayashi et al., 1972). Heavy concentrations of silver grains over the contact zone 10 min following intraventricular infusion of ³H-TRF supports the notion that specialized ependymal cells can rapidly transport substances from the CSF to the portal blood. Tight junctions between the apposed apical plasmalemmata of ependymal cells of this circumventricular organ (Brightman and Reese, 1969) would serve to prevent interstitial movement of the radiolabelled hormone. The time course and heavy

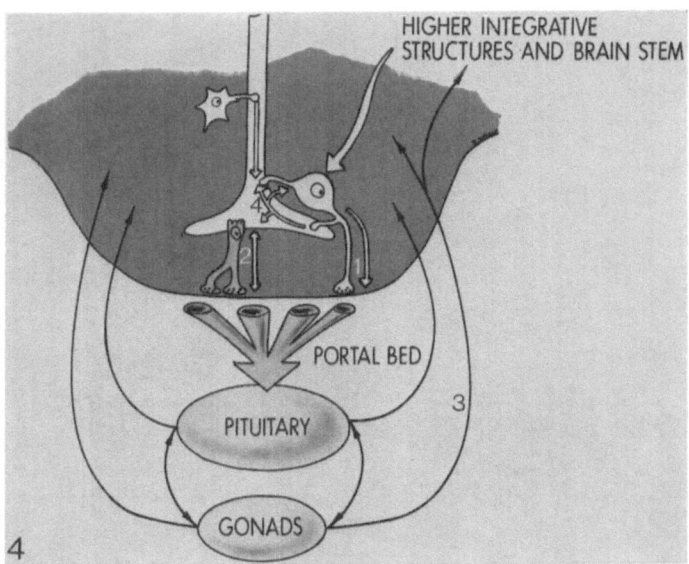

Fig. 4. Diagrammatic representation of potential modes of delivery of releasing factors to the portal bed. (*1*) represents traditional theories that involve direct tuberoinfundibular input to portal bed. (*2*) this scheme demonstrates the putative transependymal mechanisms discussed for ependyma with entry of hormone(s) into CSF via axon collaterals from arcuate neurons or other nuclei. (*3*) this represents classical concepts regarding long loop feed back from peripheral target organs to pituitary and/or brain. (*4*) this depicts the potential for ultrashort loop feed back upon arcuate neurons by releasing hormones which may gain entry into the cerebrospinal fluid

concentration of silver grains over the Palisade-contact zone argues against the systemic recirculation of ^{3}H-TRF as a mode of uptake by the median eminence.

The results of this study are in agreement with the immunohistochemical observations of Zimmerman et al. (1974) who have demonstrated localization of GNRF in tanycytes of the mouse median eminence. The time course for uptake of ^{3}H-TRF is consistent with that of another biologically active molecule. Weiner et al. (1972) and Ondo et al. (1973) have demonstrated rapid rises in plasma luteinizing hormone following intraventricular infusion of LRF.

Uptake of ^{3}H-TRF by arcuate neurons supports the hypothesis that certain subpopulations of this nuclear group may be sensitive to, and are responsible for the synthesis of this hormone. Thus uptake of ^{3}H-TRF, like that for ^{3}H-LRF in preliminary studies in this laboratory, may reflect the existence of an ultrashort loop feed back mechanism that controls secretion rates of releasing factors in the arcuate nucleus or other areas of the hypothalamus.

The uptake of ^{3}H-TRF by perivascular glial cells is an intriguing phenomenon which at this point defies plausible explanation. It can be postulated however that uptake by these cells may reflect a functional interdependence between perivascular glia and tanycytes of the median eminence.

References

Brightman, M. W., Reese, T. S.: Junctions between intimately apposed cell membranes in the vertebrate brain. J. Cell Biol. **40**, 648—677 (1969).

Green, J. D., Harris, G. W.: The neurovascular link between neurohypophysis and adenohypophysis. J. Endocr. **5**, 136—146 (1947).

Horstmann, E.: Die Faserglia des Selachiergehirns. Z. Zellforsch. **39**, 588—617 (1954).

Karnovsky, M. J.: A formaldehyde glutaraldehyde fixative of high osmolarity for use in electron microscopy. J. Cell Biol. **27**, 137A—138A (1965).

Knigge, K. M., Scott, D. E.: Structure and function of the median eminence. Amer. J. Anat. **129**, 223—243 (1970).

Knowles, F. G. W., Anand Kumar, T. C.: Structural changes related to reproduction. Part I. The hypothalamus. Part II. The pars tuberalis. Phil. Trans. B **256**, 357—375 (1969).

Kobayashi, H., Wada, M., Uemura, H.: Uptake of peroxidase from the third ventricle by ependymal cells of the median eminence. Z. Zellforsch. **127**, 545—551 (1972).

Löfgren, F.: The infundibular recess, a component in the hypothalamo-adenohypophyseal system. Acta morph. neerl.-scand. **3**, 55—78 (1959).

Löfgren, F.: On the transport mechanism between the hypothalamus and the anterior pituitary. Kungl. Fysiograf. Sallskapet. I. Lund. Fork. **30**, 115 (1960).

Löfgren, F.: The glial-vascular apparatus in the floor of the infundibular cavity. Lunds. Univ. Arsskr. N. F. **57**, 1—18 (1961).

Matsui, T.: Fine structure of the median eminence of the rat. J. Fac. Sci. Univ. Tokyo **4**, 79—96 (1966).

Mazzuca, M.: Structure fine de l'éminence médian du cobaye. J. Microscop. **4**, 225—238 (1965).

Monroe, B. G.: A comparative study of the median eminence, infundibular stem and neural lobe of the hypophysis of the rat. Z. Zellforsch. **76**, 405—432 (1967).

Ondo, J. G., Eskay, R. L., Mical, R. S., Porter, J. C.: Release of LH by LRF injected into the CSF: A transport role for the median eminence. Endocrinology **93**, 213—237 (1973).

Raisman, G., Field, P. M.: Anatomical considerations relevant to the interpretation of neuroendocrine experiments. In: Martini, L., Ganong, W. F. (Eds.): Frontiers in neuroendocrinology, pp. 3—44. New York: Oxford Univ. Press 1971.

Scott, D. E., Knigge, K. M.: Ultrastructural changes in the median eminence of the rat following deafferentation of the basal hypothalamus. Z. Zellforsch. **105**, 1—32 (1970).

Scott, D. E., Krobisch Dudley, G., Weindl, A., Joynt, R. J.: An electron microscopic autoradiographic analysis of hypothalamic magnocellular neurons. Z. Zellforsch. **138**, 421—438 (1973).

Weiner, R. I., Terkel, J., Blake, C. A., Schally, A. V., Sawyer, C. H.: Changes in serum lutenizing hormone following intraventricular and intravenous injections of lutenizing hormone in the rat. Neuroendocrinology **10**, 261 (1972).

Zimmerman, E. A.: Personal communication (1974).

Identification of Adenohypophysiotropic Neurohormone Producing Neurosecretory Cells in *Rana temporaria*

K. Dierickx

Department of Embryology and Comparative Histology, Rijksuniversiteit, Gent (Belgium)

In mammals, it has been shown that the region of the median eminence contains adenohypophysiotropic hormones. There is experimental evidence that these adenohypophysiotropic hormones (releasing factors) are released into the bloodstream of the median eminence (see Harris, 1972; Guillemin and Burgus, 1972).

But as stated by Harris (1972), Guillemin (1972), Porter et al. (1972), Knowles (1972) and others, until now: (1) the releasing factor-producing cells have not been identified; (2) their localization has not been found; (3) the way in which the releasing factors are transported is unknown. The latter could be via axons (see Harris, 1970, 1972), or via the cerebrospinal fluid (see Knigge and Scott, 1970; Porter et al., 1972; Rodriguez, 1969 and others), or even via other pathways.

In this paper, a survey is given of our investigations about the releasing factor-producing cells in *Rana temporaria*. As quoted from Herrick (1948): "The amphibian brain may be used as a pattern or template, that is, as a standard of reference in the study of all other vertebrate brains, both lower and higher in the scale". Therefore, even for the higher vertebrates, the results of these investigations must be important for the understanding of the control mechanism by which the brain regulates the activity of the pars distalis of the pituitary gland.

It has first to be noted that, although it is known that the amphibian pars distalis produces the same types of hormones as the mammalian pars distalis, none of these hormones has been isolated.

Moreover, biochemical investigations about amphibian adenohypophysiotropic hormones are lacking.

Chronologically, our investigations of the central nervous control over the pars distalis of *Rana temporaria* can be divided into four periods, which are summarized below.

1. First Period

In the first period we started from the hypothesis that the pars distalis of *Rana temporaria* might be controlled by neurohumoral substances, released into the blood vessels of the median eminence, by nerve terminals of unknown hypothalamic tracts, and that these substances could be carried to the pars distalis via the bloodstream of the hypophysial portal vessels (see Harris, 1972).

At that moment, like many other investigators, we were very impressed by the investigations of Bargmann and his school (see Bargmann, 1954) concerning the aldehyde-fuchsin positive magnocellular hypothalamo-hypophysial neurosecretory system. Hence we conceived the idea that this magnocellular neurosecretory system might also be involved in the control of the activity of the pars distalis, based on our observation that, in *Rana temporaria*, aldehyde-fuchsin positive material accumulates around the blood vessels of the median eminence and that this accumulation shows an annual cyclicity (Dierickx and van den Abeele, 1959). We decided to study the possible influence of the magnocellular preoptico-hypophysial neurosecretory system on the gonadotropic activity of the pars distalis of *Rana temporaria*.

Therefore, in a large number of animals, the magnocellular preoptic nuclei were removed during that period of the year when the development of the gonads and secondary sexual characteristics is minimal. The operated animals were kept alive together with control animals. Their nutritional condition remained excellent. The animals were killed the next year, after the period of reproduction.

The results showed that, as in the normal animals, in the operated animals normal development of the gonads and of the secondary sexual characteristics had occurred. Therefore, it was concluded that the magnocellular preoptic nuclei do not play an important role in the regulation of the gonadotropic activity of the pars distalis, as far as the seasonal development of the gonads and of the secondary sexual characteristics of *Rana temporaria* are concerned (Dierickx, 1963a and b, 1967a).

2. Second Period

After complete removal of the aldehyde-fuchsin positive magnocellular preoptic nuclei, in the median eminence and in the neural lobe, all axons of the magnocellular preoptico-hypophysial system of the operated animals disappeared. However, in the median eminence, numerous aldehyde-fuchsin negative nerve fibres of hypothalamic origin remained. We therefore decided to explore the possibility that some of these remaining aldehyde-fuchsin negative nerve fibres might be involved in the control of the gonadotropic activity of the pars distalis.

To test this possibility, in twenty-seven adult female animals, all neural connections between the brain and the median eminence-hypophysis were surgically interrupted, without disturbing the blood supply of the neurally isolated median eminence-hypophysis (Fig. 1). The operation was performed during that period of the year when the development of the gonads and of the secondary sexual characteristics is minimal.

The operated animals were kept alive together with control animals. Their nutritional condition remained excellent. The animals were killed three months after operation. In all control animals the seasonal development of the ovaries and oviducts was normal.

In the 27 operated animals a varying degree of regeneration of the interrupted nerve fibres had occurred in 19 animals; in 8 operated animals total neural isolation of the median eminence-hypophysis had persisted.

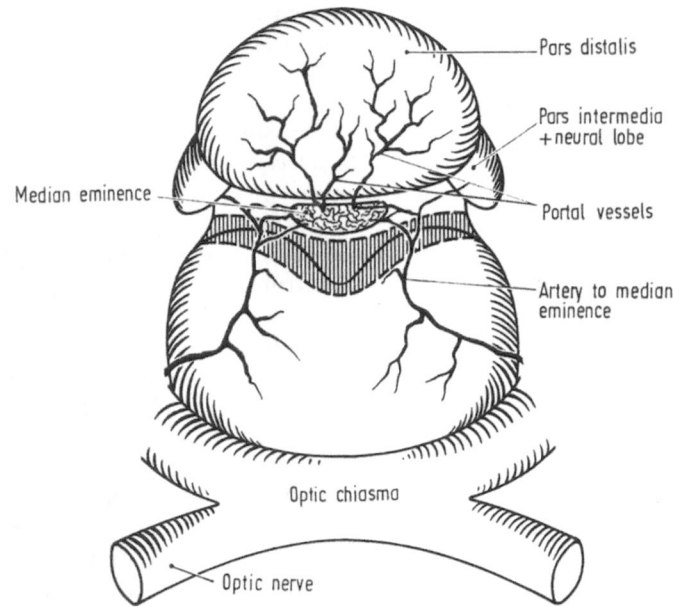

Fig. 1. Sketch of the ventral hypothalamo-hypophysial region of *Rana temporaria*. In the hatched area, at operation, all nervous tissue was removed, without interfering with the hypophysial portal vascularization [from: Dierickx, K.: Z. Zellforsch. **63**, 938—949 (1966)]

In the animals in which nerve regeneration had been observed, different degrees of development of the ovaries and of the oviducts had occurred.

In the eight animals in which total neural isolation of the median eminence-hypophysis had persisted, seasonal development of the gonads and of the oviducts was completely absent (Dierickx, 1964).

From the results of this experiment it may be concluded that, in contradiction with the hypothesis of Knigge and Scott (1970), Porter et al. (1972) and others, in *Rana temporaria*, neither the cerebrospinal fluid nor the general blood circulation play an important role in the transport of gonadotropic releasing factors to the median eminence-hypophysis.

From the comparison of these results with those of the animals in which the magnocellular preoptic nuclei had been removed it may be concluded that nerve fibres of the median eminence, which do not belong to the magnocellular preoptico-hypophysial system, are involved in the control of the gonadotropic activity of the pars distalis of *Rana temporaria*.

As the secretory cells of the pars distalis are not innervated by the brain (see Green, 1966; Harris, 1972), it may be inferred that these nerve fibres must influence the gonadotropic activity of the pars distalis by means of neuro-humoral substances (gonadotropic hormone releasing factors) released into the blood-stram of the median eminence. Also these nerve fibres could be axons of gonadotropic hormone releasing factor-producing nerve cells which must be located somewhere in the brain.

3. Third Period

In a third period we tried to determine the localization of these putative gonadotropic hormone releasing factor-producing nerve cells. Based on the fact that, in
mammals, lesions of the region of the nucleus infundibularis (arcuate nucleus),
located in the tuber cinereum, near the hypophysis, cause atrophy of the gonads
(see Spatz, 1958), we postulated that the pars ventralis of the tuber cinereum of
Rana — which in amphibia is the homologous region of the arcuate and ventromedial nuclei of mammals (see Diepen, 1962) — could be the area in which the
putative gonadotropic hormone releasing factor-producing nerve cells are located.
To test our hypothesis, we performed two kinds of operations (Fig. 2):

One kind of operation obtained animals with a hypothalamic island, consisting
of the pars ventralis tuberis cinerei + median eminence and the other parts of the
hypophysis. As it appeared that regeneration of the interrupted nervous pathways
occurred rather easily, to prevent any regeneration, a teflon barrier was inserted
into the operative gap between the island and the brain. Thus a large number of
animals was obtained of which the complete neural isolation of the hypothalamic
island persisted (= first group of operated animals (Fig. 2c).

By another kind of operation, animals were obtained in which the hypothalamic island consisted only of the median eminence-hypophysis, while the pars
ventralis of the tuber cinereum was removed (= second group of operated animals
(Fig. 2b).

The blood supply of the hypothalamic islands of both groups of animals was
carefully preserved during operation. The other parts of the brain were left intact.
The operated animals were kept alive from several months till two years after
operation. Their nutritional condition remained excellent.

The results showed that, in the first group, normal development of the gonads
and of the secondary sexual characteristics occurred, while in the second group
development of the gonads and of the secondary sexual characteristics was completely absent (Dierickx, 1965, 1966, 1967b). Moreover, as shown by the radioactive Iodine-uptake by the thyroid gland, it appeared that, in the first group, the
thyrotropic activity of the pars distalis was very significantly higher than in the
second group (Vandesande and Dierickx, 1971; Dierickx and Vandesande, to be
published). As in all operated animals the normal blood supply of the hypothalamic
islands had been preserved, the difference in gonadotropic and thyrotropic activity
of the pars distalis between the two groups cannot be explained by a difference in
the blood supply of the hypothalamic islands. Therefore, as the operative difference
between the two groups only consisted in the presence or absence of the pars
ventralis tuberis cinerei in the hypothalamic islands: (1) it may be concluded that
the pars ventralis tuberis exerts a control upon the gonadotropic and the thyrotropic activity of the pars distalis of the hypophysis; (2) it may be inferred that this
control is exerted by cells located in the pars ventralis of the tuber cinereum.

Theoretically, this control could be exerted (1) by direct innervation of the
secretory cells of the pars distalis of the hypophysis or (2) via a humoral pathway.
But, as it is generally agreed that the secretory cells of the pars distalis of the
tetrapod hypophysis are not innervated by nerve fibres of the brain (see Green,
1966; Harris, 1972), the first possibility may be discarded. Therefore it must be

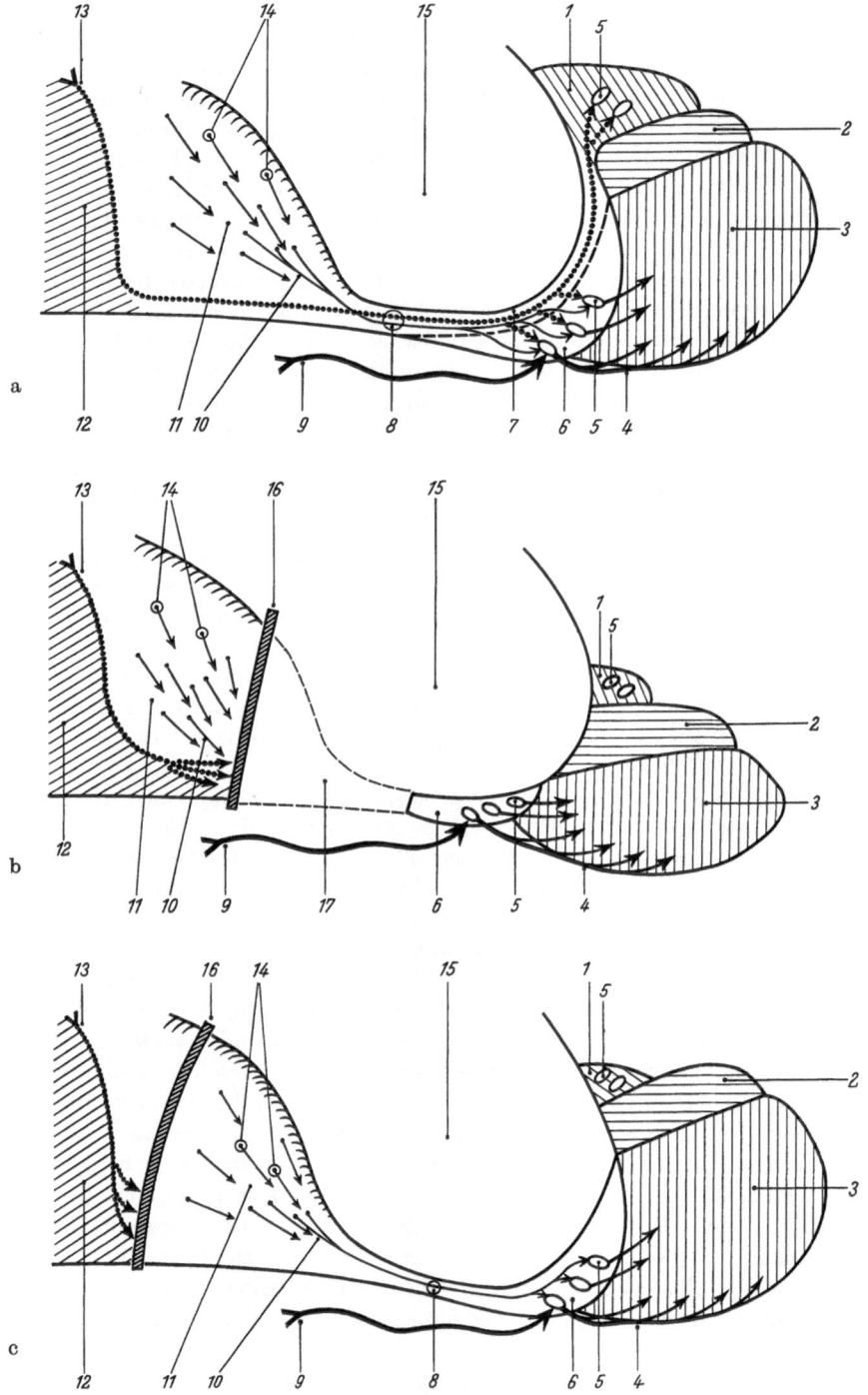

Fig. 2 a—c (Legend see p. 175)

concluded that the cells of the pars ventralis tuberis cinerei which exert this control, produce substances (so-called releasing factors or adenohypophysiotropic hormones) which reach the secretory cells of the pars distalis via a humoral pathway.

In the case of the hypothalamic islands of *Rana temporaria*, there are only two possible humoral pathways for the transport of releasing factors from the pars ventralis of the tuber cinereum to the pars distalis of the hypophysis. The first possibility is that the cerebrospinal fluid or the general blood circulation might be involved in the transport of releasing factors to the blood capillaries of the median eminence, from which they could reach the pars distalis via the hypophysial vascular portal system. The second possibility is that the releasing factors could be transported to the hypophysial portal system via axons of neurosecretory cells (located in the isolated pars ventralis tuberis cinerei) ending on the blood capillaries of the median eminence (Fig. 2).

The results already described in *Rana temporaria* with permanent interruption of all nervous connections between the pars ventralis of the tuber cinereum on the one side and the median eminence-hypophysis on the other, showed that, at least the gonadotropic releasing factors are not transported to the median eminence via the cerebrospinal fluid or via the general blood circulation. Therefore, it may be inferred that, in the hypothalamic islands of *Rana temporaria*, releasing factors produced in neurosecretory cells located in the pars ventralis tuberis cinerei are transported to the blood capillaries of the median eminence via axons of these neurosecretory cells.

4. Fourth Period

In a fourth period of our investigations we decided to attempt to identify these releasing factor-producing neurosecretory cells in the pars ventralis of the tuber cinereum. Therefore, in normal animals and in animals with a permanent complete neurally isolated hypothalamic island, (1) fluorescence microscopic and (2) electron microscopic studies of the pars ventralis tuberis cinerei and of the median eminence-hypophysis were done.

Fig. 2a—c. Sagittal section of the operative region. a Normal animal. b Animals of which the caudal part (or the whole) of the pars ventralis of the tuber cinereum was removed. Fig. 2c animals with complete neurally isolated hypothalamic island consisting of the pars ventralis tuberis cinerei + hypophysis. *1* neural lobe; *2* pars intermedia; *3* pars distalis; *4* portal vessels to the pars distalis; *5* blood capillaries (of the median eminence or of the neural lobe); *6* external zone of the median eminence; *7* internal zone of the median eminence; *8* tractus hypothalamo-hypophyseus; *9* afferent blood vessels to the median eminence; *10* A.F.-negative axons of nerve cells localized in the pars ventralis tuberis; the axons run to the blood capillaries of the median eminence; *11* pars ventralis tuberis cinerei; *12* chiasma opticum; *13* A.F.-positive neurosecretory nerve fibres to the median eminence and to the neural lobe; *14* cell bodies of nerve cells of the area periventricularis of the pars ventralis tuberis cinerei; *15* saccus infundibuli; *16* teflon barrier; *17* extirpated part of nervous tissue. In Fig. 2b the A.F.-positive and the A.F.-negative nerve fibres end at the rostral surface of the teflon barrier. Note the extreme atrophy of the median eminence and of the neural lobe. Note also the reduced volume of the pars distalis. In Fig. 2c the A.F.-positive nerve fibres end at the rostral surface of the teflon barrier. The internal zone of the median eminence has disappeared. Note the extreme atrophy of the neural lobe [from: Dierickx, K.: Z. Zellforsch. **74**, 53—79 (1966)]

4.1. Fluorescence Microscopic Studies

In the fluorescence microscopic studies (Dierickx et al., 1973b), the brain of adult *Rana temporaria* was investigated with the fluorescence microscopic technique of Falck and Owman (1965) for catecholamines and serotonin.

In this investigation, three groups of animals were used: (1) normal, untreated animals; (2) animals injected with pharmacological substances which increase the monoamine content of the brain; (3) animals with a neurally isolated hypothalamic island consisting of the pars ventralis tuberis + median eminence-hypophysis and of which the normal blood supply had been preserved.

The fluorescence microscopic observations showed that the pars ventralis tuberis cinerei, the median eminence and the pituitary pars intermedia of normal *Rana temporaria* contain numerous monoaminergic fibres. Moreover, catecholaminergic fibres accumulate around the blood capillaries of the median eminence, suggesting release of catecholamines into the bloodstream.

On the other hand, it appeared that, in the normal pars ventralis tuberis cinerei, fluorescent monoamine-containing perikarya are absent. This total absence of fluorescent monoamine-containing perikarya in the pars ventralis tuberis cinerei was confirmed by the results obtained in the drug-treated animals.

Moreover, in the animals with a hypothalamic island, not only fluorescent monoaminergic perikarya were absent, but also the fluorescent monoaminergic fibres of the pars ventralis tuberis cinerei, median eminence and pars intermedia of the hypophysis had completely disappeared. This total disappearance of monoaminergic fibres in the hypothalamic islands must be due to operative disconnection of these fibres from their cell bodies located outside the pars ventralis of the tuber cinereum.

Therefore, from these results it is concluded that:

(1) The pars ventralis of the tuber cinereum of *Rana temporaria* does not contain monoaminergic cell bodies.

(2) The monoaminergic nerve fibres which, in normal animals, are present in the pars ventralis tuberis, in the median eminence and in the pars intermedia of the hypophysis, originate from monoamine-producing cells of which the perikarya must be located outside the pars ventralis tuberis cinerei.

(3) As, in the hypothalamic islands, monoaminergic cells were absent and monoaminergic nerve fibres had completely disappeared, monoaminergic cells or fibres could not have exerted the control upon the gonadotropic and thyrotropic activity of the pars distalis of the hypophysis, which we had observed in animals with hypothalamic islands. Hence, this control must be exerted by other kinds of neurosecretory cells of the pars ventralis of the tuber cinereum.

4.2. Electron Microscopic Investigation of the Pars Ventralis Tuberis Cinerei and of the Median Eminence

As will be described now, these controlling neurosecretory cells were tentatively identified by electron microscopic investigation of the pars ventralis tuberis cinerei and of the median eminence (Dierickx et al., 1972, 1973a).

4.2.1. Identification of a Tubero-Hypophysial Neurosecretory System

In this investigation, normal animals were contrasted with animals with neurally isolated hypothalamic islands consisting of the pars ventralis tuberis cinerei + median eminence-hypophysis of which the normal blood supply had been preserved.

In this electron microscopic investigation, a tubero-hypophysial neurosecretory system has been identified, consisting of, at least, six different neurosecretory cell types, characterized by the different shape and size of their respective secretory granules (Fig. 3).

The perikarya of these neurosecretory cells are located in the area periventricularis of the pars ventralis of the tuber cinereum. They contain a varying number of secretory granules. In some perikarya of the operated animals, hundreds of secretory granules may be present. In normal animals, a maximal accumulation of granules occurs during hibernation, while the granule content of the perikarya is minimal during summer (to be published). According to the pictures observed, the secretory granules appear to be formed in the Golgi apparatus.

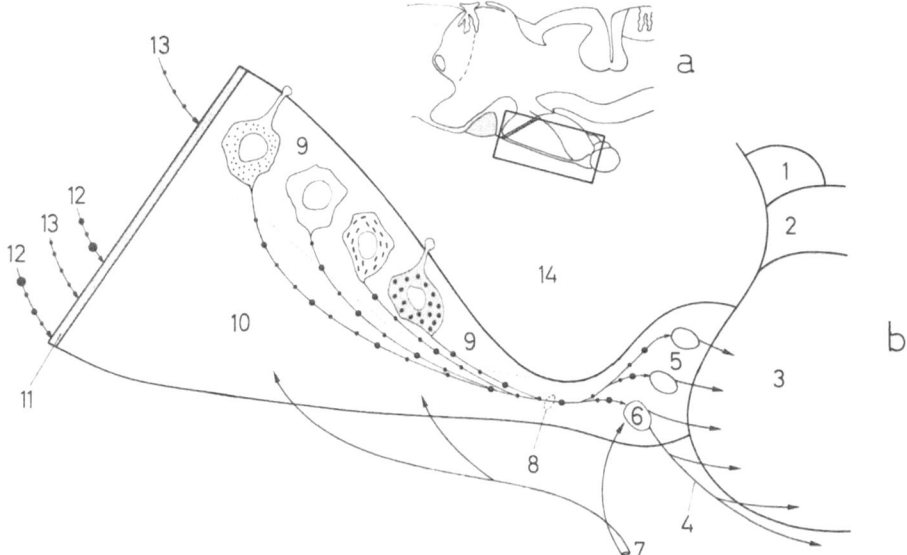

Fig. 3. a) Medio-sagittal section of the brain of an animal with hypothalamic island. The dark bar represents the location of the teflon barrier which prevents nervous regeneration. For legend see Dierickx, Goossens, De Waele: Z. Zellforsch. **109**, 328, Fig. 1 (1970). b) Oblique sagittal section of the part of Fig. 3a enclosed in the rectangle (= hypothalamic island). *1* atrophied neural lobe; *2* pars intermedia; *3* pars distalis; *4* portal vessels to the pars distalis; *5* remaining part of the external region of the median eminence; *6* blood capillaries of the median eminence; *7* intact blood vessels to the hypothalamic island; *8* tubero-hypophysial neurosecretory tract to the blood capillaries of the median eminence; *9* area periventricularis of the isolated pars ventralis tuberis cinerei, containing neurosecretory cells with large dendrite to the ventricular cavity; *10* peripheral area of the isolated pars ventralis tuberis cinerei containing the axons of the tuberal neurosecretory cells; *11* teflon barrier; *12* neurosecretory axons of magnocellular preoptico-hypophysial neurosecretory system ending at the rostral surface of the teflon barrier; *13* monoaminergic axons; *14* cavity of the saccus infundibuli

The secretory granules are transported, via the axons of the neurosecretory cells, towards the external region of the median eminence. In the axons, the secretory granules tend to accumulate. Localized accumulations of granules produce bead-like expansions of the axons. Successive granule-containing axonal varicosities are joined by thinner axonal segments that contain few or no secretory granules.

Occasionally, the size of the intra-axonal accumulations of granules may be so large that the axonal expansions resemble Herring bodies of the magnocellular preoptico-hypophysial neurosecretory system.

In the external region of the median eminence, the terminal arborizations of the neurosecretory axons end on the pericapillary space of the blood capillaries. These terminal arborizations show electron microscopic evidence of the release of neurosecretory material, via the pericapillary space, into the bloodstream of the median eminence.

In each neurosecretory cell type, the size and internal structure of the secretory granules are different from those of the monoamine-containing dense core vesicles of the central and peripheral nervous system. This observation strongly suggests that the secretory products of this tubero-hypophysial neurosecretory system are not monoamines.

Moreover, in the external region of the normal median eminence, separate mono-aminergic fibres were tentatively identified. In the median eminence of animals with a hypothalamic island these putative monoaminergic fibres completely disappeared, suggesting that the perikarya of these monoaminergic fibres are located outside the pars ventralis of the tuber cinereum. In the same hypothalamic islands, the tuberohypophysial neurosecretory system persisted.

So, according to our electron microscopic investigations, the tubero-hypophysial neurosecretory fibres and the monoaminergic tubero-hypophysial nerve fibres are separate, transporting and secreting different products.

As already described above, these inferences have been confirmed by our fluorescence microscopic study of the monoaminergic fibres of the tubero-hypophysial region.

Finally, it is worth mentioning that transmission electron micrographs showed that in a quite large number of neurosecretory cells a thick dendrite extends from the perikaryon to the infundibular cavity. This dendrite ends between the ependymal cells, while its expanded end-bulb protrudes into the ventricular cavity. This is beautifully seen on scanning electron micrographs of the ventricular surface of the pars ventralis of the tuber cinereum, on which the expanded end-bulbs of the dendrites are easily recognizable. The structural features of these dendrites plead in favour of a possible receptive role. This could explain the results obtained after intraventricular injection of monoamines (see Porter et al., 1972; McCann et al., 1972).

4.2.2. The Nature of the Secretory Products of the Tubero-Hypophysial Neurosecretory System of Rana temporaria

What could be the nature of the secretory products of this tubero-hypophysial neurosecretory system of Rana temporaria?

As already shown above, the secretory products of this system are not mono-amines. On the other hand, it is known that polypeptide hormone-producing endo-crine cells are characterized by the production of secretory granules which are formed in the Golgi-apparatus (see Bargmann, 1971; Fawcett et al., 1969; Farqu-har, 1971). Therefore, it is highly probable that, as the secretory cell types of the tubero-hypophysial neurosecretory system show close structural resemblance to polypeptide hormone-producing cells, they produce polypeptide hormones, which are released into the bloodstream of the median eminence.

On the contrary, the ultrastructure of the ependymal and glial cells of the pars ventralis tuberis cinerei and of the median eminence of *Rana temporaria*, pleads against the assumption that these cells could produce polypeptide hormones (Dierickx et al., 1973a).

Moreover, as the known releasing factors are small polypeptides, it may be assumed that the releasing factor-producing cells (like all other polypeptide hormone-producing cells) produce secretory granules.

So, as the neurosecretory cells of the tubero-hypophysial neurosecretory system are the only cell types of the pars ventralis tuberis of the hypothalamic islands which show ultrastructural evidence of polypeptide hormone-producing endocrine cells, and as they show ultrastructural evidence of a direct transport of polypeptide hormones, via axons, into the bloodstream of the median eminence: therefore it may be postulated that the tubero-hypophysial neurosecretory system of *Rana temporaria* produces peptide adenohypophysiotropic hormones.

Direct identification of releasing factors in the secretory granules of the neuro-secretory cells of the pars ventralis tuberis cinerei of *Rana temporaria* could confirm our tentative identification of releasing factor producing cells. This may be possible if antibodies against amphibian releasing factors become available.

Summary

The pars ventralis of the tuber cinereum of *Rana temporaria* is a region which controls the secretory activity of the pars distalis of the hypophysis. For the gonadotropic and thyrotropic activities of the pars distalis, this has been shown by the results obtained from two different groups of animals with hypothalamic islands of which the complete neural isolation from the brain persisted.

By means of electron microscopy, in neurally isolated and normal pars ventralis of the tuber cinereum, at least six different neurosecretory cell types, characterized by the different shape and size of their respective secretory granules, were identified. Their secretory granules, apparently formed in the Golgi apparatus, are transported, via the axons, towards the peri-vascular spaces of the external region of the median eminence. The terminal arborizations of the neurosecretory axons show electron microscopic evidence of release of neurosecretory material into the blood capillaries of the median eminence.

Fluorescence microscopy showed that the pars ventralis of the tuber cinereum does not contain monoaminergic perikarya and that the monoaminergic fibres which, in normal animals, are present in the pars ventralis tuberis and in the median eminence originate from mono-amine-producing cells of which the perikarya must be located outside the pars ventralis tuberis cinerei.

From the results, it is concluded that the fibres of the tubero-hypophysial neurosecretory system and the monoaminergic tubero-hypophysial nerve fibres are separate, transporting and secreting different products. It is inferred that the tubero-hypophysial neurosecretory cells, identified in *Rana temporaria*, must be adenohypophysiotropic neurohormone-producing cells.

References

Bargmann, W.: Das Zwischenhirn-Hypophysensystem. Berlin-Göttingen-Heidelberg: Springer 1954.

Bargmann, W.: Die funktionelle Morphologie des endokrinen Regulationssystems. In: Altmann, H.W., Büchner, F., Cottier, H., Grundmann, E., Holle, G., Letterer, E., Masshoff, W., Meessen, H., Roulet, F., Seifert, G., Siebert, G. (Eds.): Handbuch der allgemeinen Pathologie, VIII. Band: Regulationen, 1. Teil, pp. 1—106. Berlin-Heidelberg-New York: Springer 1971.

Diepen, R.: Der Hypothalamus. In: Handbuch der mikroskopischen Anatomie des Menschen, Band IV, Teil 7. Berlin-Göttingen-Heidelberg: Springer 1962.

Dierickx, K.: The total extirpation of the preoptic magnocellular nucleus of Rana temporaria. Arch. int. Pharmacodyn. 143, 268—275 (1963a).

Dierickx, K.: The extirpation of the neurosecretory preoptic nucleus and the reproduction of Rana temporaria. Arch. int. Pharmacodyn. 145, 580—589 (1963b).

Dierickx, K.: The nerve fibres controlling the gonadotropic activity of the hypophysis of Rana temporaria. Z. Zellforsch. 63, 938—949 (1964).

Dierickx, K.: The origin of the aldehyde-fuchsin-negative nerve fibres of the median eminence of the hypophysis: a gonadotropic centre. Z. Zellforsch. 66, 504—518 (1965).

Dierickx, K.: Experimental identification of a hypothalamic gonadotropic centre. Z. Zellforsch. 74, 53—79 (1966).

Dierickx, K.: The function of the hypophysis without preoptic neurosecretory control. Z. Zellforsch. 78, 114—130 (1967a).

Dierickx, K.: The gonadotropic centre of the tuber cinereum hypothalami and ovulation. Z. Zellforsch. 77, 188—203 (1967b).

Dierickx, K., Druyts, A., Vandenberghe, M.P., Goossens, N.: Identification of adenohypophysiotropic neurohormone producing neurosecretory cells in Rana temporaria. I. Ultrastructural evidence for the presence of neurosecretory cells in the tuber cinereum. Z. Zellforsch. 134, 459—504 (1972).

Dierickx, K., Goossens, N., Vandenberghe, M.P.: Identification of adenohypophysiotropic neurohormone producing neurosecretory cells in Rana temporaria. III. The tuberohypophysial monoaminergic fibres and the role of the tuberohypophysial neurosecretory system. Z. Zellforsch. 143, 93—106 (1973b).

Dierickx, K., Van den Abeele, A.: On the relations between the hypothalamus and the anterior pituitary in Rana temporaria. Z. Zellforsch. 51, 78—87 (1959).

Dierickx, K., Vandenberghe, M.P., Goossens, N.: Identification of adenohypophysiotropic neurohormone producing neurosecretory cells in Rana temporaria. II. Identification, in the median eminence, of the terminal arborizations of axons of the tubero-hypophysial neurosecretory system. Z. Zellforsch. 142, 479—513 (1973a).

Falck, B., Owman, C.: A detailed methodological description of the fluorescence method for the cellular demonstration of biogenic monoamines. Acta Univ. Lund, Sectio II, N. 7, 1965.

Farquhar, M.G.: Processing of secretory products by cells of the anterior pituitary gland. Mem. Soc. Endocrinol. N. 19. In: Heller, H., Lederis, K. (Eds.): Subcellular organization and function of endocrine tissues, pp. 79—124. Cambridge University Press 1971.

Fawcett, A.W., Long, J.A., Jones, A.L.: The ultrastructure of endocrine glands. Rec. Progr. Hormone Res. 25, 315—380 (1969).

Green, J.D.: The comparative anatomy of the portal vascular system and of the innervation of the hypophysis. In: Harris, G.W., Donovan, B.T. (Eds.): The pituitary gland. Vol. I: Anterior pituitary, pp. 127—146. London: Butterworths 1966.

Guillemin, R.: Opening remarks: In: Knigge, K.M., Scott, D.E., Weindl, A. (Eds.): Brain-endocrine interaction Median eminence: Structure and function, pp. 1—2. Basel-München-Paris-London-New York-Sydney: S. Karger 1972.

Guillemin, R., Burgus, R.: The hormones of the hypothalamus. Scientific American 227, 24—33 (1972).

Harris, G.W.: In: Knigge, K.M., Scott, D.E. (Eds.): Structure and function of the median eminence. Discussion by Harris. Amer. J. Anat. 129, 245—246 (1970).

Harris, G.W.: Humours and hormones. J. Endocr. 53, 2—23 (1972).

Herrick, C. J.: The brain of the tiger salamander. Chicago: Chicago University Press 1948.
Knigge, K. M., Scott, D. E.: Structure and function of the median eminence. Amer. J. Anat. **129**, 223—244 (1970).
Knowles, Sir F.: Ependyma of the third ventricle in relation to pituitary function. Progr. Brain Res. **38**, 255—270 (1972).
McCann, S. M., Kalra, P. S., Donoso, A. O., Bishop, W., Schneider, H. P. G., Fawcett, C. P., Krulich, L.: The role of the monoamines in the control of gonadotropin and prolactin secretion. In: Knigge, K. M., Scott, D. E., Weindl, A. (Eds.): Brain-endocrine interaction. Median eminence: Structure and function, pp. 224—235. Basel-München-Paris-London-New York-Sydney: S. Karger 1972.
Porter, J. C., Kamberi, I. A., Ondo, J. G.: Role of biogenic amines and cerebrospinal fluid in the neurovascular transmittal of hypophysiotrophic substances. In: Knigge, K. M., Scott, D. E., Weindl, A. (Eds.): Brain-endocrine interaction. Median eminence: Structure and function, pp. 245—253. Basel-München-Paris-London-New York-Sydney: S. Karger 1972.
Rodriguez, E. M.: Ependymal specializations. I. Fine structure of the neural (internal) region of the toad median eminence, with particular reference to the connection between the ependymal cells and the subependymal capillary loops. Z. Zellforsch. **102**, 153—171 (1969).
Spatz, H.: Die proximale (supra-selläre) Hypophyse, ihre Beziehungen zum Diencephalon und ihre Regenerationspotenz. In: Curri, S. B., Martini, L., Kovac, W. (Eds.): Pathophysiologia diencephalica, pp. 53—77. Wien: Springer 1958.
Vandesande, F., Dierickx, K.: Experimental identification of a hypothalamic thyrotrope centre in *Rana temporaria*. Acta endocr. (Kbh.) Suppl. **155**, 33 (1971).

Structural and Functional Aspects of Two Types of Gomori-Negative Neurosecretory Centres in the Caudal Hypothalamus of Amphibia

P. G. W. J. van Oordt, H. J. Th. Goos, J. Peute, and M. Terlou

Section for Comparative Endocrinology, Zoological Laboratory, State University, Utrecht (The Netherlands)

Combining light and electron microscopical techniques three types of paired neurosecretory centres can be identified in the hypothalamus of Amphibia. The first comprises the nucleus preopticus which consists of Gomori-positive and Falck-negative peptidergic cells containing elementary granules with a diameter of more than 1000 Å. The second type is formed by the paraventricular organ and the nucleus infundibularis dorsalis. In these nuclei the cells are Gomori-negative and Falck-positive, and are therefore labelled aminergic neurosecretory cells. They contain dense-core vesicles with a diameter not seldom less than 1000 Å. The third type is represented by the nucleus infundibularis ventralis. Its nerve cells are Gomori- as well as Falck-negative, and contain elementary granules larger than 1000 Å in diameter (Peute and van Oordt, 1974). The Gomori-negative centres are discussed in this paper.

The Paraventricular Organ (PVO; Fig. 1)

The first indication of the existence of aminergic neurosecretory centres in the caudal hypothalamus of Amphibia has been given by Goos and van Halewijn (1968) who used the method of Falck et al. (1962) in a study of neurosecretion in larvae of *Xenopus laevis*. Shortly after, Braak (1970) and Bartels (1971) confirmed the presence of such centres in *Rana esculenta* and *Rana temporaria* respectively. Recently, Terlou and Ploemacher (1973) could give a detailed description of the distribution of monoamines in the brains of *Xenopus* larvae. To that end they improved the normally weak fluorescence by keeping the larvae in a solution of iproniazide phosphate for 48–54 h prior to fixation. This solution inhibits mono-amine oxidase, the enzyme that causes the breakdown of amines. Thus, the authors observed two paired aminergic nuclei, localized in the lateral wall of the ventricle and situated behind each other. One of these, the PVO, consists of a rostral part and a latero-caudal part, which are continuous. The rostral part is found at the entrance of the infundibulum and is oriented from rostro-caudal to caudo-ventral. The latero-caudal part is localized at the lateral dilatations of the infundibular recess.

The PVO is composed of an ependymal lining and 2—4 layers of tigthly packed subependymal neurons. These neurons are pear-shaped, the apical parts projecting into the ventricle where most of the protrusions form a dense intraventricular network. In electron micrographs of the PVO, Peute (1969) could discern two

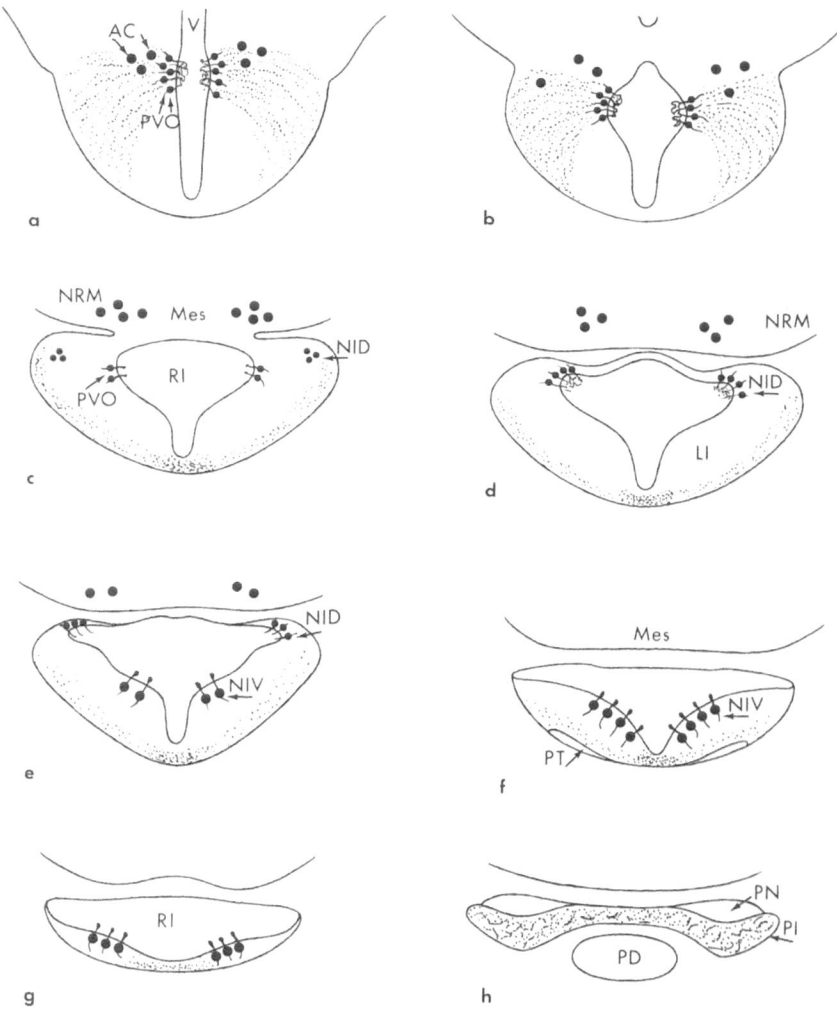

Fig. 1a—h. Diagrams of transverse sections through the hypothalamo-hypophysial region of an anuran, showing the localization and the extension of paired Gomori-negative, Falck-positive neurosecretory centres (PVO, NID), and a paired Gomori-negative, Falck-negative neurosecretory centre (NIV). Fluorescent tracts are marked by small black dots. *Abbreviations*: AC = PVO-accompanying cells; LI = lobus infundibularis; Mes = mesencephalon; NID = nucleus infundibularis dorsalis; NIV = nucleus infundibularis ventralis; NRM = nucleus reticularis mesencephali; PD = pars distalis; PI = pars intermedia; PN = pars nervosa; PT = pars tuberalis; PVO = paraventricular organ; RI = recessus infundibularis; V = third ventricle

different types of nerve cells. Both contain large dense-core vesicles in the peri-karyon as well as in the intraventricular protrusions. Those in the Type I cells have a more or less round profile, with a clear halo around the dense core. The diameter of these vesicles varies from 800–1000 Å. In the Type II cells the vesicles are often elongated and larger, i.e. from 1200–1400 Å in diameter.

Another difference between the two types of neurons in the PVO is the synaptic contact with other nerve cells. The Type II cells are innervated via axo-somatic synapses. Such synapses are suggestive of a secreto-motor innervation, probably resulting in the extrusion of amines into the cerebrospinal fluid. The intraventricular amines might influence other liquor-contacting neurons or specialized ependymal cells (cf. Knowles, 1967; Rodriguez, 1969).

The Type I cells have somato-dendritic synapses. In tissue fixed with the zinc-iodide-osmium-tetroxide mixture of Akert and Sandri (1968) the small vesicles of these synapses contain a black deposit. This phenomenon together with the pre-sence of cilia of the 8+1 type on the protrusions seems to point to a sensory func-tion of the Type I cells (Peute, 1971).

Apart from these morphological differences there may be differences in the amines produced by the two types of neurons of the PVO. With Falck's technique both cells with a green fluorescence and cells with a yellow-orange fluorescence have been observed (Terlou and Ploemacher, 1973), indicating the presence of catechol-amines and indolamines respectively. Injection of ^{3}H-DOPA and ^{3}H-5-hydroxy-tryptophan (5-HTP) not only showed the selective uptake of these precursors in the PVO, but also a relatively high incorporation of ^{3}H-DOPA in the Type I cells and of ^{3}H-5-HTP in the Type II cells (Peute and van Oordt, 1974). Thus, it is not impossible that the Type I cells produce catecholamines and the Type II cells indolamines.

Treatment of *Xenopus* larvae with para-chlorophenylalanine (Peute and van Oordt, 1974), a depletor of serotonin and catecholamine stores (Keller, 1972), resulted in the disappearance of the large granular vesicles in both types of nerve cells in the PVO. Instead they contained twice the normal amount of small agranular vesicles, with a diameter of 500–800 Å. This indicates a depletion of the amines from the storage site, i.e. the large granular vesicles. Probably, the small vesicles are formed as a result of exocytosis of the large granular vesicles. The presence of coated vesicles in the protrusions, and the regularly observed coated invaginations of the cell membrane, support this hypothesis (Nagasawa et al., 1970). In other words, the neural cells of the PVO – not only the Type II cells, but also the Type I cells – seem to release amines into the cerebrospinal fluid.

The Nucleus Infundibularis Dorsalis (NID; Fig. 1)

The NID is situated dorso-laterally of the caudal end of the PVO, and borders the dorsal wall of the recessus lateralis infundibuli (syn.: recessus mamillaris). In *Xenopus laevis* the NID is separated from the caudal parts of the PVO, but in *Rana esculenta* the NID homologue is incorporated into the PVO (Terlou and Ploemacher, 1973). The situation in *Rana temporaria* resembles that in *Xenopus* (Parent, 1973).

Fluorescence is localized in the cytoplasm and intraventricular processes of the neurons. Although Terlou and Ploemacher (1973) observed mainly green fluorescing cells, some yellow-orange fluorescing cells were found also. It is not certain that these two types of fluorescing cells are identical with the two types of nerve cells identified by Peute (1973) in electron micrographs of the NID. On ultrastructural grounds the neurons can be divided into Type I cells containing round granular vesicles with an average diameter of 800 Å, and Type II cells which contain round as well as elongated granular vesicles. The round vesicles have an average diameter of 1200 Å, and the long axis of the elongated ones measures up to 2500 Å.

The neurons of the NID bear cilia of the $8+1$ type on their intraventricular protrusions. In the rostral part of the NID these protrusions form an intraventricular plexus. In the caudal part, mainly composed of Type I cells, the protrusions are present as separate, knob-like structures. The neurons of the NID are bipolar, which might indicate a sensory function of these cells (Vigh, 1971). However a secretory function cannot be excluded, for both cell types are innervated, as follows from the presence of many axo-somatic synapses.

Bioamines Formed in PVO and NID

Several attempts have been made to identify the fluorescent material in the aminergic neurosecretory centres of *Xenopus laevis*. Goos et al. (1972) extracted the pooled midbrains of 1450 *Xenopus* larvae, separated different catecholamines and serotonin from the extract, and determined the presence of dopamine, DOPA, noradrenaline, adrenaline and serotonin in the fractions. The results justified the conclusion that dopamine is the main catecholamine in the hypothalamus of *Xenopus laevis*, but that noradrenaline may also be present. Notwithstanding the yellow-orange fluorescence of some cells in the PVO and NID mentioned above, the presence of indoles in these nuclei could not be demonstrated biochemically.

Terlou and Fennema (cf. Terlou and van Kooten, 1974) compared the excitation and emission spectra of the fluorescent material in the neurons of the PVO with those of fluorophores of the beforementioned monoamines. Their results too point to the presence of dopamine, and probably 5-hydroxytryptamine.

PVO, NID and the Pars Intermedia (PI) of the Adenohypophysis

Terlou and Ploemacher (1973) succeeded in visualizing numerous tracts of Falck-positive fibres in the brains of *Xenopus* larvae. Among these is a paired tract that originates at the lateral side of PVO and NID, first curves ventro-caudally and then ventro-caudo-medially. In the ventro-medial hypothalamus the fibres turn in a caudal direction and are combined into a single, flat tract in the bottom of the infundibulum and the median eminence (Fig. 2a). The tract does not end in the pars nervosa, but fans out into the pars intermedia (PI) where the fluorescent fibres form a network surrounding the melanophore-stimulating hormone (MSH) producing cells. This network resembles that described for *Rana temporaria*

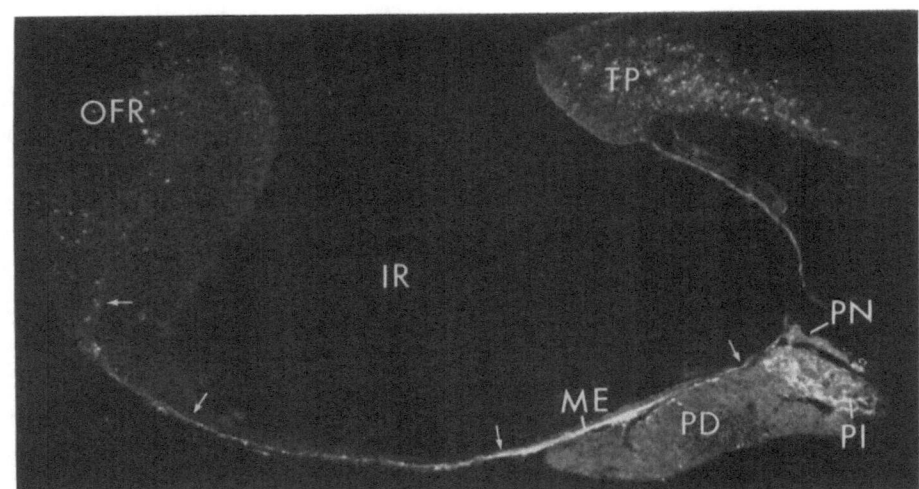

a

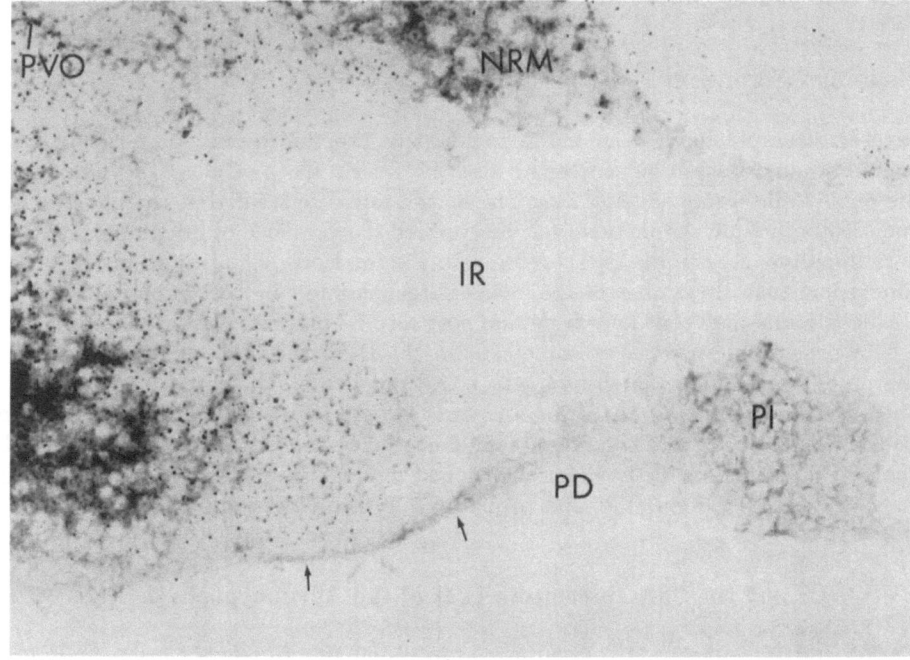

b

Fig. 2a and b. Sagittal sections through the hypothalamo-hypophysial region of *Xenopus laevis* tadpoles. (a) shows a catecholaminergic tract (↑) running from the ventromedial hypothalamus towards the developing median eminence (ME) and the pars intermedia (PI). Paraformaldehyde-treatment (× 140; after Terlou and Ploemacher, 1973). (b) Shows a monoamine oxidase-positive tract (↑) from the hypothalamus towards the pars intermedia. Note that the tract is fanning out before penetrating the pars intermedia (× 225; after Terlou and Stroband, 1973). *Abbreviations*: IR = infundibular recess; ME = median eminence; NRM = nucleus reticularis mesencephali; OFR = optic fibre region; PD = pars distalis; PI = pars intermedia; PN = pars nervosa; PVO = paraventricular organ; TP = tuberculum posterius

(Enemar and Falck, 1965; Bartels, 1971), *Bufo arenarum* (Enemar et al., 1967) and *Rana esculenta* (Braak, 1970). The entire infundibulo-hypophysial tract could also be traced with a modification of the method of Glenner et al. (1957) for the demonstration of monoamine oxidase (Terlou and Stroband, 1973; Fig. 2b). This underlines the aminergic character of the neurons. More evidence for an aminergic innervation of the PI cells in Amphibia is supplied by the electron microscopical studies of Iturriza (1964), Cohen (1967), Pehlemann (1967), Saland (1968), Nakai and Gorbman (1969), Doerr-Schott and Follenius (1969, 1970), Hopkins (1971), Ito (1971), and Imai (1971).

Among the arguments for a functional implication of the morphological connections between the aminergic centres in the caudal hypothalamus and the MSH-secreting cells in the PI are the experimental results of Goos (1969), who treated *Xenopus* larvae with reserpine. He found that reserpine not only causes a depletion of the monoaminergic centres, but at the same time results in an uncontrolled release of MSH. Moreover, Terlou and van Straaten (1973) as well as Nyholm (1972) observed in young *Xenopus* larvae a close correlation between the attainment of the ability to adapt to a white background and the development of aminergic nerve cells in the hypothalamus.

The Melanotropin Inhibiting Hormone (MIH)

Although the above morphological and experimental evidence seems to point to a relation between monoaminergic neurons and the hypothalamic regulation of the MSH production, it is not sufficient to prove that the hypothalamic MIH is a catecholamine (cf. van Oordt et al., 1972). Indeed, Nair et al. (1971) and Celis et al. (1971) isolated a tripeptide with MIH properties from hypothalami of various vertebrates including frogs. This peptide was identified as prolyl-leucyl-glycinamide (PLG). Schally and Kastin (1972) have concluded on experimental grounds that PLG is the physiological MIH.

Goos and Sangster (cf. Terlou et al., 1974) tested the MIH activity of PLG and of the catecholamines dopamine, noradrenaline and adrenaline on the PI of adult *Xenopus laevis in vitro*. In a concentration of 10^{-3} M the tripeptide remained without effect. On the contrary, the catecholamines in a concentration of 10^{-3} and 10^{-4} M considerably inhibited MSH secretion *in vitro*. This seemed to be a matter of release rather than production, for the addition of one of the catecholamines to the Ringer solution appeared to lower the loss of MSH from the PI during the incubation period. Electron micrographs of the PI cells showed that catecholamines inhibited the change of dense granules into fibrillar granules. According to Whur and Weatherhead (1971) and Hopkins (1972) in an active gland MSH can be transferred from these dense granules to the fibrillar granules. This means that the data of Goos and Sangster all point to a catecholamine and not to PLG as the physiological MIH. As PLG can potentiate the action of catecholamines and can influence the central nervous system independently of any MIH activity (Plotnikoff et al., 1971, 1973), its MIH function might be part of a general effect on the metabolism of catecholamines, including the MIH.

The Nucleus Infundibularis Ventralis (NIV; Fig. 1)

In a recent review on the hypothalamo-hypophysial relationships in Amphibia, van Oordt et al. (1972) for the first time drew attention to a paired centre of Gomori- and Falck-negative neurosecretory cells in the lateral lobes of the caudal hypothalamus of *Xenopus laevis* and *Rana esculenta*. A more detailed account of this NIV in *Rana esculenta* has been given by Peute and Mey (1973). Two types of granulated nerve cells were described (Fig. 3): the Y cells containing spheroidal and elongated elementary granules with an average diameter of about 1400 Å, and the Z cells with similar elementary granules of about 1800 Å in diameter. In the Y cells, unlike the Z cells lipid droplets can be observed as well as numerous multivesicular bodies, generally in close association with a number of granulated vesicles. Both the Y and the Z cells are bipolar neurons, the apical process or dendrite ending knob-like in the lumen of the infundibular recess and the basal process extending in a ventro-lateral direction. Thus, the two cell types can be regarded as liquor-contacting neurons. They have a well developed rough endoplasmic reticulum, many mitochondria and often a large Golgi apparatus. The cells, and especially the perikarya, are innervated by large numbers of axons. The presynaptic axon endings invariably contain small dense-core vesicles, 800 Å in diameter, and electron lucent vesicles with a diameter of 500 Å. In fact, the only important difference between classical Gomori-positive peptidergic neurons and the NIV cells is the absence in the latter of material that can be stained by chrome-hematoxylin or aldehyde-fuchsin.

Dierickx et al. (1972) described the ultrastructure of neurosecretory cells in the lateral lobes of *Rana temporaria*. Contrary to the situation in *Rana esculenta*, it appears that in *Rana temporaria* spheroidal and elongated granules are found in separate cell types. Moreover, Dierickx et al. (1972) described both pale and dark cell types, whereas in *Rana esculenta* dark cells occur that can be regarded as functional stages of the Y as well as of the Z cells (Peute and Mey, 1973).

Extrusion of neurosecretory material from the NIV may take place both into the cerebrospinal fluid and in the outer zone of the median eminence. The former follows from the presence of many granulated vesicles in the intraventricular protrusions and of coated invaginations on the cell membrane of these protrusions (cf. Nagasawa et al., 1970). On the other hand, coated membrane invaginations have also been interpreted as signs of micropinocytosis (Daems et al., 1969). Indeed, the Y and Z cells may use micropinocytosis for the incorporation of substances, such as catecholamines, from the cerebrospinal fluid.

Evidence for the transport of secretory material from the NIV to the outer zone of the median eminence and its extrusions into the portal vessels, can be derived from the fact that nerve endings with the same types of granulated vesicles as observed in the NIV are present in the outer zone of the median eminence (Rodriguez, 1969; Budtz, 1970; Peute and Mey, 1973). Moreover, Dierickx (1965) obtained evidence that Gomori-negative fibres, originating from cells in the caudal part of the lateral lobes, end near portal vessels. The material released by this route may contain one or more hypothalamic releasing factors.

With regard to the question which releasing factors are produced by the NIV, it is of interest that Stutinsky and Befort (1964) as well as Dierickx (1965) placed

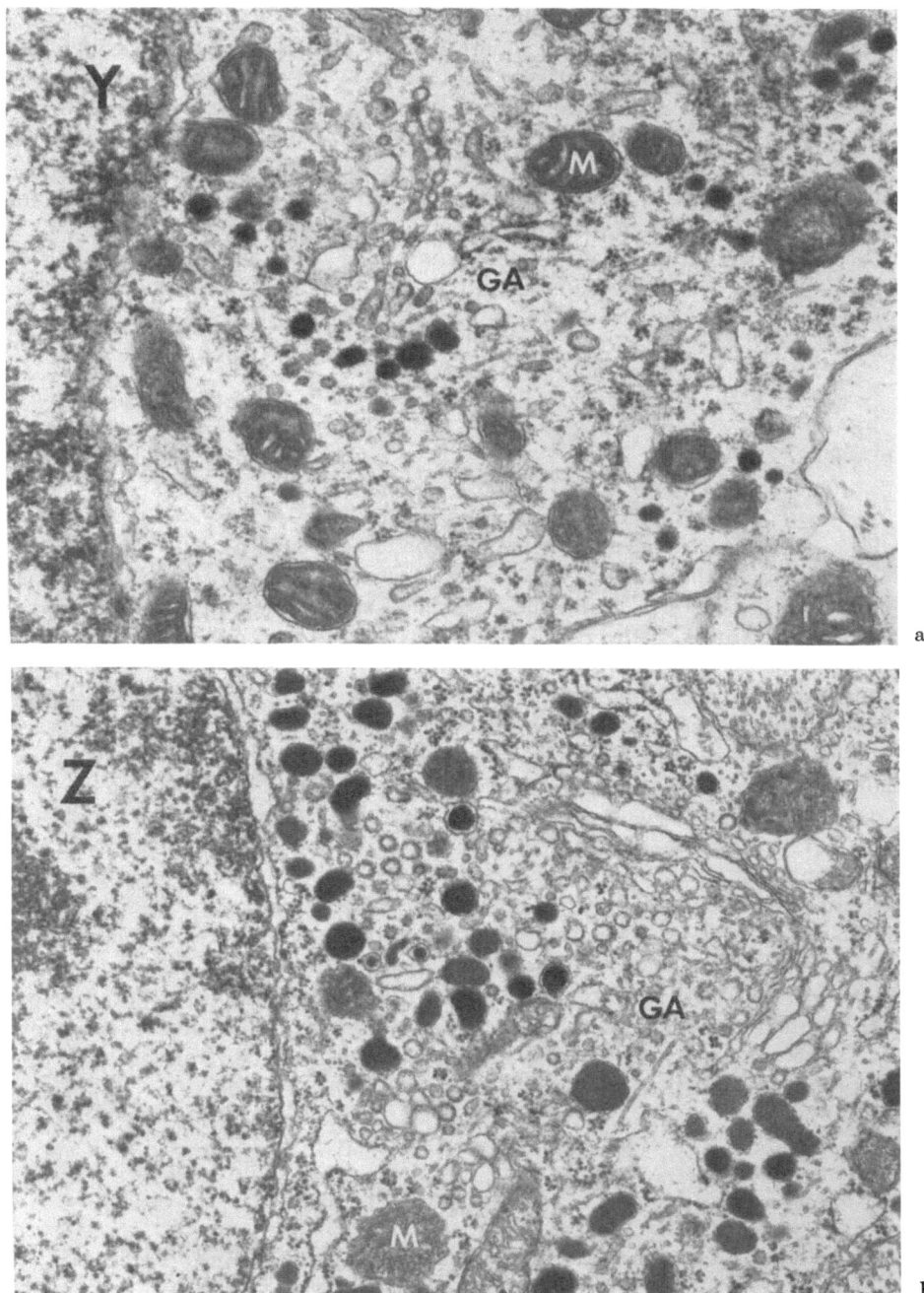

Fig. 3a and b. Part of Type Y cell and Type Z cell respectively, of the nucleus infundibularis ventralis of *Rana esculenta*. Note the difference in size between the secretory granules in the Y cells (± 1400 Å) and in the Z cells (± 1800 Å). GA = Golgi area; M = mitochondria (× 27 000)

the source of the gonadotropin releasing factor(s) in the ventro-caudal part of the lateral lobe of the infundibulum. Peute and Mey (1973) succeeded in inducing ultrastructural changes in the Y cells of the NIV in *Rana esculenta* both by castration and testosterone treatment. Two months after castration the number of granulated vesicles in the Y cells had increased, whereas in the testosterone treated animals granulated Y-cells had become scarce. Moreover, numerous Y-cells of the testosterone treated frogs contained widened cisternae of the rough endoplasmatic reticulum, filled with an heterogenous grey material. Comparing these changes with changes in the testes, the thumb pads and the gonadotropic cells of the adenohypophysis, Peute and Mey (1973) concluded that in *Rana esculenta* the Y cells of the NIV are involved in the regulation of the gonadotropic activity of the pituitary.

Summary

In the caudal hypothalamus of anurans, including *Xenopus laevis* and *Rana esculenta*, two paired monoaminergic nuclei have been found, i.e. the paraventricular organ (PVO) and the nucleus infundibularis dorsalis (NID). The PVO extends along the ventricular wall from the entrance of the infundibulum to the lateral dilatation of the infundibular recess. The NID borders the dorsal wall of the recessus lateralis infundibuli (syn. recessus mamillaris). Both nuclei contain two types of liquor-contacting neurons. In the PVO one cell type may have a sensory function, the other a secretory activity. The granular vesicles of the cells can store amines. The cell types in the NID may combine a sensory with a secretory function. In both nuclei dopamine occurs. An aminergic fibre tract links PVO and NID with the pars intermedia of the hypophysis. This tract has a function in the regulation of the MSH release. *In vitro* studies point to a catecholaminergic nature of the melanotropin inhibiting hormone.

A paired Gomori- and Falck-negative neurosecretory centre is present in the lateral lobes of the caudal hypothalamus of anurans, including *Xenopus laevis* and *Rana esculenta*. This nucleus infundibularis ventralis (NIV) contains two types of peptidergic, bipolar liquor-contacting neurons. Elementary granules are transported in axons ending in the outer zone of the median eminence. The results of castration and testosterone treatment indicate that one of the cell types is involved in the regulation of the gonadotropic activity of the adenohypophysis.

References

Akert, K., Sandri, C.: An electron-microscopic study of zinc iodide-osmium impregnation of neurons. I. Staining of synaptic vesicles at cholinergic junctions. Brain Res. **7**, 286—295 (1968).

Bartels, W.: Die Ontogenese der aminhaltigen Neuronensysteme im Gehirn von *Rana temporaria*. Z. Zellforsch. **116**, 94—118 (1971).

Braak, H.: Biogene Amine im Gehirn vom Frosch *(Rana esculenta)*. Z. Zellforsch. **106**, 269—308 (1970).

Budtz, P.E.: Effect of transection at different levels of hypothalamus on the hypothalamo-hypophysial system of the toad, *Bufo bufo*, with particular reference to the ultrastructure of the zona externa of the median eminence. Z. Zellforsch. **107**, 210—233 (1970).

Celis, M.E., Taleisnik, S., Walter, R.: Regulation of formation and proposed structure of the factor inhibiting the release of melanocyte-stimulating hormone. Proc. nat. Acad. Sci. (Wash.) **68**, 1428—1433 (1971).

Cohen, A.G.: Observations on the pars intermedia of *Xenopus laevis*. Nature (Lond.) **215**, 55—56 (1967).

Daems, W.Th., Wisse, E., Brederoo, P.: Electron microscopy of the vacuolar apparatus. In: Dingle, J.T., Fell, H.B. (Eds.): Lysosomes in biology and pathology, Vol. I, pp. 64—114. Amsterdam-London: North-Holland 1969.

Dierickx, K.: The origin of the aldehyde-fuchsin-negative nerve fibres of the median eminence of the hypophysis: a gonadotropic centre. Z. Zellforsch. **66**, 504—518 (1965).

Dierickx, K., Druyts, A., Vandenberghe, M.P., Goossens, N.: Identification of adenohypophysiotropic neurohormone producing neurosecretory cells in *Rana temporaria*. I. Ultrastructural evidence for the presence of neurosecretory cells in the tuber cinereum. Z. Zellforsch. **134**, 459—504 (1972).

Doerr-Schott, J., Follenius, E.: Localisation des fibres aminergiques dans l'hypophyse de *Rana esculenta*. Etude autoradiographique au microscope électronique. C. R. Acad. Sci. (Paris) **269**, 737—740 (1969).

Doerr-Schott, J., Follenius, E.: Innervation de l'hypophyse intermédiaire de *Rana esculenta*, et identification des fibres aminergiques par autoradiographie au microscope électronique. Z. Zellforsch. **106**, 99—108 (1970).

Enemar, A., Falck, B.: On the presence of adrenergic nerves in the pars intermedia of the frog, *Rana temporaria*. Gen. comp. Endocr. **5**, 577—583 (1965).

Enemar, A., Falck, B., Iturriza, F.C.: Adrenergic nerves in the pars intermedia of the pituitary in the toad, *Bufo arenarum*. Z. Zellforsch. **77**, 325—330 (1967).

Falck, B., Hillarp, N.-Å., Thieme, G., Torp, A.: Fluorescence of catecholamines and related compounds condensed with formaldehyde. J. Histochem. Cytochem. **10**, 348—354 (1962).

Glenner, G.G., Burtner, H.J., Brown, G.R.: The histochemical demonstration of monoamine oxidase activity by tetrazolium salts. J. Histochem. Cytochem. **5**, 591—600 (1957).

Goos, H.J.Th.: Hypothalamic control of the pars intermedia in *Xenopus laevis* tadpoles. Z. Zellforsch. **97**, 118—124 (1969).

Goos, H.J.Th., van Halewijn, R.: Biogenic amines in the hypothalamus of *Xenopus laevis* tadpoles. Naturwissenschaften **55**, 393—394 (1968).

Goos, H.J.Th., van Ree, G.E., van Oordt, P.G.W.J.: Aminergic neurosecretion in the hypothalamus of *Xenopus laevis* tadpoles. Gen. comp. Endocr. **18**, 593 (1972).

Hopkins, C.R.: Localization of adrenergic fibers in the amphibian pars intermedia by electron microscope autoradiography and their selective removal by 6-hydroxydopamine. Gen. comp. Endocr. **16**, 112—120 (1971).

Hopkins, C.R.: The biosynthesis, intracellular transport and packaging of melanocyte-stimulating peptides in the amphibian pars intermedia. J. Cell Biol. **53**, 642—653 (1972).

Imai, K.: Color change and pituitary function in *Xenopus laevis*. In: Kawamura, T., Fitzpatrick, T.B., Seiji, M. (Eds.): Biology of normal and abnormal melanocytes, pp. 17—30. Baltimore-London-Tokyo: University Park Press 1971.

Ito, T.: Changes in skin color and fine structure of the intermediate pituitary gland of the frog, *Rana nigromaculata*, after extirpation of the median eminence. Neuroendocrinology **8**, 180—197 (1971).

Iturriza, F.C.: Electronmicroscopic study of the pars intermedia of the pituitary of the toad, *Bufo arenarum*. Gen. comp. Endocr. **4**, 492—502 (1964).

Keller, H.H.: Depletion of cerebral monoamines by *p*-Chlorophenylalanine in the cat. Experientia (Basel) **28**, 177 (1972).

Knowles, F.: Neuronal properties of neurosecretory cells. In: Stutinsky, F. (Ed.): Neurosecretion, pp. 8—19. Berlin-Heidelberg-New York: Springer 1967.

Nagasawa, J., Douglas, W.W., Schulz, R.A.: Ultrastructural evidence of secretion by exocytosis and of "synaptic vesicle" formation in posterior pituitary gland. Nature (Lond.) **227**, 407—409 (1970).

Nair, R. M. G., Kastin, A. J., Schally, A. V.: Isolation and structure of hypothalamic MSH release inhibiting hormone. Biochem. biophys. Res. Commun. **43**, 1376—1381 (1971).

Nakai, Y., Gorbman, A.: Evidence for a double innervated secretory unit in the anuran pars intermedia. II. Electron microscopic studies. Gen. comp. Endocr. **13**, 108—116 (1969).

Nyholm, N. E. I.: Hypophysial activity and melanophore regulation in early *Xenopus* tadpoles. Gen. comp. Endocr. **18**, 613 (1972).

van Oordt, P. G. W. J., Goos, H. J. Th., Peute, J., Terlou, M.: Hypothalamo-hypophysial relations in amphibian larvae. Gen. comp. Endocr. Suppl. **3**, 41—50 (1972).

Parent, A.: Distribution of monoamine-containing neurons in the brain stem of the frog, *Rana temporaria*. J. Morph. **139**, 67—78 (1973).

Pehlemann, F. W.: Ultrastructure and innervation of the pars intermedia of the pituitary of *Xenopus laevis*. Gen. comp. Endocr. **9**, 481 (1967).

Peute, J.: Fine structure of the paraventricular organ of *Xenopus laevis* tadpoles. Z. Zellforsch. **97**, 564—575 (1969).

Peute, J.: Somato-dendritic synapses in the paraventricular organ of two anuran species. Z. Zellforsch. **112**, 31—41 (1971).

Peute, J.: Ultrastructural aspects of the nucleus infundibularis dorsalis in the hypothalamus of *Xenopus laevis*. Z. Zellforsch. **137**, 513—520 (1973).

Peute, J., Mey, J. C. A.: Ultrastructural and functional aspects of the nucleus infundibularis ventralis in *Rana esculenta*. Z. Zellforsch. **144**, 191—217 (1973).

Peute, J., van Oordt, P. G. W. J.: Ultrastructural and functional aspects of Gomori-negative neurosecretory cells in the caudal hypothalamus of Amphibia. Fortschr. Zool. **22**, 134—154 (1974).

Plotnikoff, N. P., Kastin, A. J., Anderson, M. S., Schally, A. V.: DOPA potentiation by a hypothalamic factor, MSH release-inhibiting hormone (MIF). Life Sci. **10**, 1279—1283 (1971).

Plotnikoff, N. P., Kastin, A. J., Anderson, M. S., Schally, A. V.: Deserpidine antagonism by a tripeptide, L-Prolyl-L-Leucylglycinamide. Neuroendocrinology **11**, 67—71 (1973).

Rodriguez, E. M.: Ependymal specializations. I. Fine structure of the neural (internal) region of the toad median eminence, with particular reference to the connections between the ependymal cells and the subependymal capillary loops. Z. Zellforsch. **102**, 153—171 (1969).

Saland, L. C.: Ultrastructure of the frog pars intermedia in the relation to hypothalamic control of hormone release. Neuroendocrinology **3**, 72—88 (1968).

Schally, A. W., Kastin, A. J.: Hypothalamic releasing and inhibiting hormones. Gen. comp. Endocr. Suppl. **3**, 76—85 (1972).

Stutinsky, F., Befort, J. J.: Effects des stimulations électriques du diencéphale de *Rana esculenta* mâle. Gen. comp. Endocr. **4**, 370—379 (1964).

Terlou, M., Goos, H. J. Th., van Oordt, P. G. W. J.: Hypothalamic regulation of pars intermedia activity in Amphibians. Fortschr. Zool. **22**, 117—133 (1974).

Terlou, M., Ploemacher, R. E.: The distribution of monoamines in the tel-, di-, and mesencephalon of *Xenopus laevis* tadpoles, with special reference to the hypothalamo-hypophysial system. Z. Zellforsch. **137**, 521—540 (1973).

Terlou, M., van Kooten, H.: Microspectrofluorometric identification of formaldehyde induced fluorescence in hypothalamic nuclei of *Xenopus laevis* tadpoles. Z. Zellforsch. **147**, 529—536 (1974).

Terlou, M., van Straaten, H. W. M.: The development of a hypothalamic monoaminergic system for the regulation of the pars intermedia activity in *Xenopus laevis*. Z. Zellforsch. **143**, 229—238 (1973).

Terlou, M., Stroband, H. W. J.: The distribution of monoamine oxidase and acetylcholinesterase in the brain of *Xenopus laevis* tadpoles. Z. Zellforsch. **140**, 261—275 (1973).

Vigh, B.: Das Paraventrikularorgan und das zirkumventrikuläre System des Gehirns. Studia Biol. Acad. Scient. Hung., Vol. 10 (Ed. J. Szentágothai). Budapest 1971.

Whur, P., Weatherhead, B.: Rates of incorporation of ³H-leucine into protein of the pars intermedia of the pituitary in the amphibian *Xenopus laevis* after change of background colour. J. Endocr. **51**, 521—532 (1971).

Control of Prolactin Secretion in the Goldfish, *Carassius auratus**

R. E. PETER and B. A. McKEOWN

Department of Zoology, University of Alberta, Edmonton (Canada) and
Department of Zoology, University of Guelph, Guelph (Canada)

The osmoregulatory function of prolactin in teleost fishes has been extensively studied (e.g., Lam, 1972; Utida et al., 1972). However, relatively little is known about the control of prolactin secretion in teleosts.

In organ culture, prolactin cells of the trout *Salmo fario* appear active histologically (Baker, 1963). Cultured prolactin cells from *Fundulus heteroclitus* have been shown by Emmart and Mossakowski (1967) to spontaneously synthesize prolactin in amounts detectable by the fluorescent-antibody technique. These findings suggest that teleost prolactin cells are spontaneously active independent of hypothalamic influence.

Sage (1968) observed that dilution of the organ culture medium stimulated the secretory activity of prolactin cells of *Xiphophorus* sp. He suggested that activity of prolactin cells in teleosts may normally be controlled by osmotic stimuli. In view of the osmoregulatory function of prolactin, such a control mechanism would have great functional significance. However, there is no evidence to support the existence of such a control mechanism *in vivo*.

In pituitary transplant studies done on a variety of teleosts, the prolactin cells surviving in the grafts generally appeared hyperactive histologically (for review: Ball et al., 1972; Peter, 1973). This was interpreted to indicate that the hypothalamus normally inhibits their spontaneous activity. This suggests the presence of a prolactin inhibitory factor (PIF) in teleosts.

The present study was designed to determine the regions of the hypothalamus that are involved in the control of prolactin secretion in goldfish. Electrolytic lesions were stereotaxically placed in various locations of the hypothalamus and thalamus, and the effects of destruction of various nuclei on serum and pituitary prolactin levels determined.

Materials and Methods

Goldfish were acclimated to laboratory conditions for at least 14 days before starting each experiment. At the end of the acclimation period the fish were divided

---
* This study was supported by grant A-6371 to R.E. Peter and grant A-6978 to B.A. McKeown from the National Research Council of Canada.

into four groups: a normal control group, a sham-operated group, and two groups in which lesions were stereotaxically placed. Lesion and sham operations were performed according to the procedure of Peter (1970) as modified by Peter and Gill (1974). At 26 days post-operatively the fish were killed. A blood sample was taken from each fish, and a serum sample frozen for subsequent prolactin determination. The brain from each fish was dissected out and fixed in Bouin's solution. The brains were subsequently histologically examined and the exact lesion location plotted on a diagram. The pituitary was also dissected out, weighed, and frozen.

Serum and pituitary prolactin levels were measured by radioimmunoassay according to the technique of Leatherland and McKeown (1973, 1974) and Leatherland et al. (1974). Prolactin levels of the sham-operated animals and the normal control animals were similar in each experiment. Within an experiment, the serum and pituitary prolactin values, respectively, of animals with lesions in a common location were grouped for comparison to the normal and sham control groups. Significance was tested by Student's t test.

Results and Discussion

Lesions that completely destroyed the nucleus preopticus and partially destroyed adjoining periventricular nuclei had no effect on serum or pituitary prolactin levels. Lesions in the nucleus anterior tuberis of the dorsal hypothalamus also had no effect. Similarly lesions in the nucleus lateralis tuberis (NLT) pars anterior, NLT pars inferior, or the NLT pars posterior had no effect on serum or pituitary prolactin levels. Complete bilateral destruction of the nucleus lateralis tuberis pars lateralis (NLTl, see Fig. 1) caused a significant elevation in serum prolactin levels, but had no effect on pituitary prolactin content. Animals with only unilateral destruction of the NLTl had serum prolactin levels similar to the control values. Animals with large lesions involving the anterior and dorsal hypothalamic-medial thalamic region (see Fig. 2) had significantly lower serum prolactin levels than either of the two control groups. Pituitary prolactin content of this lesioned group was not significantly different from values for the control groups, but showed a tendency to be higher. No other lesioned group had a similar deviation from control values in pituitary prolactin content.

The increase in serum prolactin following complete bilateral destruction of the NLTl indicates that this region has an inhibitory effect on prolactin secretion. Lesions in other locations, all around the NLTl, did not cause a significant increase in serum prolactin. Thus, the results support the idea of a PIF in teleosts and indicate that it originates from the NLTl.

In various mammals, lesions in the basal tuberal hypothalamus, and in the paraventricular nucleus region, result in increased prolactin secretion (for review: Pasteels, 1970). PIF in mammals may therefore originate, at least in part, from the basal tuberal region. This suggests that to some extent homologous regions of the hypothalamus may be involved in regulation of prolactin secretion in mammals and teleosts.

The decrease in serum prolactin due to the large lesions in the anterior and dorsal hypothalamic-medial thalamic region cannot be easily interpreted. The

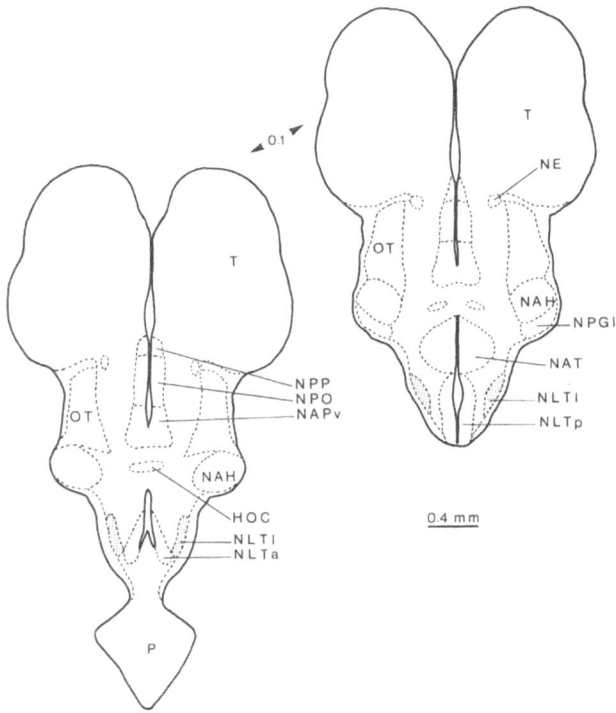

Fig. 1. Diagrammatic cross-sections through the forebrain of the goldfish. The shaded area is the nucleus lateralis tuberis pars lateralis (NLTl). The region of destruction of the lesions included the NLTl and adjacent tissues within a radius of not more than 0.1 mm. The distance between the two cross-sections is given in mm. HOC = horizontal commissure; NAH = nucleus anterioris hypothalami; NAPv = nucleus anterioris periventricularis; NAT = nucleus anterior tuberis; NE = nucleus entopeduncularis; NLTa = nucleus lateralis tuberis pars anterioris; NLTp = nucleus lateralis tuberis pars posterior; NPGl = nucleus preglomerulosus pars lateralis; NPO = nucleus preopticus; NPP = nucleus preopticus periventricularis; OT = optic tract; P = pituitary, T = telencephalon

result could have been due to the destruction of a center that is the origin of a prolactin releasing factor (PRF). However, there is no firm evidence to support the presence of a PRF in teleosts (see Peter, 1973). Probably a more reasonable explanation is that the large lesions interrupted neural afferents to the NLTl that normally inhibit the secretion of PIF. Destruction of such inhibitory afferents would allow for more PIF secretion and cause a decrease in prolactin secretion. Pathways that have a similar function as hypothesized above have been demonstrated in the rabbit by Tindal and Knaggs (1972). They found that electrical stimulation of medio-dorsal and preoptic hypothalamic regions, amongst other locations, caused an increase in prolactin secretion. Stimulation of these centers presumably caused the increase in prolactin secretion by activation of pathways that resulted in inhibition of PIF secretion.

Although no significant changes in pituitary prolactin content were observed in the study, there was a trend to a higher level in the anterior and dorsal hypo-

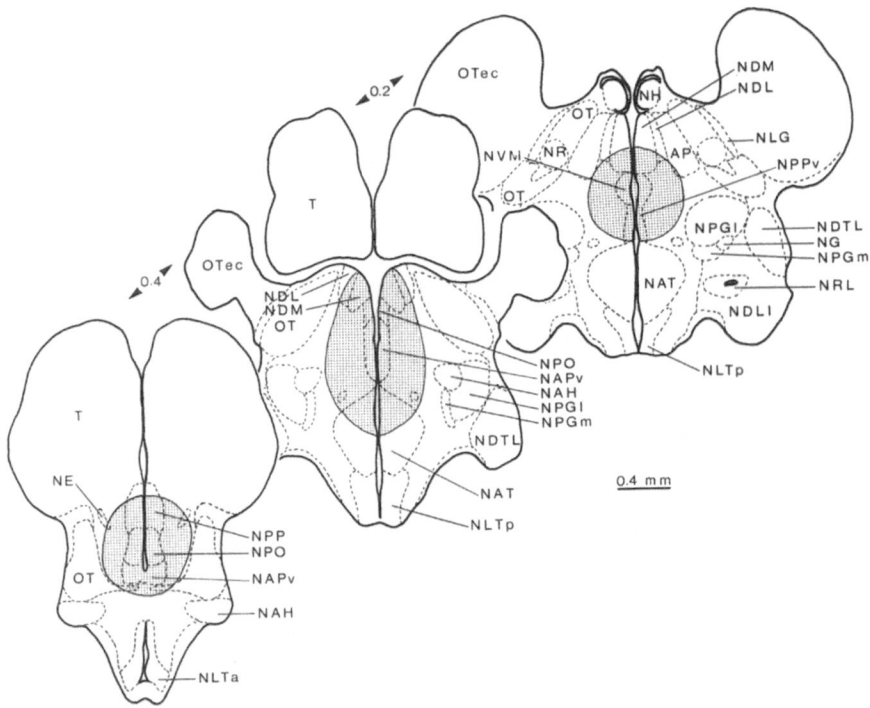

Fig. 2. Diagrammatic cross-sections through the forebrain of the goldfish. The shaded area represents the general region of destruction of the lesions. The distance between the cross-sections is given in mm. AP = area pretectalis; NAH = nucleus anterioris hypothalami; NAPv = nucleus anterioris periventricularis; NAT = nucleus anterior tuberis; NDL = nucleus dorsolateralis thalami; NDM = nucleus dorsomedialis thalami; NDLI = nucleus diffusus lobi inferioris; NDTL = nucleus diffusus tori lateralis; NE = nucleus entopeduncularis; NG = nucleus glomerulosus; NH = nucleus habenularis; NLG = nucleus lateralis geniculatus; NLTa = nucleus lateralis tuberis pars anterior; NLTp = nucleus lateralis tuberis pars posterior; NPGl = nucleus preglomerulosus pars lateralis; NPGm = nucleus preglomerulosus pars medialis; NPO = nucleus preopticus; NPP = nucleus preopticus periventricularis; NPPv = nucleus posterioris periventricularis; NR = nucleus rotundus; NRL = nucleus recessus lateralis; NVM = nucleus ventromedialis thalami; OT = optic tract; OTec = optic tectum; T = telencephalon

thalamic-medial thalamic lesioned animals. This was accompanied by a significant decrease in serum prolactin. It may be that under conditions of low prolactin secretion, pituitary content of the hormone increases. The relationship between pituitary content and the secretion rate of prolactin in teleosts deserves further investigation.

Summary

Electrolytic lesions were stereotaxically placed in various regions of the hypothalamus and thalamus of goldfish, and the effects of destruction of various nuclei on serum and pituitary prolactin levels determined. Lesions in only the nucleus lateralis tuberis pars lateralis caused a significant increase in serum prolactin levels, indicating that this region has an inhibitory effect on prolactin secretion. This supports the idea of a prolactin inhibitory factor in teleosts. Large lesions in the anterior and dorsal hypothalamic-medial thalamic region caused a significant decrease in serum prolactin levels and tended to cause an increase in pituitary prolactin content. These lesions may have interrupted neural pathways that normally inhibit the secretion of prolactin inhibitory factor.

References

Baker, B. I.: Comportement en culture organotypique des cellules de la truite. C. R. Acad. Sci. (Paris) **256**, 3356—3358 (1963).

Ball, J. N., Baker, B. I., Olivereau, M., Peter, R. E.: Investigations on hypothalamic control of adenohypophysial functions in teleost fishes. Gen. comp. Endocr. Suppl. **3**, 11—21 (1972).

Emmart, E. W., Mossakowski, M. J.: The localization of prolactin in cultured cells of the rostral pars distalis of the pituitary of *Fundulus heteroclitus* (Linnaeus). Gen. comp. Endocr. **9**, 391—400 (1967).

Lam, T. J.: Prolactin and hydromineral regulation in fishes. Gen. comp. Endocr. Suppl. **3**, 328—338 (1972).

Leatherland, J. F., McKeown, B. A., John, T. M.: Circadian rhythm of plasma prolactin, growth hormone, glucose and free fatty acid in juvenile kokanee salmon, *Oncorhynchus nerka*. Comp. Biochem. Physiol. **47 A**, 821—828 (1974).

Leatherland, J. F., McKeown, B. A.: Circadian rhythm in plasma levels of prolactin in goldfish, *Carassius auratus*. J. interdiscipl. Cycle Res. **4**, 137—143 (1973).

Leatherland, J. F., McKeown, B. A.: Effect of ambient salinity on prolactin and growth hormone secretion and on hydro-mineral regulation in kokanee salmon smolts *(Oncorhynchus nerka)*. J. comp. Physiol. **89**, 215—226 (1974).

Pasteels, J. L.: Control of prolactin secretion. In: Martini, L., Motta, M., Fraschini, F. (Eds.): The hypothalamus, p. 385. New York-London: Academic Press 1970.

Peter, R. E.: Hypothalamic control of thyroid gland activity and gonadal activity in the goldfish, *Carassius auratus*. Gen. comp. Endocr. **14**, 334—356 (1970).

Peter, R. E.: Neuroendocrinology of teleosts. Amer. Zool. **13**, 743—755 (1973).

Peter, R. E., Gill, V. E.: A stereotaxic atlas and technique for forebrain nuclei of the goldfish, *Carassius auratus*. J. comp. Neurol. In press (1974).

Sage, M.: Responses to osmotic stimuli of *Xiphophorus* prolactin cells in organ culture. Gen. comp. Endocr. **10**, 70—74 (1968).

Tindal, J. S., Knaggs, G. S.: Pathways in the forebrain of the rabbit concerned with the release of prolactin. J. Endocr. **52**, 253—262 (1972).

Utida, S., Hirano, T., Oide, H., Ando, M., Johnson, D. W., Bern, H. A.: Hormonal control of the intestine and urinary bladder in teleost osmoregulation. Gen. comp. Endocr. Suppl. **3**, 317—327 (1972).

Pars Intermedia Control with and without Innervation — Studies in Elasmobranchs and a Lizard*

PATRICK MEURLING and LEONARD LARSSON

Department of Zoology, University of Lund, LUND (Sweden)

In recent years the structure and function of the pituitary pars intermedia of vertebrates have attracted a great deal of interest (see reviews by Etkin, 1967; Dodd et al., 1971; Rodriguez and Gimenez, 1972; Bagnara and Hadley, 1973). Apart from mammals, in which the function of the intermedia is still enigmatic, the Amphibia have, for a number of reasons, been the most thoroughly investigated. This report will deal chiefly with work from our laboratory on the control of the pars intermedia in Elasmobranchs and in the lizard *Anolis carolinensis*.

Elasmobranchs

Twenty years ago, Ernst Scharrer (1952) applied the chrome-alum hematoxylin technique to the hypothalamus and pituitary of the spotted dogfish, *Scyliorhinus stellaris*, and described the neurosecretory hypothalamo-hypophysial system. In contrast to higher vertebrates, the endings of the tract did not form a distinct neural lobe, but were dispersed within the pars intermedia.

Scharrer's interest was, then, mainly to determine how the neural lobe hormones reached the blood stream; but the question soon arose: Do the neurosecretory fibres have any functional significance to the pars intermedia ? Bargmann (1955) observed conditions similar to those of *Scyliorhinus* to be present in some other Elasmobranch species.

Studies with light microscopical methods in various species (Meurling, 1962, 1963, 1967 a) indicated that the hypothalamo-hypophysial tract besides neurosecretory fibres contained fibres of other kinds, which were stainable with silver methods. This was also the case with the neuro-intermediate lobe of *Scyliorhinus*, *Pristiurus*, *Mustelus*, and *Raja*. In these cases silver-stained fibres accompanied the neurosecretory fibres into the intermedia parenchyma. But in *Etmopterus spinax* the neural and intermediate lobes were separated by a vascular membrane, and neurosecretory nerve endings in the intermedia were rather scanty. On the other hand, non-neurosecretory silver-stained fibres penetrated the entire lobe and formed a plexus among the secretory poles of the cells. Lastly, in the spiny dogfish, *Squalus acanthias*, the two lobes were distinct, and with the light micro-

---

* Supported by grants from the Swedish Natural Science Research Council.

scope only some occasional silver-stained fibres could be observed to enter the intermedia. There thus appears to be a considerable variation in the morphological picture of the neural lobe – pars intermedia interrelationship.

Studies of the vascular system of the pituitary region of *Scyliorhinus* (Mellinger, 1960, 1963a; Meurling, 1960, 1967a) and several other species (Meurling, 1967a and b) revealed distinct vascular pathways linking the hypothalamus with the neuro-intermediate lobe (apart from those supplying the rostral and median lobes).

In all Elasmobranchs the basic blood system of the neuro-intermediate lobe is a plexus (corresponding to the plexus intermedius of higher vertebrates) that is interposed between the neural and intermediate components, but is modified in those cases when the lobes are fused. Arising from this plexus is a rich supply of vessels penetrating the intermedia. In striking contrast to amphibians and mammals there is a very rich blood supply of the intermedia in Elasmobranchs – not surprising, however, considering the large size of the organ.

Considerable variations in the vascular arrangement exist between different species, but as a generalization it may be stated that there is usually some kind of hypothalamo-intermedia vascular connection (rather insignificant in *Squalus*) and that in those species in which the innervation of the intermedia is feeble *(Squalus, Etmopterus)* the vascular neural lobe-intermedia connections are well developed: such connections are, however, prominent also in other cases, e.g. *Raja*.

The experimental work by Mellinger (1963b) showed that after lesions in the hypothalamus – stalk region in *Scyliorhinus*, there was an irreversible darkening of the fish. The neurosecretory fibres, being the most evident component of the neuro-intermedia innervation at this time, were suggested as being responsible for inhibiting MSH release.

But Knowles (1965), also in *Scyliorhinus*, confirmed with the electron microscope that in this species not only neurosecretory fibres but also other kinds were present in the neuro-intermediate lobe. Type-A fibres, i.e. classical neurosecretory fibres, made close contacts with the synthetic poles of the intermedia cells, and B fibres, suspected to be aminergic, were observed to connect with the release poles. Later work has modified this picture somewhat, so that both types of fibres, and perhaps some other types, may be found in association with various parts of the intermedia cells (Knowles, personal communication).

Raja radiata

Knowles (1965) suggested that A fibres were involved in the control of hormone synthesis and B fibres in hormone release. We had the opportunity to test this hypothesis in the skate *Raja radiata*, whose neuro-intermediate lobe is rather similar to that of *Scyliorhinus*. In the skates both A and B fibres make synapselike contacts with intermedia cells, but with no special polarity (Chevins, 1972).

The hypophysial stem in *Raja radiata* is very broad and is covered with vessels, many of which run from the posterior hypothalamus to the neuro-intermediate lobe. In this stem the neurosecretory fibres were found to be present almost exclusively in a narrow median tract, whereas the lateral parts were almost devoid of them (Meurling, 1967a). An electron microscopic study (Meurling, 1967c) confirmed this and revealed B-Type fibres in the lateral parts.

When applying the Falck-Hillarp technique for biogenic amines to the neuro-intermediate lobe of the skate (Meurling and Björklund, 1971), we found many specific fluorescent nerve endings (with the characteristics of catecholamines) among the intermedia cells, especially around the release poles close to the vessels.

Since the adrenergic, MSH release-inhibiting innervation of amphibians is rather well established (Enemar and Falck, 1965; Enemar et al., 1967; Iturriza, 1967, 1969; Goos, 1969; Doerr-Schott and Follenius, 1970) it was natural to suspect the observed adrenergic innervation to be involved in intermedia control. An experimental study of the skate (Meurling et al., 1969; Meurling and Fremberg, 1974) first showed that reserpine treatment gave results similar to what is obtained in Amphibia, i.e. darkening of the skin owing to uninhibited MSH release. This did not occur in neurointermediate lobectomized specimens.

Discrete transections were then made in the stem region so as to compare the effect of severing the median and lateral parts. When the median tract, which contains most of the neurosecretory fibres bound for the neuro-intermediate lobe, was transected there was usually no observable effect on colour change: the specimens were able to respond to changes in background as accurately as before the operation.

But when the lateral parts, which are believed to carry most of the B fibres to the neuro-intermediate lobe, were severed, an irreversible darkening usually occurred. However, some specimens responded in the opposite manner; and Chevins and Dodd (1970) reported darkening after transecting the neurosecretory tract. But all of these discrepancies are readily explained by the disposition of the fibres: the tract appears to be mixed in the hypothalamus and to a varying degree in the stem; the separation of fibres occurs gradually (Meurling and Fremberg, 1974). Therefore, lesions at a slightly anteriorly situated level will cause severance of both kinds of fibres.

It should be pointed out that in the lateral lesions not only nerve fibres but also blood vessels are damaged. The interruption of the hypothetical neurovascular connection between the hypothalamus and the intermedia might be of some significance.

To sum up, the experiments with *Raja radiata* gave evidence that adrenergic fibres were responsible for the release inhibition of MSH secretion. Further investigations in *Scyliorhinus* by Wilson and Dodd (1973a and b) have also clearly elucidated a similar role for adrenergic fibres in this species. On the other hand, the role of the Type A neurosecretory fibres remained obscure. It may be recalled that Dierickx (1967) has provided evidence that neurosecretory fibres are not essential for normal colour change in *Rana temporaria*.

Squalus acanthias

To obtain some suggestions of the possible role of the neurosecretory A fibres in intermedia regulation, we turned to a species in which such fibres are absent in this gland to determine whether there was any difference in intermediate lobe function. The species is the previously mentioned *Squalus acanthias*, in which the neural and intermediate lobes are separated by a continuous vascular membrane (Meurling, 1962).

Adult *Squalus acanthias* are on account of their size not practicable for experimental work, but nearly full-term yolk-sac embryos, taken from the mothers by simple "Caesarean" section, appeared to be a suitable material, at least for short-term experiments. They survived well in aquaria and exhibited rapid and distinct colour changes when exposed to different backgrounds.

The histology of the neuro-intermediate lobe at this early stage is very similar to that of the adult, with strongly staining intermedia cells. The electron microscope revealed nerve endings of various kinds in the neural lobe and granule-containing endocrine cells in the intermedia manifesting secretory activity. The vascular membrane between the two lobes seemed to be continuous, but evidently nerve fibres pass through it to some degree, for small B-Type nerve profiles were discerned in the intermedia, especially located around the synthetic poles of the endocrine cells. Typical A-Type fibres have as yet not been observed in the intermedia.

The Falck-Hillarp fluorescence method revealed strong specific fluorescence in the neural lobe and small varicosities within the intermedia in positions similar to those of the B fibres observed with the electron microscope. It thus seemed likely that adrenergic fibres would be involved in intermedia control. A precise control mechanism could be postulated from the rapid and distinct colourchanging behaviour.

A series of experiments, including reserpine treatment, pituitary stalk transection, and neuro-intermediate lobe transplantation, provided evidence that the intermedia is regulated by an adrenergic inhibitory mechanism (Meurling, 1972; Meurling et al., 1973). Hence, the function and control of the pars intermedia in this species resembles – in spite of the considerable differences in structure – that of other Elasmobranchs which have been studied.

Although we have no positive evidence of the participation of neurosecretory fibres in pars intermedia control in Elasmobranchs, this possibility is not ruled out, especially since the vascular connections seem to allow neuro-intermediate connections. Bearing this in mind, the function of a pars intermedia that lacks innervation but which exhibits distinct vascular connections evokes interest. In order to find such a material, however, we have to turn to the Reptiles.

Anolis carolinensis

A number of lizard species have been found to lack intermedia innervation (Rodriguez and La Pointe, 1970; Pandalai and Sheela, 1969; Weatherhead, this volume), and this is also true for the lizard *Anolis carolinensis* (Forbes, 1972; Weatherhead, op. cit.).

The distinct and rapid colour changes of *Anolis* are regulated by purely hormonal mechanisms (Kleinholz, 1938a and b; Hadley and Goldman, 1969), with the intermedia responsible for the dark phase, and the disappearance of MSH from the circulation leading to pallor under normal conditions.

The neural lobe is the end-point for various kinds of nerve fibres, including peptidergic and adrenergic ones, and this lobe is in close contact with vessels of the plexus intermedius. This plexus in turn gives rise to the vascular supply of the intermedia, but there is also a vascular connection from the median eminence to the neurointermediate lobe (Meurling and Willstedt, 1970). Accordingly, it seems likely that substances released from the neurohypophysis act in intermedia control (Nayar and Pandalai, 1963; Sheela and Pandalai, 1965; Rodriguez, La Pointe, and Dellman, 1971; Rodriguez and Gimenez, 1972). To gain some knowledge of the nature of these substances and their actions, we have performed some experimental studies – partly of a preliminary nature – in *Anolis carolinensis* (cf. Larsson, 1973; Meurling et al., 1973).

The colour reactions of intact *Anolis* in the terrarium and on black and white illuminated backgrounds, and the conditions under which colour responses could be elicited, were carefully studied in long-term experiments (Larsson and Meurling, in preparation).

In order to minimize stress effects, which are of short duration, an adaptation time of 30 min was chosen, and for the experiments lizards were selected whose capacity to change colour in response to changes of background had been thoroughly tested.

In an experimental series with reserpine injections it was found that very high doses, around 30 mg/kg, were necessary to induce a disappearance of the specific amine fluorescence (Falck-Hillarp technique) in the hypothalamus and neural lobe. Even so, the only effect on colour change was a temporary loss of the ability to respond to a black background, contrary to what occurs in amphibians (Iturriza, 1966) and Elasmobranchs (Meurling and Fremberg, 1974), though this might have been a non-specific or peripheral effect. The lizards could still become brown in the terrarium.

In a second experiment, 9 lizards were neuro-intermediate lobectomized, and after a postoperative period of up to 60 days received grafts under the dorsal skin, one being the neuro-intermediate lobe and the other the rostral pars distalis, both from a fresh specimen. The immediate effect of the transplantation was usually an overall body darkening with a duration of about 1 day, but after that only a dark brown spot remained, overlying the transplanted neuro-intermedia, and a smaller spot above the rostral pars distalis. The latter, probably due to ACTH, was not affected by the treatment mentioned below.

Very minute amounts of MSH are sufficient to give rise to such a spot, as judged from in vitro studies (Hadley and Goldman, 1969). It may well be that this small amount of MSH leaks out passively and that the transplant is not actively secreting MSH (as the amphibian and Elasmobranch glands do under these conditions). This view is strengthened by the fact that when the animal is subjected to stress (intense handling for 1 min) the neuro-intermedia patch enlarges and becomes darker – i.e., there occurs a release of stored MSH (Fig. 1). In the intact lizard handling results in pallor.

It seems possible, however, that the effect of the handling on the transplant is due to increased levels of circulating catecholamines and/or other substances, released as a response to the stress. If this is the case, the MSH secretion must be

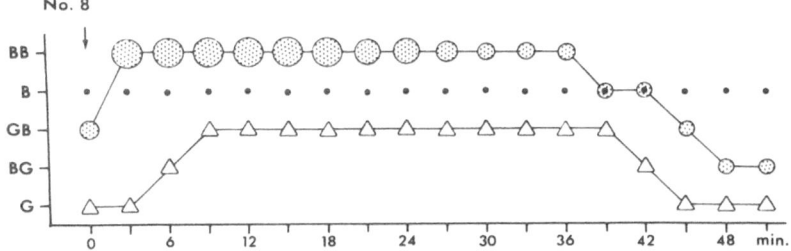

Fig. 1. *Anolis carolinensis*. Reactions which the dark skin patches overlying the transplanted neuro-intermediate lobe (open circles with dots) and rostral pars distalis (solid circles) undergo when the specimen is subjected to 1 min. stress (intense handling). The size of the circles is proportionate to their true size. The triangles denote overall body colour. Colour of skin (ordinate): G = green; BG = brownish green; GB = greenish brown; B = brown; BB = blackish brown (supernormal)

abundant to override the inhibitory action of the catecholamines on the effect of MSH on the melanophores.

We do not at this time propose that aminergic fibres promote MSH secretion in the intact pituitary in situ. The conditions under which adrenergic nerve endings affect secretory cells by synaptic transmission need not be the same as when circulating amines affect a transplant. So far we are only taking the results as an indication that the transplanted neuro-intermediate lobe contains stored MSH but that some kind of stimulus is required for its release.

To compare these effects with the activity of the disconnected neuro-intermediate lobe in situ, the pituitary stalk was transected in 49 specimens. The immediate effect of the operation (Fig. 2), here designated as Phase I, is a loss of

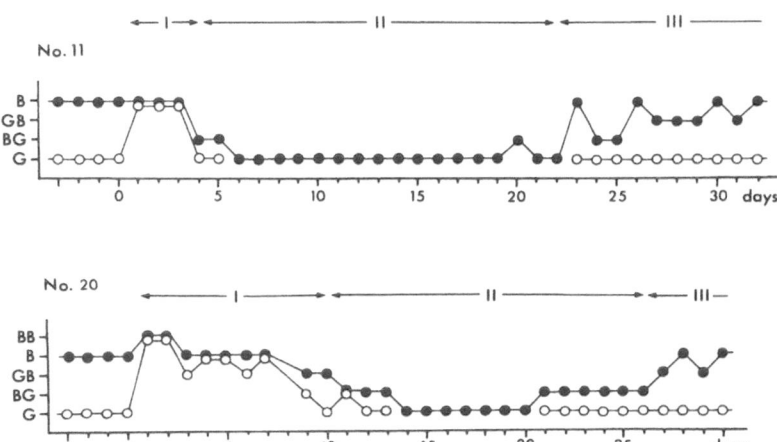

Fig. 2. *Anolis carolinensis*. Colour reactions of two specimens after pituitary stalk section on day O. Ordinate: colour of skin, see Fig. 1. Solid circles: skin colour after 30 min on a black background; open circles: skin colour after 30 min on a white background. Phases I—III are indicated

the ability to respond to a white background, usually lasting for about 3 days (mean 2.9 days; range 1–9 days). This phase may be comparable to the darkening obtained by Rodriguez et al. (1971) after stalk-section in *Klauberina*. Phase II is conversely characterized by the loss of the dark background response. This condition may last for a very variable period (mean 33 days; range 7–47 days), but is then followed by Phase III, during which normal colour reactions gradually reoccur. This latter phase is apparently accompanied by regeneration of nerve fibres – with the light microscope neurosecretory fibres may be seen entering the severed lobe. The latter finding is in contrast to the Amphibia, in which the disconnected neural lobe is not reinnervated (Rodriguez and Dellman, 1970). In the latter investigation, however, the transection was placed rostral to the median eminence.

It is too early to give a satisfactory explanation of the sequence of colour-change events that occur after pituitary-stalk section. It is hoped that work presently in progress on the ultrastructure and hormone content of the lobe in the different phases will, however, provide some clues.

Pandalai and Sheela (1969) suggested that MSH secretion in the lizard *Calotes* was controlled by stimulatory action of neurosecretory peptides, perhaps in combination with an adrenergic inhibitory system. A dual control system, as discussed above for Elasmobranchs, has also been suggested for the Amphibia (Oshima and Gorbman, 1969; Nakai and Gorbman, 1969; Jørgensen and Vijayakumar, 1971, and others). But there seems to be no agreement as to the nature of the non-adrenergic counterpart, although some type of peptidergic action seems likely.

Our present results could be made to fit the dual regulatory hypothesis by assuming that Phase I is the result of the withdrawal of both components in a double control system; that Phase II would signify the reappearance of one of these (inhibitory); and that Phase III would mark the return of the second component (stimulatory). But the results of the transplantation experiment could be interpreted to contradict this hypothesis: the transplanted lobe, in spite of an apparently healthy condition, did not seem to secrete, as the disconnected lobe in situ does for a time. This in turn could, however, be due to the difference in vascular arrangement: the transplanted neuro-intermediate lobe, when revascularized, cannot be expected to acquire the distinct vascular connections between neural lobe and intermedia that the lobe in situ will retain.

Another important consideration is that depriving the gland of its normal influences could lead to a sensitization or other kinds of modification of receptor properties. This also could be valid for the melanophores.

Thus there are still too many unknown variables, and a serious interpretation of these experiments will have to await the acquisition of further data. For the time being it may suffice to state that the control mechanisms of the pars intermedia of the lizard seem to be different from those of other vertebrates.

References

Bagnara, J. T., Hadley, M. E.: Chromatophores and color change. New Jersey: Prentice-Hall 1973.

Bargmann, W.: Weitere Untersuchungen am neurosekretorischen Zwischenhirn-Hypophysensystem. Z. Zellforsch. **42**, 247—272 (1955).

Chevins, P. F. D.: Ultrastructure of the pituitary complex in the genus *Raia* (Elasmobranchii). I. The pars neurointermedia. Z. Zellforsch. **130**, 193—204 (1972).

Chevins, P. F. D., Dodd, J. M.: Pituitary innervation and control of colour change in the skates *Raia naevus, R. clavata, R. montagui,* and *R. radiata.* Gen. comp. Endocr. **15**, 232—241 (1970).

Dierickx, K.: The function of the hypophysis without preoptic neurosecretory control. Z. Zellforsch. **78**, 114—130 (1967).

Dodd, J. M., Follett, B. K., Sharp, P. J.: Hypothalamic control of pituitary function in submammalian vertebrates. Adv. comp. Physiol. Biochem. **4**, 113—223 (1971).

Doerr-Schott, J., Follenius, E.: Innervation de l'hypophyse intermédiaire de *Rana esculenta,* et identification des fibres aminergiques par autoradiographie au microscope électronique. Z. Zellforsch. **106**, 99—118 (1970).

Enemar, A., Falck, B.: On the presence of adrenergic nerves in the pars intermedia of the frog, *Rana temporaria.* Gen. comp. Endocr. **5**, 577—583 (1965).

Enemar, A., Falck, B., Iturriza, F. C.: Adrenergic nerves in the pars intermedia of the pituitary in the toad, *Bufo arenarum.* Z. Zellforsch. **77**, 325—330 (1967).

Etkin, W.: Relation of the pars intermedia to the hypothalamus. In: Neuroendocrinology, Vol 2, pp. 261—282. New York: Academic Press 1967.

Forbes, M. S.: Observations on the fine structure of the pars intermedia in the lizard *Anolis carolinensis.* Gen. comp. Endocr. **18**, 146—161 (1972).

Goos, H. J.: Hypothalamic control of the pars intermedia in *Xenopus laevis* tadpoles. Z. Zellforsch. **97**, 118—124 (1969).

Hadley, M. E., Goldman, J. M.: Physiological color change in reptiles. Amer. Zoologist **9**, 489—504 (1969).

Iturriza, F. C.: Monoamines and control of the pars intermedia of the toad pituitary. Gen. comp. Endocr. **6**, 19—25 (1966).

Iturriza, F. C.: The secretion of intermedin in autotransplants of pars intermedia growing in the anterior chamber of intact and sympathectomized eyes of the toad. Neuroendocrinology **2**, 11—18 (1967).

Iturriza, F. C.: Further evidence for the blocking effect of catecholamines on the secretion of melanocyte-stimulating hormone in toads. Gen. comp. Endocr. **12**, 417—426 (1969).

Jørgensen, C. B., Vijayakumar, S.: Is the toad pars intermedia under both excitatory and inhibitory nervous control? Gen. comp. Endocr. **17**, 575—577 (1971).

Kleinholz, L. H.: Studies in reptilian colour changes. II. The pituitary and adrenal glands in the regulation of the melanophores of *Anolis carolinensis.* J. exp. Biol. **15**, 474—491 (1938a).

Kleinholz, L. H.: Studies in reptilian colour changes. III. Control of the light phase and behaviour of isolated skin. J. exp. Biol. **15**, 492—499 (1938b).

Knowles, F.: Evidence for a dual control, by neurosecretion, of hormone synthesis and hormone release in the pituitary of the dogfish, *Scylliorhinus stellaris.* Phil. Trans. B **249**, 435—456 (1965).

Larsson, L.: Background adaptation after total denervation of the pituitary in the lizard, *Anolis carolinensis.* In: Szentagothai, J., Hajos, F. (Eds.): VII. Conf. Europ. Comp. Endocrinol. Budapest 1973.

Mellinger, J. C. A.: Contribution à l'étude de la vascularisation et du développement de la région hypophysaire d'un sélacien, *Scyliorhinus caniculus* (L.) Bull. Soc. zool. France **85**, 123—139 (1960).

Mellinger, J. C. A.: Les relations neuro-vasculo-glandulaires dans l'appareil hypophysaire de la rousette, *Scyliorhinus caniculus* (L.). Thèse Strasbourg (Fac. Sci. Univ. Strasb. 238, Ser. E.) 1963a.

Mellinger, J. C. A.: Etude histophysiologique du système hypothalamo-hypophysaire de *Scyliorhinus caniculus* (L.) en état de mélanodispersion permanente. Gen. comp. Endocr. **3**, 26—45 (1963b).

Meurling, P.: Presence of a pituitary portal system in elasmobranchs. Nature (Lond.) **187**, 336—337 (1960).

Meurling, P.: The relations between neural and intermediate lobes in the pituitary of *Squalus acanthias*. Z. Zellforsch. **58**, 51—69 (1962).

Meurling, P.: Nerves of the neuro-intermediate lobe of *Etmopterus spinax* (Elasmobranchi). Z. Zellforsch. **61**, 183—201 (1963).

Meurling, P.: The vascularization of the pituitary in elasmobranchs. Sarsia **28**, 1—104 (1967a).

Meurling, P.: The vascularization of the pituitary in *Chimaera Monstrosa* (Holocephali). Sarsia **30**, 83—106 (1967b).

Meurling, P.: Observations of nerve-types in the hypophysial stem of *Raja radiata*. Acta Univ. Lund. II. **19**, 1—20 (1967).

Meurling, P.: Control of pars intermedia in large embryos of the spiny dogfish, *Squalus acanthias*. Gen. comp. Endocr. **18**, Abstract no 120 (1972).

Meurling, P., Björklund, A.: The arrangement of neurosecretory and catecholamine fibres in relation to the pituitary intermedia cells of the skate, *Raja radiata*. Z. Zellforsch. **108**, 81—92 (1970).

Meurling, P., Fremberg, M.: Effects of partial denervations of the neuro-intermediate lobe in the skate, *Raja radiata*. Acta Zool. **55**, 7—15 (1974).

Meurling, P., Fremberg, M., Björklund, A.: Control of MSH release in the intermediate lobe of *Raja radiata* (Elasmobranchii). Gen. comp. Endocr. **13**, Abstract no 99 (1969).

Meurling, P., Klefbohm, B., Larsson, L.: Transplantation of the pars intermedia in an elasmobranch and a lizard. In: Szentagothai, J., Hajos, F. (Eds.): VII. Conf. Europ. Comp. Endocrinol. Budapest 1973.

Meurling, P., Willstedt, A.: Vascular connections in the pituitary of *Anolis carolinensis* with special reference to the pars intermedia. Acta Zool. **51**, 211—218 (1970).

Nakai, Y., Gorbman, A.: Evidence for a doubly innervated secretory unit in the anuran pars intermedia. II. Electronmicroscopic studies. Gen. comp. Endocr. **13**, 108—116 (1969).

Nayar, S., Pandalai, K. R.: Pars intermedia of the pituitary gland and integumentary colour changes in the garden lizard *Calotes versicolor*. Z. Zellforsch. **58**, 837—845 (1963).

Oshima, K., Gorbman, A.: Evidence for a doubly innervated secretory unit in the anuran pars intermedia. I. Electrophysiologic studies. Gen. comp. Endocr. **13**, 98—107 (1969).

Pandalai, K. R., Sheela, R.: Hypothalamic control of the pars intermedia of the pituitary gland in the garden lizard, *Calotes versicolor*. Gen. comp. Endocr. Supp. **2**, 477—484 (1969).

Rodriguez, E. M., Dellmann, H.-D.: Hormonal content and ultrastructure of the disconnected neural lobe of the grass frog (*Rana pipiens*). Gen. comp. Endocr. **15**, 272—288 (1970).

Rodriguez, E. M., La Pointe, J.: Light and electron microscopic study of the pars intermedia of the lizard, *Klauberina riversiana*. Z. Zellforsch. **104**, 1—13 (1970).

Rodriguez, E. M., La Pointe, J., Dellmann, H.-D.: The nervous control of the pars intermedia of an amphibian and a reptilian species. Mem. Soc. Endocr. **19**, 827—837 (1971).

Rodriguez, E. M., Gimenez, A.: Comparative aspects of nervous control of pars intermedia. Gen. comp. Endocr. Suppl. **3**, 97—107 (1972).

Scharrer, E.: Das Hypophysen-Zwischenhirnsystem von *Scyllium stellare*. Z. Zellforsch. **37**, 196—204 (1952).

Sheela, R., Pandalai, K. R.: Blood supply of the pituitary gland with particular reference to pars intermedia control in the garden lizard, *Calotes versicolor*. Neuroendocrinology **1**, 303—311 (1965).

Wilson, J. F., Dodd, J. M.: Distribution of monoamines in the diencephalon and pituitary of the dogfish, *Scyliorhinus canicula* L. Z. Zellforsch. **137**, 451—470 (1973a).

Wilson, J. F., Dodd, J. M.: Effects of pharmacological agents on the *in vivo* release of melanophore-stimulating hormone in the dogfish, *Scyliorhinus canicula*. Gen. comp. Endocr. **20**, 556—566 (1973b).

Wilson, J. F., Goos, H. J. Th., Dodd, J. M.: Neuronal mechanisms in the colour change response of the dogfish. *Scyliorhinus canicula*. In: Szentagothai, J., Hajos, F. (Eds.): VII. Conf. Europ. Comp. Endocrinol. Budapest 1973.

III. Aminergic Mechanisms in Neuroendocrine Control

Organization of the Dopamine and Noradrenaline Innervations of the Median Eminence-Pituitary Region in the Rat

Anders Björklund, Bengt Falck, Anders Nobin, and Ulf Stenevi

Department of Histology, University of Lund, Lund (Sweden)

Introduction

In studies of hypothalamic regulation of pituitary function the interest has mainly been focussed on two classes of substances: the hypothalamic releasing and inhibiting factors (which are peptides) and the biogenic monoamines. There is now much experimental evidence that catecholamines (CA) participate importantly in the regulation of the release of hypothalamic hormones (see Lichtensteiger, 1970; McCann et al., 1972; Hökfelt and Fuxe, 1972; Porter et al., 1972 for reviews) and special attention has been devoted to the role of CAs in the function of the median eminence. This was initiated by the observations by Carlsson et al. (1962) and by Fuxe (1963, 1964) of a massive supply of CA fibres to the median eminence of various mammalian species. In later studies, Fuxe and Hökfelt (1966) and Lichtensteiger and Langemann (1966) provided evidence in the rat and mouse that at least part of this innervation originated in the arcuate nuclei, constituting a tubero-infundibular CA (probably DA-containing) system. It soon became clear, however, that the CA innervation of the infundibular region is very complex and since it was felt that a detailed neuroanatomical knowledge would be indispensable for correct interpretations of functional and experimental data, a series of studies has been carried out in our laboratory, aiming at a more detailed picture of the topography and organization of the dopamine (DA) and noradrenaline (NA) producing neurons innervating the pituitary-median eminence complex. These studies have chiefly been carried out in the rat, and the following description will therefore deal primarily with this species. Comparisons with other mammalian species will be made to the extent that such information is available.

Occurrence of Biogenic Amines in the Median Eminence-Pituitary Region

The presence of both DA and NA in the mammalian pituitary complex and its various subdivisions has been reported in a number of papers, and the concentrations obtained by the several authors are summarized in Table 1. In most species studied DA occurs in high or very high concentrations throughout the neurohypophysis and in the pars intermedia; NA tends to be more unevenly distributed

Table 1. Content of CA and 5-HT in the pituitary gland and its various subdivisions. Values are given as ng/mg of wet tissue. References within brackets

Compound	Species[a]	Median eminence plus infundibular stem		Neural lobe		Pars intermedia[b]		Pars distalis	
DA	rat	0.73	[1]			4.8	[1]	—	
		2.3—3.8	[2]			1.6—2.0	[2]		
		2.20	[3]						
		10.3	[4]						
	cat	1.3—8.7	[5]			0.78	[6]		
	pig	0.85	[7]	0.32	[8]	0.18—0.62	[8]	0.01	[8]
	horse	0.24	[1]	1.3	[1]	0.37	[1]	—	
	cow[c]	0.43	[7]						
	sheep[c]	5.05	[5]						
	goat[c]	2.0	[5]						
	man	0.24	[7]						
NA	rat	2.8	[1]			0.7	[1]	—	
		3.8—4.4	[2]			0.74	[2]		
		4.52	[3]						
		4.1	[4]						
	cat	1.1—2.9	[5]			0.29	[6]		
	pig	0.78	[7]	0.04	[8]	0.01—0.03	[8]	0.01	[8]
	horse	0.28	[1]	0.13	[1]	0.05	[1]		
	cow	0.91	[7]						
	sheep	0.32	[5]						
	goat	0.16	[5]						
	man	1.66	[7]						
5-HT	rat[d]	—		0.15	[9]	0.25	[9]	0.11	[9]
	cat	—				0.94	[6]		
	pig	—		0.05	[8]	0.08	[8]	0.09	[8]
	cow	0.9—3.1 (median eminence)[e]	[10]	5.4—6.7	[10][e]	4.5—5.1	[10][e]	1.7—1.9	[10][e]
		5.3—6.0 (infund. stem)[e]	[10]						

[a] The postmortem time varies considerably and is longest for the human specimens.
[b] Due to the difficulties to dissect the pars intermedia free, this preparation can be expected to contain also neural lobe tissue.
[c] Mast cells of ruminant species (cow and sheep at least) contain high concentrations of DA (Falck et al., 1964).
[d] Rat mast cells contain high concentrations of 5-HT.
[e] Two different assay procedures were used.

1. Iwata and Ishii (1969).
2. Björklund et al. (1970).
3. Brown et al. (1972).
4. Cuello et al. (1973a).
5. Laverty and Sharman (1965).
6. Björklund and Falck (1969).
7. Rinne and Sonninen (1968).
8. Björklund et al. (1967).
9. Piezzi and Wurtman (1970).
10. Piezzi et al. (1970).

and the highest concentrations of this amine have been found in the median eminence and the infundibular stem. In the pars distalis – so far studied only in the pig (Björklund et al., 1967) – both these CAs occur in very low concentrations. Laverty and Sharman (1965) reported also traces of adrenaline in the cat median eminence and infundibular stem. Other investigators, using fluorimetric techniques, failed to detect adrenaline (Björklund et al., 1967; Björklund and Falck, 1969; Iwata and Ishii, 1969; Björklund et al., 1970); it thus seems that if adrenaline is present intraneuronally in the pituitary complex it is probably in very low concentrations.

The rat has been the most extensively studied species and the CAs in the median eminence-pituitary region of this animal have been subjected to special investigations by Iwata and Ishii (1969), Björklund et al. (1970), Brown et al. (1972), and Cuello et al. (1973a). In this species appreciable concentrations of NA occur both in median eminence-infundibular stem preparations and in neural lobe-pars intermedia preparations (Table 1). In preparations of the median eminence including part of the arcuate nuclei (1–2.5 mg of tissue) the concentration of NA exceeds that of DA (Björklund et al., 1970; Brown et al., 1972), whereas in a more restricted median eminence preparation (averageing 0.3 mg of tissue) Cuello et al. (1973a) found that the DA concentration was approximately twice as high as that of NA. Still, the NA concentration reported by Cuello et al. (1973a) (4.1 ng/mg) is higher than has so far been found in any other brain region.

Notably high concentrations of what appeared to be serotonin have been detected fluorometrically in the pituitaries of cat (0.9 ng/g; Björklund and Falck, 1969a) and cow (Piezzi et al., 1970) (see Table 1). In the cow, the highest concentrations (about 5–6 ng/mg) occurred in the neural lobe, the infundibular stem and the pars intermedia. Lower serotonin concentrations (1.7–1.9 ng/g) were found in the pars distalis (Piezzi et al., 1970). The identity of the assayed material as serotonin has not been fully secured, and it seems possible that also other indolamines could be present (cf. Björklund et al., 1970). Besides serotonin, the occurrence of tryptamine in low concentrations (about 0.05 ng/mg) in extracts from steer pituitary has also been reported (Martin et al., 1972).

In addition to CAs and indolamines also histamine is present in the mammalian pituitary (Harris et al., 1951; Adam and Hye, 1966). This histamine is partly mast cell bound, but there is good evidence in the cat that, at least in the pars distalis, histamine is localized in other cells than mast cells (Adam and Hye, 1966). Being outside the scope of the present review, the interesting problem of pituitary indolamines and histamine will not be further considered.

Distribution and Origin of the Pituitary CA Innervation

Fluorescence histochemical studies have demonstrated that the CA in the median eminence-pituitary region is located in axons and axon terminals and in most laboratory mammals the pituitary CA seems to be exclusively neuronal. Mast cells of ruminant species (at least in cow and sheep; cf. Falck et al., 1964), contain a high concentration of DA. Such DA-containing mast cells are abundant in the neurohypophysis (Björklund, unpublished) and in these animals a significant proportion of the pituitary DA is thus non-neuronal.

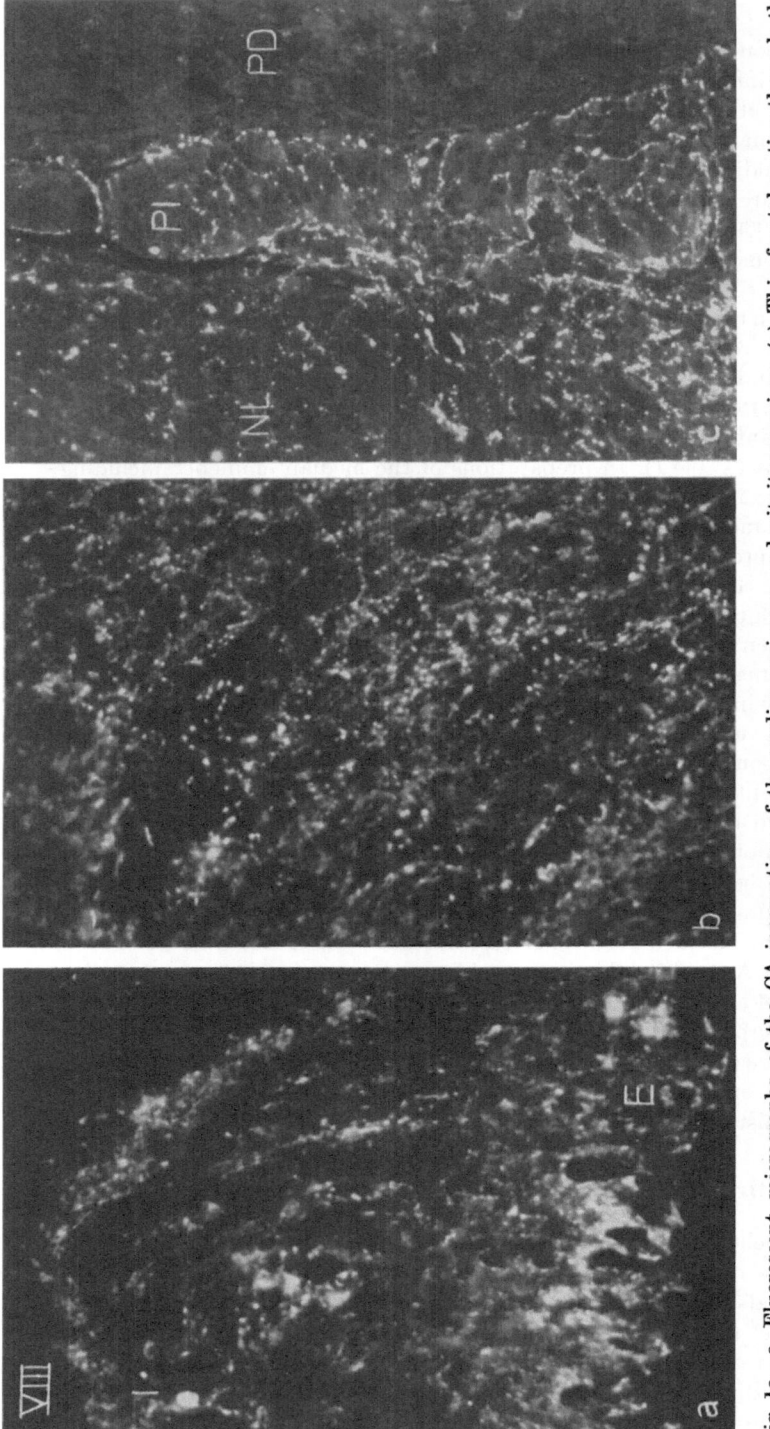

Fig. 1a—c. Fluorescent micrographs of the CA innervation of the median eminence and pituitary regions. (a) Thin frontal section through the median eminence of an adult mouse. The catecholamines in the zona externa (E) are localized in delicate varicose fibres with terminal swellings or droplets. Fluorescent varicose fibres and droplets also occur in the zona interna (I) close to the deep vessels. VIII third ventricle. × 500. From Björklund et al. (1968). (b) The CA innervation of the proximal part of the neural lobe of pig. The rich plexus of thin, varicose fluorescent fibres is seen. × 280. From Björklund (1968). (c) Frontal section from the pituitary of an adult, normal rat. A plexus of thin, varicose fluorescent fibres is seen both in the neural lobe (NL) and pars intermedia (PI). The pars distalis (PD) is devoid of fluorescent nerve fibres. × 160

CA innervation occurs in all subdivisions of the median eminence (Fig. 1a), the infundibular stem and the neural lobe (Fig. 1b), and in the pars intermedia (Fig. 1c), and seems to be a common feature of all mammalian species studied, including man (Fuxe, 1964; Enemar and Falck, 1965; Dahlström and Fuxe, 1966; Odake, 1967; Björklund, 1968; Björklund et al., 1968, 1970, 1973b; Björklund and Falck, 1969; Nobin and Björklund, 1973; Weman and Nobin, 1973). An exception is the neural lobe of the mouse where a parenchymal CA fibre supply has so far not been demonstrated (Björklund et al., 1968).

A special feature of the CA-containing structures of the median eminence-pituitary region is that the amines or their formaldehyde-induced fluorophores have a strong tendency to diffuse, and the fluorophores in some of the fibre systems are easily extracted from their tissue sites by xylene or hot paraffin (Björklund and Falck, 1968) two media used in the preparation of the specimen for fluorescence microscopy according to the Falck-Hillarp method. By reducing the exposure of the specimen to these media the precision of the fluorescence histochemical picture is improved and with such precautions the previously unknown system of CA-containing parenchymal fibres was discovered in the neural lobe of the rat and pig (Björklund, 1968), cat (Björklund and Falck, 1969), monkey (Nobin and Björklund, unpublished) and human fetus (Nobin and Björklund, 1973).

The distribution and morphology of the CA innervation, as revealed in the rat, are illustrated schematically in Fig. 2. It has been shown (Björklund, 1968; Björklund et al., 1973b) that this innervation is mainly of central origin. The neural lobe receives in addition a supply of peripheral sympathetic NA fibres to some of its larger vessels, especially those situated at the junction between the neural lobe and pars intermedia. These vascular fibres are removed by a bilateral extirpation of the superior cervical ganglia (Björklund, 1968; Björklund et al., 1973b).

The origin and course of the central DA and NA innervation of the median eminence-pituitary region were investigated using stereotaxic lesions in combination with fluorescence histochemistry and microspectrofluorometric analysis (Björklund et al., 1970, 1973b). The results are summarized schematically in Fig. 3. One system of fibres was found to originate outside the medio-basal hypothalamus. This system – which was designated *the reticulo-infundibular system* – is in all

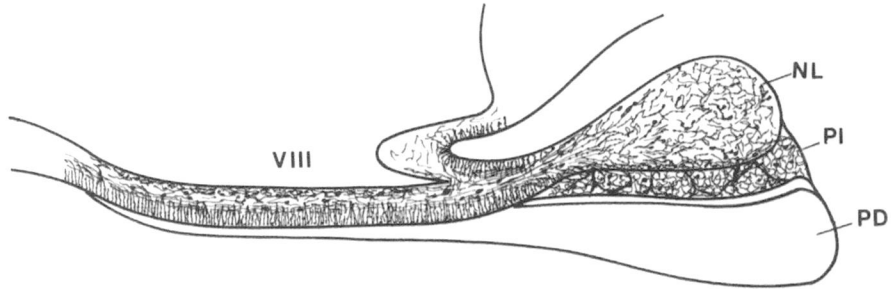

Fig. 2. Semischematic drawing of the morphology and distribution of the CA innervation of the median eminence-pituitary region as seen in a sagittal plane. NL = neural lobe; PI = pars intermedia; PD = pars distalis; VIII = third ventricle

probability NA-containing, originating in cell bodies of the pontine or medullary reticular formation. The exact location of the cells of origin has so far not been established, but from the combined observations it appears that the fibres ascend in the medial forebrain bundle up to the level of the rostral median eminence. Here, they turn sharply medially along the ventral surface to enter the most rostral median eminence from the lateral side (Björklund et al., 1970). Within the infundibulum these fibres are distributed (probably bilaterally) primarily to the internal and subependymal layers of the median eminence and the stem. Destruction of this input through a bilateral lesion in the caudal mesencephalon removes only part of the fibres in the internal and subependymal layers (Björklund et al., 1973b), a finding that is in agreement with the microspectrofluorometric observations of DA-containing fibres in these layers (Björklund et al., 1970). The fluorescent terminals in the deeper layers have an irregular morphology with varicosities that vary notably in size, some of them having the appearance of large droplet-like swellings (see below). These fibres are particularly abundant close to the ependyma of the third ventricle, and many occur in close relation to the deep capillary loops of the portal vessels (see Fig. 1a).

The reticulo-infundibular NA system is the only central NA projection to the median eminence-pituitary region identified so far. The question whether this system projects also to the external layer of the median eminence is not entirely clear. It is obvious that minor projections to such a densely innervated area are difficult to establish with certainty in denervation experiments such as those performed by Björklund et al. (1970, 1973b) and Jonsson et al. (1972). Following deafferentation of the medio-basal hypothalamus Réthely and Halász (1970) failed to detect any degenerating terminals in the external layer, at the electron microscopical level, whereas Cuello et al. (1973b) found such degeneration in some fibres of this layer. Moreover, Fuxe et al. (this volume, pp. 223) using immunofluorescence technique have reported the presence of the NA-synthesizing enzyme dopamine-β-hydroxylase not only in fibres of the deeper layers, but also in some few fibres of the external zone, pointing to a minor NA input to this region.

Remaining components of the median eminence-pituitary CA innervation are removed only by lesions involving the arcuate or anterior periventricular nuclei of the medio-basal hypothalamus (Björklund et al., 1973b; Jonsson et al., 1972; Smith and Fink, 1972). Microspectrofluorometrically, only DA-containing cells have been detected in these nuclei (Björklund and Nobin, 1973), which is in agreement with the pharmacological observations of Carlsson et al. (1962), Fuxe (1964) and Fuxe et al. (1966) indicating that these cells constitute a system of *tubero-hypophyseal DA neurons*.

DA-containing fibres have been detected by microspectrofluorometric analysis both around the endocrine cells of the pars intermedia, and in the neural lobe and the median eminence of the rat (Björklund et al., 1970). In the *neuro-intermediate lobe* it seems likely that the NA detected chemically (see Table 1) derives from the peripheral sympathetic vascular supply, and that the central innervation is exclusively dopaminergic. Experiments with small, partial lesions of the arcuate nuclei (Björklund et al., 1973b) have provided evidence that the DA fibres of the neuro-intermediate lobe – as well as part of the DA fibres in the median eminence – originate in the rostral portion of the arcuate nucleus, the cells innervating the pars intermedia lying immediately rostral to those innervating the neural lobe (Fig. 3).

The DA fibres of the neuro-intermediate lobe are predominantly of a fine varicose type distributed throughout the parenchyma of the neural lobe and around the endocrine cells of the pars intermedia (Fig. 1b and c). These fibres form the densest pattern in the vascular border zone between the two lobes and at the outer margins of the lobules formed by the intermedia cells. From here, the fibres penetrate between the intermedia cells to form a plexus inside the lobules. The abundance of this plexus of fluorescent fibres varies notably from animal to animal (Björklund et al., 1968). In optimal specimens, or in specimens treated with exogenous CA, the plexus is seen to cover the whole pars intermedia, and it seems quite possible that all intermedia cells could be in contact with the DA terminals.

The ultrastructural arrangement of the CA terminals in the neural lobe and pars intermedia was subjected to a combined electron microscopic and fluorescence microscopic study in the rat by Baumgarten et al. (1972), using the DA analogues, 5-hydroxydopamine and 6-hydroxydopamine, for their ultrastructural identification. The fibre type that was identified as CA-containing was ultrastructurally chiefly characterized by dense-cored vesicles, $500-1200$ Å in diameter, intermingled with varying numbers of small empty vesicles. 5-Hydroxydopamine was selectively accumulated in these fibres and caused an increased electron density of the granular vesicles as well as of some small normally agranular vesicles, and systemically administered 6-hydroxydopamine caused a selective degeneration of these fibres, most prominently within the neural lobe. This fibre type in the mammalian neuro-intermediate lobe has also been described by Bargmann et al. (1967), Wittkowski (1967), Vincent and Anand Kumar (1969), Cannata and Tramezzani (1969) and Naik (1972).

The dopaminergic terminals of the neural lobe identified in this way showed frequent close contacts ($80-120$ Å), without real membrane thickenings, to neurosecretory axons and to pituicyte processes. It is suggested that these close contacts might signify a direct dopaminergic influence on the neurosecretory axons and/or on the pituicytes. The central CA fibres were found to make close contacts also on the pars intermedia cells, whereas — in the rat — the innervation by neurosecretory fibres was very rare in the pars intermedia. Close contacts of probable CA-containing fibres with intermedia cells have also been observed by Naik (1972) and Weman and Nobin (1973) in mouse and mink. This suggests that the direct central nervous control of the rat pars intermedia is exerted by the tubero-hypophyseal DA system. Enemar and Falck (1965) and Iturriza (1966, 1969) have, in fact, obtained experimental evidence for a direct inhibitory action of the CA innervation on the pituitary MSH-secretion in anuran species, and preliminary observations on the MSH release from electrically stimulated pituitaries in vitro indicate that this might be the case also in the rat (Nobin and Björklund, unpublished).

A special feature of the DA fibres in the pituitary complex is the occurrence of peculiar, large DA-filled droplet-like swellings (Björklund, 1968). Electron microscopically, such large axonal swellings (more than 2μ in diameter) were found to contain, in addition to the characteristic vesicles and organelles, strongly osmiophilic lamellated membrane complexes resembling myelin bodies and multivesicular bodies encircling disintegrated vesicles, suggesting that these "droplet fibres" represent dilated stumps of spontaneously degenerating dopaminergic axons. It is proposed that the dopaminergic neural lobe fibres are undergoing continuous reorganization through degeneration-regeneration cycles, a phenomenon previously suggested by Dellmann and Rodriguez (1971) for the neurosecretory axons of the neural lobe. An indirect support for this idea is the observation that DA-containing droplet-like swellings increase in number in animals treated with 6-hydroxydopamine, i.e. in a situation when extensive terminal degeneration of the DA fibres has been induced (Baumgarten et al., 1972).

The DA innervation of *the median eminence and the stem* originates in cell bodies situated in the arcuate nucleus and in the part of the periventricular nucleus lying dorsal to the arcuate nucleus (Björklund et al., 1970, 1973b). From the lesion experiments, these tubero-infundibular DA neurons could be distinguished as two groups on the basis of their mode of projection (see Fig. 3). One group, situated in the rostral part of the arcuate nuclei, projects more diffusely to all levels of the median eminence and the stem (as well as to the pars intermedia and the neural lobe as mentioned above). The second group, having a more regular dorsoventrally oriented projection, appears to connect each portion of the arcuate nucleus (i.e. the rostral, middle, or caudal portion) with a corresponding part of the ventrally situated median eminence.

The tubero-infundibular DA neurons project to all layers of the median eminence and the stem. The terminals are more abundant in the external layer where they are very densely packed in a palisade-like manner, close to the capillaries of the portal vessels. The fibres have a regular, finely-varicose appearance, often ending with a strongly fluorescent droplet-like enlargement (cf. Fig. 1a). In the internal layer it is likely that part of the fibres are of preterminal nature running parallel to one another in the sagittal and frontal planes. However, part of the fibres appear to ramify with the reticulo-infundibular NA fibres to form irregular patterns in the deeper layers, partly in association with the capillary loops of the portal vessels.

The Incerto-Hypothalamic DA System

Hypothalamic DA is known to occur in significant amounts also outside the arcuate nucleus-pituitary region. However, the cellular localization of this extratuberal DA has not been possible to identify with the standard Falck-Hillarp formaldehyde histofluorescence method. With the introduction of the glyoxylic acid method (Lindvall and Björklund, 1974) a previously unknown CA system was discovered in the zona incerta and the dorsal and anterior hypothalamus, as illustrated schematically in Fig. 3 (Björklund et al., 1973a). These delicate fibres, having a characteristic finely-varicose appearance, were followed in a loosely arranged bundle from the region of the fluorescent cell bodies of the so-called A11 and A13 cell groups (Dahlström and Fuxe, 1965; Björklund and Nobin, 1973) in the parafascicular thalamic nucleus and the medial zona incerta. As the bundle passed rostrally, the A11 and A13 cell bodies most probably contributed fibres to the bundle, and at the level of the A13 cell group the system became abundant. From here the fibres extended rostrally and ventrally into the dorsomedial nucleus and the dorsal and anterior hypothalamic areas, and laterally and rostrally in the zona incerta. From the micro-spectrofluorometric analysis of the cell bodies (Björklund and Nobin, 1973) it seems highly probable that this incerto-hypothalamic system is DA-containing. These observations thus provide evidence for a second, short intradiencephalic DA system, having their cell bodies in the caudal thalamus and the medial zona incerta and projecting to the zona incerta and to dorsal and anterior hypothalamic regions, i.e. to areas of importance in hypothalamic neuroendocrine functions.

Discussion

The DA- and NA-producing neurons innervating the median eminence-pituitary region may be classified as three different neuronal systems: peripheral sympathetic NA neurons probably located in the superior cervical ganglion; reticulo-infundibular NA neurons located in the pontine or medullary reticular formation; and tubero-

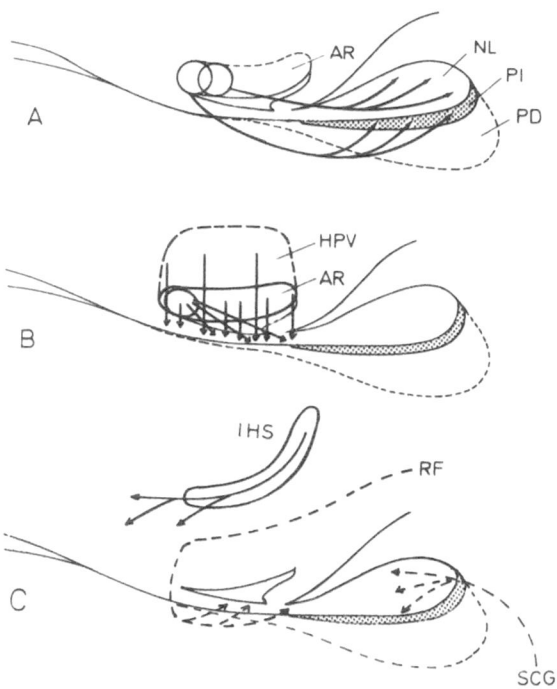

Fig. 3 A—C. Schematic illustration of the different CA neuron systems of the median eminence-pituitary region of the rat. A The tubero-hypophyseal DA neurons are illustrated by solid arrows. B The principal organization of the tubero-infundibular DA neurons is indicated by solid arrows. C The reticulo-infundibular NA neurons and the peripheral sympathetic NA neurons (probably from the superior cervical ganglion) are illustrated by dashed arrows. The incerto-hypothalamic DA neuron system is also indicated (solid arrows). AR = arcuate nucleus; HPV = periventricular nucleus; IHS = incerto-hypothalamic system; NL = neural lobe; PD = pars distalis; PI = pars intermedia; RF = reticular formation; SCG = superior cervical ganglion

hypophyseal DA neurons located in the arcuate and periventricular nuclei of the hypothalamus.

From the present studies it appears that the DA of the whole median eminence-pituitary complex is entirely confined to the tubero-hypophyseal neuronal systems. In terms of projection of these DA cell bodies they can be distinguished as two principal groups (see Fig. 3). One group of neurons, situated in the rostral arcuate nuclei projects in a diffuse manner to the whole median eminence-pituitary region. At least with respect to the neural lobe and pars intermedia (Björklund et al., 1973 b) there is evidence that the different subdivisions are supplied by separate sets of neurons. The second group, probably distributed throughout the arcuate nuclei and the part of the periventricular nucleus lying dorsal to the arcuate nuclei, appeared to have a more regular, dorso-ventrally oriented projection to the median eminence and the stem. In addition, there are periventricular DA-containing cell bodies, located rostrally to the arcuate nucleus, that do not seem to have any significant projection to the median eminence-pituitary region (Björklund et al., 1973 b). It has not so far been possible to identify the terminals of these rostral periventricular DA neurons (designated group A14 by Björklund and Nobin, 1973).

It is therefore evident that the tubero-hypophyseal DA cell group is a heterogenous system of neurons. Tentatively, one might be able to distinguish at least four different cell types on morphological grounds: cells with a regionally ordered projection to the median eminence and the stem; cells with a diffuse projection to the median eminence and the stem; cells with a projection to the neural lobe; and cells with a projection to the pars intermedia. It is also conceivable that one and the same cell in the rostral arcuate nucleus might have its terminals both in the median eminence and the neuro-intermediate lobe.

From a neuroanatomical point of view the tubero-hypophyseal dopaminergic system is only one component of a more extensive and heterogenous system of tubero-hypophyseal neural connections. The best known part of this system, called the parvicellular neurosecretory system by Szentágothai (1964), is the axonal connections between the arcuate nuclei and the external layer of the median eminence; the DA neurons thus form an important part of Szentágothai's parvicellular system. Also other hypothalamic nuclei probably contribute to the tubero-hypophyseal system but the knowledge of these connections is very incomplete (for references, see Björklund et al., 1970). The tubero-hypophyseal system has often been regarded as the "final common path" for the neuroendocrine control of pituitary functions (see Nauta, 1963), being concerned with the production and release of hypothalamic hypophysiotrophic hormones. It appears unlikely that DA itself could act as a releasing or inhibiting factor at the level of the anterior pituitary (see Hökfelt and Fuxe, 1972; McCann et al., 1972; Porter et al., 1972) and thus the arrangement of the dopaminergic component of the tubero-hypophysial system should rather allow for a DA-mediated control at the sites where the hypothalamic hormones are known to be released, i.e. in the several subdivisions of the neurohypophysis, as well as in the pars intermedia. In addition, the studies with the glyoxylic acid method (Björklund et al., 1973 a) have provided evidence for a dopaminergic supply also to the anterior and dorsal hypothalamus, which are parts of the so-called hypophysiotrophic area (Halász et al., 1962; Flament-Durand and Desclin, 1970). This area is thought to be the site of production of several hypophysiotrophic hormones, and it is evident that the arrangement of the incerto-hypothalamic DA system provides morphological possibilities for a dopaminergic influence also at these higher levels of hypothalamic neuroendocrine regulation: such a possibility has also been suggested by Porter et al. (1972) on the basis of experiments with DA perfusions of the median eminence.

The reticulo-infundibular NA system projects primarily to the deeper layers of the median eminence where the NA terminals intermingle with terminals of the tubero-hypophyseal DA system and form dense patterns close to the capillary loops of the portal vessels and close to the ependyma of the third ventricle. It seems probable that the NA fibres of the median eminence are the projections of the same reticular neuron system that innervates also many other hypothalamic areas, e.g. the paraventricular, dorsomedial, periventricular and arcuate nuclei (see Ungerstedt, 1971; Maeda and Shimizu, 1972; Olson and Fuxe, 1972). Thus, in contrast to the probably highly ordered DA neurons, the NA neurons – being a component of the ascending reticular projections – appear to be more diffusely organized and to have wide-spread projections. It seems possible that one and the same NA neuron – or one and the same group of neurons – has its terminals both in the median eminence and in hypothalamic nuclei involved in neuroendocrine functions.

The role of hypothalamic monoamines in the central nervous control of pituitary functions has been extensively studied during recent years. This research was initiated and much stimulated by the studies of Sawyer et al. (for review, see Sawyer, 1963) on the blocking of the ovulation trigger mechanism with an adrenergic α-receptor blocker, dibenamin, and by the findings that amine-depleting drugs, such as reserpine, exert multiple endocrine effects via the hypothalamo-hypophyseal system (for reviews, see Gaunt et al., 1962; Gold and Ganong. 1967). From the experimental data available today it is clear that interference with the function of central NA, DA or 5-HT neurons will affect practically all known endocrine functions of the pituitary gland. A role of CA neurons has been postulated in the control of the release of many hypothalamic hypophyseotrophic hormones from the median eminence, including LRF, FRF, PIF, TRF, and GRF (see reviews by Lichtensteiger, 1970; Hökfelt and Fuxe, 1972; McCann et al., 1972; Porter et al., 1972). There is also experimental evidence that monoamines might play a role in ADH secretion (Chaudhury et al., 1962; Fang et al., 1962; Moses, 1964; Mills and Wang, 1964; deWied and László, 1967) and oxytocin secretion (Grosvenor and Turner, 1957; Mizuno et al., 1967) from the posterior pituitary. In amphibia, pharmacological and physiological experiments indicate that the central CA innervation of the intermedia cells exerts an inhibitory control of the MSH-production (Enemar and Falck, 1965; Iturriza, 1966, 1969).

From these various functional and experimental data it seems clear that the complex organization of the NA and DA innervations could reflect a complex involvement of CAs in the control of the secretion of several hypothalamic and pituitary hormones. From the structural point of view there are possibilities for DA and NA neurons to exert influences at several different levels of the hypothalamo-hypophyseal system. Moreover, the sub-organization of the CA neuron systems could allow both for coordination and for separate and independent control of different hormonal systems through neurons operating with the same neurotransmitter.

Acknowledgements. The studies were supported by grants from the Ford Foundation, from the Swedish Medical Research Council (grants No. 04X-4493 and 04X-712), and from the Magnus Bergwall and Harald and Greta Jeansson foundations.

References

Adam, H. M., Hye, H. K. A.: Concentration of histamine in different parts of brain and hypophysis of cat and its modification by drugs. Brit. J. Pharmacol. **28**, 137—152 (1966).

Bargmann, W., Lindner, E., Andres, K. H.: Über Synapsen an endokrinen Epithelzellen und die Definition sekretorischer Neurone. Untersuchungen am Zwischenlappen der Katzenhypophyse. Z. Zellforsch. **77**, 282—298 (1967).

Baumgarten, H. G., Björklund, A., Holstein, A. F., Nobin, A.: Organization and ultrastructural identification of the catecholamine nerve terminals in the neural lobe and pars intermedia of the rat pituitary. Z. Zellforsch. **126**, 483—517 (1972).

Björklund, A.: Monoamine-containing fibres in the neurointermediate lobe of the pig and rat. Z. Zellforsch. **89**, 573—589 (1968).

Björklund, A., Enemar, A., Falck, B.: Monoamines in the hypothalamohypophyseal system of the mouse with special reference to the ontogenetic aspects. Z. Zellforsch. **89**, 590—607 (1968).

Björklund, A., Falck, B.: An improvement of the histochemical fluorescence method for monoamines. Observations on varying extractability of fluorophores in different nerve fibres. J. Histochem. Cytochem. **16**, 717—720 (1968).

Björklund, A., Falck, B.: Pituitary monoamines of the cat with special reference to the presence of an unidentified monoamine-like substance in the adenohypophysis. Z. Zellforsch. **93**, 254—264 (1969).

Björklund, A., Falck, B., Hromek, F., Owman, Ch., West, K. A.: Identification and terminal distribution of the tubero-hypophyseal monoamine fibre systems in the rat by means of stereotaxic and microspectrofluorimetric techniques. Brain Res. **17**, 1—23 (1970).

Björklund, A., Falck, B., Rosengren, E.: Monoamines in the pituitary gland of the pig. Life Sci. **6**, 2103—2110 (1967).

Björklund, A., Lindvall, O., Nobin, A., Stenevi, U.: The adrenergic innervation of the thalamus as revealed by the glyoxylic acid fluorescence method. Comm. Dept. Anat., Univ. Lund, No. 4 (1973a).

Björklund, A., Moore, R. Y., Nobin, A., Stenevi, U.: The organization of tubero-hypophyseal and reticulo-infundibular catecholamine neuron systems in the rat brain. Brain Res. **51**, 171—191 (1973b).

Björklund, A., Nobin, A.: Fluorescence histochemical and microspectrofluorometric mapping of dopamine and noradrenaline cell groups in the rat diencephalon. Brain Res. **51**, 193—205 (1973).

Brown, G. M., Krigstein, E., Dankova, J., Hornykiewicz, O.: Relationship between hypothalamic and median eminence catecholamines and thyroid function. Neuroendocrinology **10**, 207—217 (1972).

Cannata, M. A., Tramezzani, J. H.: The neural lobe of the neurohypophysis of the rat: Several types of nerve endings. Experientia (Basel) **25**, 1281—1282 (1969).

Carlsson, A., Falck, B., Hillarp, N.-Å.: Cellular localization of brain monoamines. Acta physiol. scand. **56**, Suppl. 196 (1962).

Chaudhury, R. R., Chaudhury, M. R., Lu, F. C.: The mechanism of the reserpine-induced antidiuresis in the rat. Can. J. Biochem. Physiol. **40**, 1465—1472 (1962).

Cuello, A. C., Horn, A. S., Mackay, A. V. P., Iversen, L. L.: Catecholamines in the median eminence: new evidence for a major noradrenergic input. Nature (Lond.) **243**, 465—467 (1973a).

Cuello, A. C., Weiner, R. I., Ganong, W. F.: Effect of lateral deafferentation of the morphology and catecholamine content of the mediobasal hypothalamus. Brain Res. **59**, 191—200 (1973b).

Dahlström, A., Fuxe, K.: Evidence for the existence of monoamine-containing neurons in the central nervous system. I Demonstration of monoamines in the cell bodies of brain stem neurons. Acta physiol. scand. Suppl. 232 (1964).

Dahlström, A., Fuxe, K.: Monoamines and the pituitary gland. Acta endocr. (Kbh.) **51**, 301—314 (1966).

Dellmann, H.-D., Rodriguez, E. M.: Herring bodies; an electron microscopic study of local degeneration and regeneration of neurosecretory axons. Z. Zellforsch. **111**, 293—315 (1970).

De Wied, D., Laszlo, F. A.: Effect of autonomic blocking agents on ADH-release induced by hyperosmoticity. J. Endocr. **37**, XVI (1967).

Enemar, A., Falck, B.: In: Owman, Ch., Falck, B. (Eds.): Localization of neuronal monoamines at the cellular level, Vol. **3**, pp. 165—183. Paper presented at Proc. Second. Int. Pharmacol. Meeting, Prague 1963. Oxford: Pergamon Press 1965.

Falck, B., Nystedt, T., Rosengren, E., Stenflo, J.: Dopamine and mast cells in ruminants, Acta pharmacol. (Kbh.) **21**, 51—58 (1964).

Fang, H. S., Liu, H. M., Wang, S. C.: Liberation of antidiuretic hormone following hypothalamic stimulation in the dog. Amer. J. Physiol. **202**, 212—216 (1962).

Flament-Durand, J., Desclin, L.: The hypophysiotropic area. In: Martini, L., Motta, M., Fraschini, F., (Eds.): The Hypothalamus, pp. 245—257. New York, London: Academic Press (1970).

Fuxe, K.: Cellular localization of monoamines in the median eminence and in the infundibular stem of some mammals. Acta physiol. scand. **58**, 383—384 (1963).

Fuxe, K.: Cellular localization of monoamines in the median eminence and infundibular stem of some mammals. Z. Zellforsch. **61**, 710—724 (1964).

Fuxe, K., Hamberger, B., Malmfors, T.: Inhibition of amine uptake in tubero-infundibular dopamine neurones and in catecholamine cell bodies of the area postrema. J. Pharm. Pharmacol. **18**, 543—544 (1966).

Fuxe, K., Hökfelt, T.: Further evidence for the existence of tubero-infundibular dopamine neurons. Acta physiol. scand. **66**, 245—246 (1966).

Gaunt, R., Renzi, A. A., Chart, J. J.: Endocrine pharmacology of methyl reserpate derivatives. Endocrinology **71**, 527—535 (1962).

Gold, E. M., Ganong, W. F.: Effects of drugs on neuroendocrine processes. In: Martini, L., Ganong, W. F. (Eds.): Neuroendocrinology, Vol. **2**, pp. 377—437. New York, London: Academic Press (1967).

Grosvenor, C. E., Turner, C. W.: Evidence for adrenergic and cholinergic components in milk let-down reflex in lactating rat. Proc. Soc. exp. Biol. (N. Y.) **95**, 719—722 (1957).

Halász, B., Pupp, L., Uhlarik, S.: Hypophysiotropic area in the hypothalamus. J. Endocr. **25**, 147—154 (1962).

Harris, G. W., Jacobsohn, D., Kahlson, G.: The occurrence of histamine in cerebral regions related to the hypophysis. Acta physiol. scand. **24**, 186—194 (1951).

Hökfelt, T., Fuxe, K.: On the morphology and the neuroendocrine role of the hypothalamic catecholamine neurons. In: Brain-endocrine interaction, median eminence: Structure and function. Int. Symp., Munich 1971, pp. 181—223. Basel: Karger (1972).

Iturriza, F. C.: Monoamines and control of the pars intermedia of the toad pituitary. Gen. comp. Endocr. **6**, 19—25 (1966).

Iturriza, F. C.: Further evidence for the blocking effect of catecholamines on the secretion of melanocyte-stimulating hormone in toads. Gen. comp. Endocr. **12**, 417—426 (1969).

Iwata, T., Ishii, S.: Chemical isolation and determination of catecholamines in the median eminence and pars nervosa of the rat and horse. Neuroendocrinology **5**, 140—148 (1969).

Jonsson, G., Fuxe, K., Hökfelt, T.: On the catecholamine innervation of the hypothalamus, with special reference to the median eminence. Brain Res. **40**, 271—281 (1972).

Laverty, R., Sharman, D. F.: The estimation of small quantities of 3,4-dihydroxyphenylethylamine in tissues. Brit. J. Pharmacol. **24**, 538—548 (1965).

Lichtensteiger, W.: Katecholaminhaltige Neurone in der neuroendokrinen Steuerung. Progr. Histochem. Cytochem. **1**, 185—276 (1970).

Lichtensteiger, W., Langemann, H.: Uptake of exogenous catecholamines by monoamine-containing neurons of the central nervous system: uptake of catecholamines by arcuato-infundibular neurons. J. Pharmacol. exp. Ther. **151**, 400—408 (1966).

Lindvall, O., Björklund, A.: The glyoxylic acid fluorescence histochemical method: a detailed account of the methodology for the visualization of central catecholamine neurons. Histochemistry **39**, 97—127 (1974).

Maeda, T., Shimizu, N.: Projections ascendentes du locus coeruleus et d'autres neurones aminergiques pontiques au niveau du prosencéphale du rat. Brain Res. 36, 19—35 (1972).

Martin, W. R., Sloan, J. W., Christian, S. T., Clements, T. H.: Brain levels of tryptamine. Psychopharmacologia (Berl.) 24, 331—346 (1972).

McCann, S. M., Kalra, P. S., Donoso, A. O., Bishop, W., Schneider, H. P. G., Fawcett, C. P., Krulich, L.: The role of monoamines in the control of gonado-tropin and prolactin secretion. In: Brain-endocrine-interaction, median eminence: Structure and function. Int. Symp. Munich 1971, pp. 224—235. Basel: Karger (1972).

Mills, E., Wang, S. C.: Liberation of antidiuretic hormone: Pharmacologic blockade of ascending pathways. Amer. J. Physiol. 207, 1405—1410 (1964).

Mizuno, H., Talwalker, P. K., Meites, J.: Inhibition of mammary secretion in rats by iproniazid. Proc. Soc. exp. Biol. (N. Y.) 115, 604—607 (1964).

Moses, A. M.: Inhibition of vasopressin release in rats by chlorpromazine and reserpine. Endocrinology 74, 889—893 (1964).

Naik, D. V.: Electron microscopic studies on the pars intermedia in normal and in mice with hereditary nephrogenic diabetes insipidus. Z. Zellforsch. 133, 415—425 (1972).

Nauta, W. J. H.: Central nervous organization and the endocrine motor system. In: Nalbandov, A. V. (Ed.): Advances in neuroendocrinology. Urbana: Univ. of Illinois Press (1963).

Nobin, A., Björklund, A.: Topography of the monoamine neuron systems in the human brain as revealed in fetuses. Acta physiol. scand. Suppl. 388 (1973).

Odake, G.: Fluorescence microscopy of the catecholamine-containing neurons of the hypothalamohypophyseal system. Z. Zellforsch. 82, 46—64 (1967).

Olson, L., Fuxe, K.: Further mapping out of central noradrenaline neuron systems: Projections of the "subcoeruleus" area. Brain Res. 43, 289—295 (1972).

Piezzi, R. S., Larin, F., Wurtman, R. J.: Serotonin, 5-hydroxyindoleacetic acid (5-HIAA), and monoamine oxidase in the bovine median eminence and pituitary gland. Endocrinology 86, 1460—1462 (1970).

Piezzi, R. S., Wurtman, R. J.: Pituitary serotonin content: Effects of melatonin or deprivation of water. Science 169, 285—286 (1970).

Porter, J. C., Kamberi, I. A., Ondo, J. G.: Role of biogenic amines and cerebrospinal fluid in the neurovascular transmittal of hypophysiotrophic substances. In: Brain-endocrine interaction, median eminence: Structure and function, Int. Symp. Munich 1971, pp. 245—253. Basel: Karger (1972).

Réthelyi, M., Halász, B.: Origin of the nerve endings in the surface zone of the median eminence of the rat hypothalamus. Exp. Brain Res. 11, 145—158 (1970).

Rinne, U. K., Sonninen, V.: The occurrence of dopamine and noradrenaline in the tubero-hypophyseal system. Experientia (Basel) 24, 177—178 (1968).

Sawyer, C. H.: Mechanisms by which drugs and hormones activate and block release of pituitary gonadotropins. In: Proc. 1st Intern. Pharmacol. Meeting. Oxford: Pergamon Press (1963).

Smith, G. C., Fink, G.: Experimental studies on the origin of monoamine-containing fibres in the hypothalamo-hypophyseal complex of the rat. Brain Res. 43, 37—51 (1972).

Szentágothai, J.: The parvicellular neurosecretory system. In: Bargmann, W., Schadé, J. P. (Eds.): Lectures on the diencephalon. Progr. Brain Res. 5, 135—146 (1964).

Ungerstedt, U.: Stereotaxic mapping of the monoamine pathway in the rat brain. Acta physiol. scand. Suppl. 367 (1971).

Vincent, D. S., Anand Kumar, T. C.: Electron microscopic study on the pars intermedia of the ferret. Z. Zellforsch. 99, 185—197 (1969).

Weman, B., Nobin, A.: The pars intermedia of the mink, *Mustela vison*. Fluorescence, light and electron microscopical studies. Z. Zellforsch. 276, 1—15 (1973).

Wittkowski, W.: Kapillaren und perikapilläre Räume im Hypothalamo-Hypophysen-System und ihre Beziehungen zum Nervengewebe. Z. Zellforsch. 81, 344—360 (1967).

New Aspects on the Catecholamine Innervation
of the Hypothalamus and the Limbic System

Kjell Fuxe, Menek Goldstein, Tomas Hökfelt, Gösta Jonsson, and Anders Löfström

Department of Histology, Karolinska Institute, Stockholm (Sweden)
Department of Psychiatry, New York University Medical Center, New York (USA)

Since the last symposium on neurosecretion in Kiel (1970) new information on the catecholamine (CA) innervation of the hypothalamus and the limbic system has been obtained mainly with the use of immunohistofluorescence techniques (antibodies against CA synthesizing enzymes) (Goldstein et al., 1972; Goldstein et al., 1973; Hökfelt et al., 1973 b and c; Hökfelt et al., 1973; Hökfelt et al., 1974) and microspectrofluorometry usually in combination with stereotaxic surgery (Jonsson et al., 1972; Björklund and Nobin, 1973; Björklund et al., 1973; Löfström et al., 1974 and this volume, pp. 313 The article will mainly review the work that has been performed in our laboratory.

I. Immunohistofluorescence Studies

A. Antibodies against Dopadecarboxylase (see Hökfelt et al., 1973 b−d)

Studies with antibodies against dopadecarboxylase (DDC) have revealed that strong fluorescence is found in dopamine (DA) cell bodies, whereas only a weak fluorescence is found in noradrenaline (NA) cell bodies. DDC immunofluorescence (IF) can also be found in the DA nerve terminals but not in the NA nerve terminals which could be explained on the basis that too low amounts of DDC are present in the NA nerve terminals.

Using antibodies against DDC it was possible to confirm the existence of tubero-infundibular DA neurons. Nerve cell bodies with specific DDC immunofluorescence were found in the arcuate nucleus and the anterior periventricular nucleus with the same characteristics and distribution as the DA cell bodies, and IF was found in the external layer of the rat median eminence. These results support the view that most of the CA nerve terminals in the external layer are DA terminals. Also the CA cell group A13 exhibited strong IF, indicating that it was a DA cell group (see Björklund and Nobin, 1973). In addition, new groups of nerve cell bodies were discovered in the hypothalamus and preoptic area which had IF but lacked any detectable endogenous amine fluorescence. These cell bodies were localized especially in the medial preoptic area but also in the premammillary area. They could also be demonstrated with the Falck-Hillarp technique after exogenous administration of dopa in combination with a peripheral decarboxylase inhibitor (Butcher et al., 1972; Lidbrink et al., 1974) or intraventricular injections of CA. These nerve cells may contain a monoamine-like transmitter or may represent peptide-containing neurons, since DDC has been found to be associated with hormone producing gland cells in endocrine tissue (see i.a. Sundler, 1973). The projections of these nerve cells are unknown as are those of the DA cell bodies of group A13.

B. Antibodies against DA-β-Hydroxylase (see Hartmann and Udenfriend, 1970; Hökfelt et al., 1973c and d)

A plexus of DA-β-hydroxylase (DBH) containing nerve terminals was found in the subependymal layer and the internal layer similar in morphology and distribution to that found using the Falck-Hillarp technique. In the external layer a thin band of nerve terminals with IF was found in the lateral part lying very superficially close to the pericapillary space. These results provide further support for the view that most of the CA nerve terminals in the inner layers contain NA. However, they also give evidence for the existence of a certain number of NA terminals in the external layer, lying in an excellent position to influence the secretion of the peptide hormones from the median eminence. The distribution of the DBH containing nerve terminals in the rest of the hypothalamus is similar to that of the CA nerve terminals as visualized with the Falck-Hillarp technique. No DBH containing nerve cell bodies were found in the hypothalamus and the preoptic area nor at the telencephalic level, supporting the view that all NA nerve terminals derive from NA cell bodies in the rhombencephalon.

C. Antibodies against Phenylethanolamine-N-Methyltransferase (Goldstein et al., 1972, 1973; Hökfelt et al., 1974)

No phenylethanolamine-N-methyltransferase (PNMT) positive terminals could be observed in the median eminence itself. PNMT containing terminals were mainly found in the perifornical area, parts of the nuc. dorsomedialis hypothalami and in the magnocellular nucleus of nuc. paraventricularis. Some PNMT-positive terminals were also found in the ventrolateral region of nuc. arcuatus. The available evidence clearly indicate that these terminals are adrenaline (A) containing terminals which arise from a special A containing nerve cell group in the medulla oblongata (see Hökfelt et al., 1974). Thus, there may exist not only a reticular NA but also a reticular A afferent input into the hypothalamus which may control for example oxytocin secretion in view of the A innervation of the paraventricular nucleus.

II. Amine Fluorescence Histochemistry According to Falck-Hillarp

A. Studies Involving Stereotaxic Surgery

After making complete hypothalamic islands (see Halász, 1969) it could be demonstrated that all the CA nerve terminals in the islands disappeared except those in the external layer of the median eminence which remained intact (Jonsson et al., 1972). With the exception of group A12 no CA cell groups were present in the island. This was correlated with the disappearance of NA levels, whereas DA levels in the islands remain unchanged (Weiner et al., 1972) giving further evidence for the view that the main monoaminergic input into the external layer is dopaminergic. This view has been confirmed by the work of Björklund et al. (1973) who, however, in their first study (Björklund et al., 1970) claimed that vast numbers of NA terminals existed in the external layer. The lesions or cuts made in that study, however, probably involved also the DA axons from the arcuate nucleus. From the work of Björklund et al. (1973) it seems as if the most anterior part of the DA cell group A12 projects to the intermediate lobe and the neural lobe of the hypophysis, whereas the rest of the cell group projects to the median eminence. Ultrastructural analysis of the external layer (Ajika and Hökfelt, 1973) has revealed that the highest density of monoamine nerve terminals in the brain is found in the lateral external layer, in which area 33% of all boutons are monoaminergic (mainly dopaminergic). It may be pointed out that a greater amount of nerve terminals actually reach the capillary basement membrane in the medial than in the lateral palisade zone (Wittkowski, 1973, and this symposium). In view of this the functional importance of the medial CA nerve terminals should not be underestimated in spite of their considerably lower frequency compared with those in the lateral part. Most of the monoamine boutons lie in close relation to glial processes (tanycytes) or to non-monoamine boutons making possible axo-axonic interactions with peptide-containing neurons e.g. LRF containing boutons. Some DA boutons are also found directly in contact with the pericapillary space making secretion into the primary capillary plexus a possible event, and a DA receptor on the prolactin cells may exist.

It has been suggested at previous meetings that a joint storage of CA and peptide hormones may occur. However, in view of the recent work of Barry and Dubois (see this volume, p. 148) demonstrating that most of the luteinizing hormone releasing factor containing nerve cell bodies are present in the preoptic region this possibility seems to be excluded. Furthermore, 2/3 of the boutons in the lateral external layer do not contain CA.

B. Pharmacological Studies

The early pharmacological work giving evidence for the dopaminergic nature of the CA nerve terminals in the external layer is summarized in Fuxe and Hökfelt (1969) and Jonsson et al. (1972). With the help of microspectrofluorometry an attempt has been made to obtain more detailed information as to the ratio DA versus NA nerve terminals in the various parts of the median eminence. Using DBH inhibitors such as FLA-63 and diethyldithiocarbamate, microfluorimetric measurements revealed a 65% decrease of the fluorescence intensity in the CA terminals of the subependymal layer, a 10% decrease in the lateral external layer and a 30—40% decrease in the medial external layer (Löfström et al., 1974, see also abstract this symposium). More than a 70% decrease is not obtained in a NA nerve terminal system after treatment with DBH inhibitors (Corrodi et al., 1970; Andén and Fuxe, 1971), and the CA nerve terminals of the subependymal layer therefore probably represent a relatively pure NA system. The 10% decrease obtained in the lateral external layer is in good agreement with the IF studies on DBH suggesting a small proportion of NA terminals in this region. The 30—40% decrease obtained in the medial external layer, however, do not agree with the IF studies on the localization of DBH. Thus, only a few DBH-containing terminals could be found. There are several ways of explaining this discrepancy, either that the IF technique is not sensitive enough to demonstrate DBH in this region or that the effect of the DBH inhibitors is unspecific and due to toxic effects. It should be underlined, however, that the DBH inhibitors had no significant effect on the fluorescence in the neostriatum and only little effect on the fluorescence in the lateral external layer. In support of the view that some NA nerve terminals may exist in the medial external layer is the fact that some CA terminals in this region have a relatively low CA turnover similar to that in the subependymal layer (Hökfelt et al., 1973a). In spite of this the turnover of the CA in the medial part is higher than that in the lateral part (Löfström et al., 1974, see also this volume p. 313). This difference in amine turnover may therefore be explained on the basis that there exist two types of tubero-infundibular DA neurons, a medial and a lateral system. However, Björklund et al. (1973) have suggested another sub-division based on lesion experiments i.e. one diffuse system innervating the whole median eminence and several subsystems innervating only the area of median eminence lying immediately ventral of it.

When discussing DA systems involved in neuroendocrine control, it should be emphasized, however, that there exists a relatively extensive subcortical (Fuxe, 1965; Carlsson et al., 1965) and cortical DA innervation of the limbic system. The DA nerve terminals of the limbic cortex were only recently discovered (Hökfelt et al., 1973; Lidbrink et al., 1974). This has been partly due to the introduction of a modification of the Falck-Hillarp technique using Vibratome sections (unembedded sections) of brains from rats perfused with glyoxylic acid (Hökfelt and Ljungdahl, 1972; Axelsson et al., 1972; Lindvall et al., 1973) and partly due to new pharmacological models to demonstrate selectively DA terminals (Fuxe et al., 1974; Lidbrink et al., 1974).

In summary, the CA innervation of areas involved in the control of neuroendocrine events is complex. The organization of the CA systems strongly indicate an interplay of hormones, neurotransmitters and releasing factors.

Several systems are involved:

1) The ventral reticular ascending NA bundle innervating most hypothalamic nuclei, the subependymal, internal and, to some extent, the external layer of the median eminence.

2) The tubero-infundibular DA system innervating mainly the external layer of the median eminence (see also Björklund et al., this volume p. 210).

3) The ascending limbic DA systems innervating subcortical and cortical limbic structures.

4) The ascending reticulo-hypothalamic A system innervating *inter alia* the paraventricular magnocellular nuclei and parts of the arcuate nucleus.

Acknowledgements. This study has been supported by grants from the Swedish Medical Research Council (04X-715; 04X-2887; 04X-2295) and by grants from the Population Council (M73.73), from Svenska livförsäkringsbolags nämnd för medicinsk forskning and from Magn. Bergvalls stiftelse. For skilful technical assistance we thank Mrs. K. Andreasson, Mrs. M. Baidins, Mrs. A. Eliason and Miss B. Hagman.

References

Ajika, K., Hökfelt, T.: Ultrastructural identification of catecholamine neurones in the hypothalamic periventricular-arcuate nucleus-median eminence complex with special reference to quantitative aspects. Brain Res. **57**, 97 (1973).

Andén, N.-E., Fuxe, K.: A new dopamine-β-hydroxylase inhibitor: Effects on the noradrenaline concentration and on the action of L-DOPA in the spinal cord. Brit. J. Pharmacol. **43**, 747 (1971).

Axelsson, S., Björklund, A., Falck, B., Lindvall, O., Svensson, L. Å.: Glyoxylic acid condensation: A new fluorescence method for the histochemical demonstration of biogenic monoamines. Acta physiol. scand. **87**, 57 (1972).

Björklund, A., Falck, B., Hromek, F., Owman, Ch., West, K. A.: Identification and terminal distribution of the tubero-hypophyseal monoamine fibre systems in the rat by means of stereotaxic and microspectrofluorimetric technique. Brain Res. **17**, 1 (1970).

Björklund, A., Moore, R. Y., Nobin, A., Stenevi, U.: The organization of tubero-hypophyseal and reticulo-infundibular catecholamine neuron systems in the rat brain. Brain Res. **51**, 171 (1973).

Björklund, A., Nobin, A.: Fluorescence histochemical and microspectrofluorometric mapping of dopamine and noradrenaline cell groups in the rat diencephalon. Brain Res. **51**, 193 (1973).

Butcher, L. L., Engel, J., Fuxe, K.: Behavioral, biochemical, and histochemical analysis of the central effects of monoamine precursors after peripheral decarboxylase inhibition. Brain Res. **41**, 387 (1972).

Carlsson, A., Dahlström, A., Fuxe, K., Hillarp, N.-Å.: Failure of reserpine to deplete noradrenaline neurons of α-methyl-noradrenaline formed from α-methyl-DOPA. Acta pharmacol. (Kbh.) **22**, 270 (1965).

Corrodi, H., Fuxe, K., Hamberger, B., Ljungdahl, Å.: Studies on central and peripheral noradrenaline neurons using a new dopamine-β-hydroxylase inhibitor. Europ. J. Pharmacol. **12**, 145 (1970).

Fuxe, K.: Evidence for the existence of monoamine neurons in the central nervous system. IV. The distribution of monoamine nerve terminals in the central nervous system. Acta physiol. scand. **64**, Suppl. **247**, 39 (1965).

Fuxe, K., Goldstein, M., Hökfelt, T., Jonsson, G., Lidbrink, P.: Dopaminergic involvement in hypothalamic function: Extrahypothalamic and hypothalamic control. A neuroanatomical analysis. Parkinson's Disease, Vol. 5, p. 405. New York: Raven Press 1974.

Fuxe, K., Hökfelt, T.: Catecholamines in the hypothalamus and the pituitary gland. In: Ganong, W. F., Martini, L. (Eds.): Frontiers in Neuroendocrinology, p. 47. New York: Oxford University Press 1969.

Goldstein, M., Anagnoste, B., Freedman, L. S., Roffman, M., Ebstein, R. P., Park, D. H., Fuxe, K., Hökfelt, T.: Characterization, localization and regulation of catecholamine synthesizing enzymes. In: Usdin, E., Snyder, S. (Eds.): Frontiers in catecholamine research, p. 69. New York: Pergamon Press 1973.

Goldstein, M., Fuxe, K., Hökfelt, T.: Characterization and tissue localization of catecholamine synthesizing enzymes. Pharmacol. Rev. **24**, 293 (1972).

Halász, B.: The endocrine effects of isolation of the hypothalamus from the rest of the brain. In: Ganong, W. F., Martini, L. (Eds.): Frontiers in Neuroendocrinology, p. 307. New York: Oxford University Press 1969.

Hartman, B. K., Udenfriend, S.: Immunofluorescent localization of dopamine-β-hydroxylase in tissue. Molec. Pharmacol. **6**, 85 (1970).

Hökfelt, T., Fuxe, K., Ajika, K., Löfström, A.: Central catecholamine neurons and gonadotropin secretion. In: Proc. IV Intern. Congr. Endocrinol. held in Washington 1972. Intern.
Congr. Ser. No. 273, p. 138 (1973).

Hökfelt, T., Fuxe, K., Goldstein, M.: Immunohistochemical localization of aromatic L-amino
acid decarboxylase (DOPA decarboxylase) in central dopamine and 5-hydroxytryptamine
nerve cell bodies of the rat. Brain Res. **53**, 175 (1973b).

Hökfelt, T., Fuxe, K., Goldstein, M.: Immunohistochemical studies on monoamine-containing
cell systems. Brain Res. **62**, 461 (1973c).

Hökfelt, T., Fuxe, K., Goldstein, M., Joh, T. H.: Immunohistochemical localization of three
catecholamine synthesizing enzymes: Aspects on methodology. Histochemie **33**, 231 (1973d).

Hökfelt, T., Fuxe, K., Goldstein, M., Johansson, O.: Immunohistochemical evidence for the
existence of adrenaline neurons in the rat brain. Brain Res. **66**, 235 (1974).

Hökfelt, T., Fuxe, K., Johansson, O., Ljungdahl, Å.: Pharmaco-histochemical evidence of the
existence of dopamine nerve terminals in the limbic cortex. Europ. J. Pharmacol. **25**, 108
(1973e).

Hökfelt, T., Ljungdahl, Å.: Modification of the Falck-Hillarp formaldehyde fluorescence
method using the Vibratome®: Simple, rapid and sensitive localization of catecholamines
in sections of unfixed or formalin fixed brain tissue. Histochemie **29**, 324 (1972).

Johnsson, G., Fuxe, K., Hökfelt, T.: On the catecholamine innervation of the hypothalamus,
with special reference to the median eminence. Brain Res. **40**, 271 (1972).

Lidbrink, P., Jonsson, G., Fuxe, K.: Selective reserpine-resistant accumulation of catecholamines in central dopamine neurons after dopa administration. Brain Res. **67**, 439 (1974).

Lindvall, O., Björklund, A., Hökfelt, T., Ljungdahl, Å.: Application of the glyoxylic acid
method to Vibratome sections for the improved visualization of central catecholamine
neurons. Histochemie **35**, 31 (1973).

Löfström, A., Jonsson, G., Fuxe, K.: Microfluorimetric quantitation of catecholamines in rat
median eminence. In: Proceedings VI: International Symposium on Neurosecretion.
Berlin-Heidelberg-New York: Springer 1974.

Löfström, A., Jonsson, G., Fuxe, K.: A quantitative fluorescence analysis of catecholamine
terminals of the median eminence. To be published (1974).

Sundler, F.: M. D. Thesis, Lund 1973.

Weiner, R. I., Gorski, R. A., Sawyer, C. H.: Hypothalamic catecholamines and pituitary
gonadotropic function. In: Brain-endocrine interaction. Median eminence: Structure and
function, p. 236. Basel-München-Paris-London-New York-Sydney: Karger 1972.

Wittkowski, W.: Elektronenmikroskopische Untersuchungen zur funktionellen Morphologie
des Tubero-hypophysären Systems der Ratte. Z. Zellforsch. **139**, 101 (1973).

Extrahypothalamic Influences on the Tubero-Infundibular Dopamine Neurones and the Secretion of Luteinizing Hormone (LH) and Prolactin*

W. Lichtensteiger[1]

Department of Pharmacology, University of Zürich, Zürich (Switzerland)

Introduction

On structural grounds, a role of noradrenergic and serotoninergic projection systems in neuroendocrine control seems to be very plausible, since their projections to a large number of brain regions should enable them to favour or inhibit the establishment of complex response patterns consisting of both endocrine and behavioural processes. The local tubero-infundibular dopamine (DA) system introduces an additional dimension into this picture. Most of the available evidence indicates that these neurones act indirectly by modulating the release of releasing or inhibiting factors, but their position within neuroendocrine organization is far from being understood. We have tried to approach this question by investigating the neural input to the tuberal DA neurones. As a tool to disclose possible influences from other brain areas, we used a characteristic change in the fluorescence intensity of the cell bodies that can be detected by histochemical microfluorometry after local electrical or trans-synaptic stimulation as well as after various treatments known to be accompanied by an increase in catecholamine turnover (Lichtensteiger, 1969b, 1971; Heinrich et al., 1971; Lienhart et al., 1973). When a representative population of DA neurones is studied, such treatments can be shown to result in a fast increase in mean fluorescence intensity which, at least in some of the experiments, was found to be part of a biphasic intensity change. The biochemical background of this acute reaction is not yet fully understood; so far, it has been shown that the initial increase in intensity depends upon tyrosine hydroxylase activity, but it remains to be determined whether DA alone or in combination with DOPA is responsible for the increase in intensity. Since the magnitude of this response is rather constant and its initial phase almost linear, it appeared to be suitable for use as an evoked response.

* Supported by SNSF grant 3.691.71, the Hartmann-Müller Stiftung, the Barell Stiftung and the Jubiläumsspende of the University of Zürich.

[1] Address: Pharmakologisches Institut der Universität Zürich, Gloriastraße 32, CH-8006 Zürich, Switzerland.

Effect of Extrahypothalamic Stimulation and Interaction with Cholinergic Systems

We were primarily interested in possible influences from limbic structures. In such areas, intermittent electrical stimulation was applied unilaterally for 10 min (30 min in some cases). Using a microfluorometric technique based on the histochemical fluorescence method of Falck and Hillarp, the fluorescence intensity of the tuberal DA nerve cells was subsequently recorded at 15 levels through the antero-posterior extension of the arcuate nucleus by means of a semi-automatic equipment with off-line computer data analysis (Lichtensteiger, 1969a, 1970; Lichtensteiger et al., in preparation). In most cases, ovariectomized rats pretreated for one day with oestradiol-dipropionate (5 µg s.c.) and progesterone (2 mg s.c.) were studied, but it should be noted that at least with regard to the amygdala (cf. below), similar changes in fluorescence intensity were also observed in cycling rats stimulated on the first day of diestrus (Lichtensteiger, 1973a). Luteinizing hormone and prolactin served as indicators for effects on anterior pituitary function. It is quite evident that a more elaborate picture of the interaction of the DA system with pituitary function could be given if additional hormones of the anterior

Table 1. *Effect of electrical stimulation and treatment with atropine, methylatropine or α-methyltyrosine on the fluorescence intensity of tuberal dopamine nerve cells.* Mean (m) and variance (s^2) of lognormal two-parameter distributions (natural logarithms), mean relative intensity (I_r as percentage of noradrenaline standard) of non-transformed distributions and cell count (n, with number of rats in brackets)[*]

Electrode position, duration of stimulation[**]	Drug[***]	m	s^2	n	$I_r\%$
med. preoptic area sham-operated	none	3.324	0.1744	1048 (5)	30.2
med. preoptic area 10 min stimulated	none	3.772[a]	0.1544	681 (5)	46.9
med. preoptic area 10 min stimulated	methyl-atropine 10.5 mg/kg	3.701[a]	0.1742	963 (5)	44.2
arcuate nucleus 10 min stimulated	atropine 10 mg/kg	3.850[a]	0.1725	896 (5)	51.2
diagonal tract nuc. 10 min stimulated	none	3.705[a]	0.1539	514 (3)	43.9
bed nuc. of stria terminalis, ventrolateral part 10 min stimulated	none	3.759[a]	0.1577	280 (2)	46.4
med. amygdaloid nuc. 10 min stimulated	none	3.596[a]	0.1412	703 (4)	39.1
ventromedial midbrain tegmentum 10 min stimulated	none	3.630[a]	0.1818	663 (4)	41.2
ventral hippocampus sham-operated	α-methyl-tyrosine	3.048[a]	0.1979	512 (4)	23.2
ventral hippocampus 30 min stimulated	α-methyl-tyrosine	3.129[a]	0.1928	415 (4)	27.5
med. preoptic area 30 min stimulated	α-methyl-tyrosine	2.994[d]	0.2034	326	22.1

Table 1 (Continuation)

Electrode position, duration of stimulation**	Drug***	m	s^2	n	$I_r\%$
med. preoptic area sham-operated	atropine 10 mg/kg	3.269	0.2212[e]	1053 (5)	29.2
med. preoptic area 10 min stimulated	atropine 10 mg/kg	3.353[b]	0.2065[e]	955 (5)	31.6
med. preoptic area 10 min stimulated	atropine 2 mg/kg	3.423[b]	0.2003[c]	953 (5)	33.8
med. preoptic area 10 min stimulated	atropine 0.4 mg/kg	3.590	0.1797[f]	894 (5)	39.5
diagonal tract nuc. 10 min stimulated	atropine 10 mg/kg	3.254[b]	0.1601	580 (3)	28.1
bed nuc. of stria terminalis, ventrolateral part 10 min stimulated	atropine 10 mg/kg	3.429[c]	0.2040[f]	625 (3)	34.2
med. amygdaloid nuc. 10 min stimulated	atropine 10 mg/kg	3.480[c]	0.1626[f]	580 (3)	35.3
ventromedial midbrain tegmentum 10 min stimulated	atropine 10 mg/kg	3.472	0.1841	642 (4)	35.3
med. preoptic area 30 min stimulated	atropine 10 mg/kg	3.411[b]	0.2036[e]	1172 (5)	33.5

[a] Values of individual cells are obtained by relating their absolute intensity to that of a noradrenaline-containing standard worked up together with the tissue, after correction for non-specific fluorescence of tissue and standard. $I_r\%$ = mean of non-transformed distributions. Since these are closely approximated by lognormal two-parameter distributions, the statistical analysis is based on mean and variance of logarithmically transformed distributions. Differences between means: a = different from sham-operated, untreated controls for $p < 0.001$; b = different for $p < 0.001$ or c = different for $p < 0.05$ from group with same stimulation site not treated with atropine; d = two groups different for $p < 0.05$. —Differences between variances of groups stimulated in the same area with or without atropine; e = for $p < 0.01$, f = for $p < 0.05$.

[b] Unilateral stimulation, monophasic positive pulses, 0.5 msec, 100 Hz, 100 μA, 15 sec on/off.

[c] Atropine or methylatropine were administered s. c. 15 min, α-methyl-tyrosine methyl ester (H 44/68, 250 mg/kg) i. p. 30 min before the onset of stimulation.

and intermediate lobes were assayed (cf. Müller, this symposium; Collu et al., 1972; Björklund et al., 1973; Taleisnik et al., 1972).

Ten minutes of electrical stimulation resulted in a rapid increase in the fluorescence intensity of the tuberal DA neurones when current was applied to the *nucleus of the diagonal tract*, ventrolateral part of the ventral half of the *bed nucleus of stria terminalis*, *medial amygdaloid nucleus* and certain sites of the *ventromedial tegmentum* of the anterior *midbrain* (Table 1, Lichtensteiger, 1973; Lichtensteiger and Keller, 1974). In the latter case, stimulation in the ventromedial tegmental area of Tsai appeared to be most effective. Although more variable in magnitude, the response was of the type induced by medial preoptic stimulation (10 min, Table 1; Lichtensteiger, 1971), which appears to indicate that the bulk of the DA neurones were influenced in a similar way from these various regions. Since the same rapid increase in fluorescence intensity had earlier been noted in the DA neurones after local electrical stimulation of the arcuate nucleus (Lichtensteiger, 1971) and in several DA neurone groups in situations linked with an enhanced catecholamine turnover (Lichtensteiger, 1969b; Heinrich et al., 1971; Lienhart et al., 1973), we assume that the majority of the DA neurones probably were activated under these conditions. The effect of acute stimulation in the *ventral hippocampus*, close to the subiculum, was studied in another experimental arrangement, i.e., after short-term inhibition of catecholamine synthesis by α-methyl-tyrosine (250 mg/kg i.p. 30 min before the onset of stimulation). Under these conditions, hippocampal stimulation (30 min) resulted in a slight retardation of the decrease in the fluorescence intensity of the DA neurones that was caused by synthesis inhibition. This change in fluorescence intensity differed from the result of preoptic stimulation (30 min, Table 1), which suggests that the effect elicited by ventral hippocampal stimulation was opposed to that of preoptic stimulation. It appears then that rapid responses can be elicited in the tubero-infundibular DA neurones by stimulation of various *limbic structures* and *ascending brainstem systems*. In consequence, one might expect that the DA system could serve as an intermediary between those brain areas and releasing or inhibiting factors in a variety of functional situations.

It seemed of interest to investigate which neurotransmitter systems might possibly be involved in the transmission of the effects of stimulation. In view of earlier reports on the role of cholinergic systems in the control of ovulation (Sawyer et al., 1949a; Sawyer et al., 1949b; Aron et al., 1966; Zarrow and Quinn, 1963), we first studied the effect of atropine (Table 1, Lichtensteiger, 1972, 1973a and b). Wherever we looked for a possible influence of this drug, it was found to exert a marked effect on the response of the DA neurones to electrical stimulation. It thereby appeared to act as a specific antagonist at one or several *central cholinergic synapses*, insofar as 1) local electrical stimulation in the arcuate nucleus was effective despite atropine treatment, 2) the reduction of the intensity response by the drug was dose-dependent (0.4–10 mg/kg s.c.) and 3) methylatropine which has much more difficulties to cross the blood-brain barrier, was ineffective. The effectiveness of atropine with stimulation in a variety of brain regions suggests that the cholinergic influence might perhaps be brought about by a modulatory effect of a cholinergic projection system rather than by the presence of a cholinergic link in a specific neuroendocrine pathway.

Response of Tuberal DA Neurones as Related to Changes in Serum Levels of Luteinizing Hormone (LH) and Prolactin

Stimulation in the various areas resulted in different patterns of hormonal changes which depended markedly upon the presence or absence of atropine. Moreover, there appeared to exist a considerable *interdependence* between changes in the two hormones (Table 2). Two *main patterns* emerge from the various experiments (Lichtensteiger and Keller, 1974): Preoptic stimulation (10 min) in the absence of atropine (as well as arcuate stimulation after atropine) induced a rise in LH while prolactin did not change (if anything it decreased). Atropine reduced the rise in LH after preoptic stimulation (10 min) but

Table 2. *Correlation between fluorescence intensity of the tuberal dopamine neurones and serum concentrations of luteinizing hormone (LH) and prolactin.* Correlation between means (*m*) of logarithmically transformed intensity distributions and hormone concentrations of individual rats of 10 min stimulated groups related to sham-operated groups[a]

Group related to sham-operated group	Correlation coefficients			Partial correlation	
	m vs. LH (r_{12})	*m* vs. prolactin (r_{13})	LH vs. prolactin (r_{23})	*m* vs. LH ($r_{12.3}$)	*m* vs. prolactin ($r_{13.2}$)
preoptic no drug	0.6395[b]	—0.3266	—0.4662	0.5827	—0.0419
preoptic methyl-atropine	0.6308[b]	0.0758	—0.3502	0.7038	0.4082
arcuate nucleus atropine	0.6335[b]	0.1791	0.0179	0.6408	0.2169
diagonal no drug	0.3488	0.4506	—0.5772	0.8352[b]	0.8518[b]
stria bed nucleus[c] no drug	—0.1131	0.6860	—0.7276[b]	0.7734	0.8857[b]
amygdaloid no drug	0.0220	0.5239	—0.6990[b]	0.6373	0.7543[b]
midbrain no drug	0.3240	0.5248	—0.2030	0.5165	0.6375

Group related to sham-operated group	Correlation coefficients			Partial correlation	
	m vs. LH (r_{12})	*m* vs. prolactin (r_{13})	LH vs prolactin (r_{23})	*m* vs. LH ($r_{12.3}$)	*m* vs. prolactin ($r_{13.2}$)
preoptic atropine 10 mg/kg	0.6275[b]	0.7123[b]	0.6639[b]	0.2946	0.5078
preoptic atropine 2 mg/kg	0.7340[b]	0.4896	0.3956	0.6747	0.3194
preoptic atropine 0.4 mg/kg	0.7093[b]	0.6319[b]	0.5650	0.5509	0.3974
diagonal tr. atropine	0.3821	0.5289	—0.0052	0.4535	0.5745
stria bed nucleus atropine	0.0456	0.5320	0.6340[b]	—0.4455	0.6512
amygdaloid atropine[d]	0.6802[b]	0.7751[b]			
midbrain atropine	0.4033	0.7572[b]	0.4663	0.0869	0.7031

[a] As it was necessary to consider the various stimulation sites separately, means and hormone concentrations of individual rats of a stimulated group were combined, for calculation of correlation coefficients, with the corresponding sham-operated group (with or without atropine). Mean intensities were those of the whole tuberal DA group. The values are tabulated in Lichtensteiger and Keller (1974). — Within the sham-operated groups, the correlation between LH and prolactin is $r = —0.9543$ without atropine and $r = 0.6825$ after atropine.

[b] r different from zero for $p < 0.05$. It should be noted that with the small number of rats assembled in each comparison, the addition or subtraction of one rat would considerably influence the level of significance, especially with the reduction of degrees of freedom in the calculation of partial correlation coefficients.

[c] These values refer to two rats with ventrolateral electrode placement in the bed nucleus, the combined mean of which is shown in Table 1. This stimulation site corresponds to that of the atropine-treated group.

[d] Since there was only one rat in this group with simultaneous determination of both hormones, no partial correlation coefficient is given.

at the same time, prolactin increased. With the other stimulation sites, no consistent rise in LH was noted in the absence of atropine, while prolactin levels were generally elevated. Atropine treatment then resulted in an increase in LH. Prolactin reached about the same levels as without atropine (Hippocampal effects are excluded from this consideration because they were studied under different experimental conditions). If we take medial amygdaloid stimulation as an example, several reasons may be put forward to explain these divergent findings: On one hand, it is known that electrophysiological responses in preoptic region and hypothalamus depend upon the *frequency* of amygdaloid stimulation (Murphy et al., 1968; Ellendorff and Wuttke, 1973) and stimulation with comparatively high frequency (150 Hz) blocked ovulation in acute experiments (Ellendorff et al., 1973). The short duration of our experiments would probably not have allowed to detect a decrease in serum LH. On the other hand, *urethane anesthesia* – which was used in the present experiments – has been found to block the induction of ovulation by (electrochemical) stimulation of the medial amygdala (Velasco and Taleisnik, 1969) and to interfere with spontaneous unit activity in the preoptico-hypothalamic region only if the connections with the remainder of the brain were intact (Cross and Dyer, 1971). Thus, the transmission of signals from the medial amygdala and possibly other areas to the preoptico-hypothalamic region appears to be influenced by urethane. This anesthetic affects peripheral cholinergic and adrenergic systems (Barrett, 1971). There, its effect differs from that of pentobarbital, e.g., with respect to atropine which increased heart rate after urethane but not after pentobarbital. It is then interesting to note that in contrast to pentobarbital (Ajika et al., 1972), urethane did not markedly depress prolactin in our experiments, whereas it interfered with the induction of LH secretion from regions such as the medial amygdala. With such stimulation sites, atropine counteracted the effect of urethane on LH but remained without a clear-cut effect on changes in prolactin levels. It becomes evident from these considerations that atropine exerted not only quantitative but also qualitative effects, a fact that is further illustrated by the change in the correlation between LH and prolactin (Table 2).

The main patterns of hormonal changes have no direct counterpart in the response of the tuberal DA neurones, as the latter responded to, for example, preoptic and amygdaloid stimulation basically in the same way. When correlations between mean fluorescence intensity and hormone levels of individual rats are calculated, there necessarily results a complex picture (Table 2). Several factors may be responsible for these discrepancies:

a) *Other neural inputs* that reach releasing factor-containing neurones either at the level of their cell bodies or at the level of the median eminence, may interfere with the action of DA on release of releasing factors. An involvement of noradrenergic and serotoninergic projection systems is highly probable (Anton-Tay et al., 1969; Bapna et al., 1971; Donoso and de Gutierrez Moyano, 1970; Donoso et al., 1971; Collu et al., 1972; Kalra and McCann, 1972; Kordon, 1969, 1972). It is to be expected from their topography that they act at various levels of neuroendocrine integration, i.e., they may exert effects that "bypass" the tubero-infundibular DA neurones but also influence the functional state of the latter. On the other hand, the role played by cholinergic systems (Sawyer et al., 1949a and b; Aron et al., 1966; Zarrow and Quinn, 1963; Blake and Sawyer, 1972) need not be limited to their effect on the tuberal DA neurones. Urethane anesthesia appears to cause a certain type of balance between various neurotransmitter systems (Barrett, 1971; Reinert, 1964) and in this way could affect the result of stimulation.

b) Differences in the *threshold* for DA action on the hormonal axes may result either from neural inputs as suggested above or, possibly, from direct hormonal feedback actions on releasing factor neurones or the pituitary. Findings such as variations in the effectiveness of intraventricular DA on LH release during the oestrous cycle (Schneider and McCann, 1970) or blockade of l-DOPA-induced ovulation by an anti-oestrogen (Raziano et al., 1971) suggest such a possibility although they do not allow to specify the site of action of the hormone or the antagonist.

c) Even if significant correlations (Table 2) indicate the existence of some parallel influence on the tuberal DA neurones and LH or prolactin, the response of these neurones need not in every case be causally related to the hormonal change but might sometimes have been linked with closely related processes that involved *other pituitary hormones*. DA neurones most probably play a role also in the regulation i.a., of growth hormone and MSH (Björklund et al., 1973; Collu et al., 1972; Müller and Cocchi, this volume; Taleisnik et al., 1972), yet, the relative importance of dopaminergic and noradrenergic neurones is not clear. In the control of ACTH, the involvement of the latter appears to be more prominent (Scapagnini et al., 1972).

d) Although an influence of the tuberal DA neurones on several hormonal axes is compatible with a common state of activity of the whole DA system (cf. Lichtensteiger, 1970), there may exist a certain functional *heterogeneity* within this group. The differences in the variance of logarithmically transformed intensity distributions (both between groups of rats or individual animals, Table 1, Fig. 1) appear to support this idea. In the present material, such differences were mainly related to the presence or absence of atropine: This drug provoked an increase in variance in almost all experimental groups. Since atropine influenced the direction of the changes in LH and prolactin (Table 2), the differences in variance can also be considered with respect to the relationship between the two hormones: It appears that an inverse relation between LH and prolactin (with a rise of either LH or prolactin) was accompanied rather by lower variances than a positive correlation between these hormones (Fig. 1). It is not possible to decide whether such differences resulted from a change in the proportion of responsive DA neurones or from a change in their response characteristics. Despite the difficulty of interpreting differences in variance in functional terms, they indicate, however, that even with similar mean intensities (cf. sham-operated controls) the distribution of individual intensity values was not always the same within the population. When the intensity response to stimulation was studied at 15 different levels through the anteroposterior extension of the arcuate nucleus, the magnitude of the intensity change was found to vary, but it became evident that neurones with quantitatively or qualitatively different responses were intermingled to a considerable degree (Keller and Lichtensteiger, 1974).

When account is taken for the interdependence of the changes in LH and prolactin by calculating partial correlation coefficients (Table 2), a rather consistent relationship between intensity changes in the tuberal DA neurones and changes in *both* hormones becomes apparent. The various relations can be arranged into a

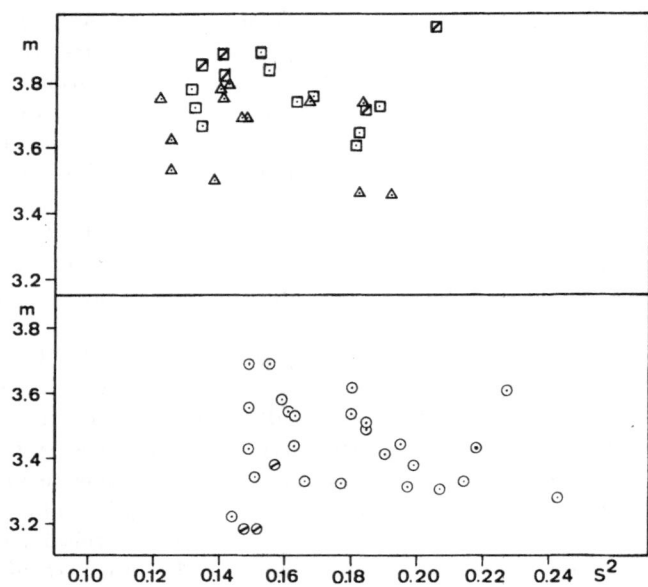

Fig. 1. Distribution of individual intensity values within the tuberal DA neurone population: Variance (s^2) plotted against mean (m) of logarithmically transformed distributions of relative fluorescence intensity of individual rats. — *Upper part:* Rats from untreated stimulated groups with a negative correlation between LH and prolactin as related to control levels (first part of Table 2. □: rise in LH, △: rise in prolactin; ◩: arcuate nucleus (atropine without effect on intensity response) $r = 0$). — *Lower part:* Rats from atropine-treated stimulated groups with positive correlation between hormones as related to control levels (second part in Table 2. ⊘: diagonal tract $r = 0$). Values are tabulated in Lichtensteiger and Keller, 1974

fairly coherent *scheme*, if only the possibilities of additional neural inputs to releasing factor neurones and of a (functional) heterogeneity of the DA neurone population are considered. A relation between DA neurones and prolactin is evident in our material. From the negative correlation between fluorescence intensity and increased prolactin levels in α-methyl-tyrosine-treated, sham-operated rats as compared to untreated, sham-operated animals (not shown), it would appear that the DA neurones exert an inhibitory influence, which agrees with earlier reports (Donoso et al., 1971; Hökfelt and Fuxe, 1972; Kamberi et al., 1970; Lu and Meites, 1971). On the other hand, the consistent correlation between intensity response of the tuberal DA neurones and rise in LH after preoptic stimulation still suggests a facilitatory role with respect to this hormone. Reports in the literature are conflicting with regard to LH (Ahrén et al., 1971; Fuxe et al., 1969; Fuxe et al., 1972; Kamberi et al., 1970a; Keller and Lichtensteiger, 1971; Kordon, 1971; Schneider and McCann, 1970). It is evident that the possibility of a false correlation simulated by some closely related process that was beyond our control, needs to be considered. Yet, the rather obvious possibility of a parallel stimulation of cell bodies containing luteinizing hormone-releasing hormone (LRH) — recently observed in the preoptic region (Barry et al., 1973) — is not sufficient to explain all our data, especially those related to DA response and prolactin secretion after stimulation in various areas. An explanation for the discrepancies between the various findings should rather be sought in the interaction between different neurotransmitter systems. Some of the observations related to catecholamines, e.g., may result from the activity of noradrenergic terminals innervating the median eminence (cf. Björklund et al., 1970). Moreover, one should keep in mind that the situation may also be more complex on the side of the releasing factors: While an appropriate interpretation of most of the results related to monoamines is possible on the basis of effects on prolactin inhibiting — factor (PIF) and LRH, additional factors such as prolactin releasing factor (Valverde et al., 1972) or thyrotropin releasing hormone may come into play, and very fast feedback effects may mask the original actions.

Returning to our recent data, I should like to emphasize that they were obtained under a special type of neurotransmitter balance that resulted from urethane anesthesia, as well as from the special neuroendocrine state of the animal. Under these conditions, LH and prolactin were inversely related in *sham-operated controls* in the absence of atropine (Table 2) which suggests a parallel relase of LRH and PIF. Atropine abolished this relation and at the same time induced an increase in the variance of the DA neurone population (Table 1). One possible explanation of this phenomenon might be sought in a loss of a common influence exerted on DA neurones related to LRH and PIF in the absence of atropine. Similar factors may have been responsible for the changes in the variance of stimulated rats. *Medial preoptic stimulation* appears to have caused an activation of DA neurones accompanied by release of LRH and, possibly, PIF. The latter is suggested by the inverse relation of the two hormones (as compared to control levels, Table 2). Prolactin levels were not definitely reduced, but the duration of the experiment (10 min) would probably not have allowed a detectable reduction in prolactin concentration. The effect of atropine could be explained by a reduction of the effect of preoptic stimulation on DA neurones related to both hormones, preventing a release of LRH above control levels and removing a stimulatory effect on PIF release. As the residual increase in mean fluorescence intensity was correlated with increased prolactin levels, this correlation became positive. When the rats were *stimulated in other regions (med. amygdala)* in the absence of atropine, it seems as if the activation of DA neurones had remained ineffective with regard to LRH or PIF release. This could have happened if the effect of DA had been counteracted by the activation of other projections to releasing factor neurones. Such a possibility can certainly not be disregarded, especially with the relatively high frequency of stimulation. In order to explain our data, one would have to assume an increased inhibitory tone on both LRH and PIF. This task could be fulfilled with respect to both hormones by serotoninergic projections (Kamberi et al., 1970a; Kordon, 1969, 1972). Atropine again affected the response of the DA neurones, but most probably, this was not its unique effect: It seems conceivable that other projections to releasing factor neurones were also influenced by the drug, possibly also those additionally activated by stimulation in areas such as the medial amygdala. Yet, it is certainly premature to attempt at any detailed interpretation of the changes induced by atropine under these conditions.

Conclusions

It appears from these stimulation experiments that the tubero-infundibular DA neurones can be influenced from various extrahypothalamic areas, notably from limbic structures. They are thus probably subject to a variety of modulatory influences. Clearly nothing can be said about the pathways involved and it is possible that other brain areas are intercalated. Yet, it seems rather certain that in most cases the transmission depends upon the activity of central cholinergic systems. The stimulation-induced changes in the fluorescence intensity of the DA neurones were correlated with both LH and prolactin but the rather complex pattern of response of DA neurones and hormones strongly suggests an interaction of these neurones with other projections to releasing factor neurones. The time course of the events may be of some importance, too: It should be mentioned that in animals stimulated for 30 min in the preoptic region after atropine treatment, LH was elevated while the mean intensity remained depressed (Table 1). This could mean either that atropine blockade of the DA system was not sufficiently complete or else, that other central systems were engaged for a slower LH response. In this context, it should be recalled that reflex ovulation in rats seems to be more easily blocked by atropine than spontaneous ovulation (Aron et al., 1966) and also, that not all processes releasing prolactin have been found to depend on the same degree on cholinergic systems (Blake and Sawyer, 1972). There may well exist different patterns of central control for one hormone axis. The DA system need not be of the same importance for all of these. This could explain in part the difficulties of defining the action of the DA neurones or even to visualize their involvement under certain experimental conditions.

References

Ahrén, K., Fuxe, K., Hamberger, L., Hökfelt, T.: Turnover changes in the tubero-infundibular dopamine neurons during the ovarian cycle of the rat. Endocrinology 88, 1415—1424 (1971).

Ajika, K., Krulich, L., McCann, S. M.: The effect of pentobarbital (Nembutal) on prolactin release in the rat. Proc. Soc. exp. Biol. (N. Y.) 141, 203—205 (1972).

Anton-Tay, F., Pelham, R. W., Wurtman, R. J.: Increased turnover of ³H-norepinephrine in rat brain following castration or treatment with ovine follicle-stimulation hormone. Endocrinology 84, 1489—1492 (1969).

Aron, C., Asch, G., Roos, J.: Triggering of ovulation by coitus in the rat. Int. Rev. Cytol. 20, 139—172 (1966).

Bapna, J., Neff, N. H., Costa, E.: A method for studying norepinephrine and serotonin metabolism in small regions of rat brain: Effect of ovariectomy on amine metabolism in anterior and posterior hypothalamus. Endocrinology 89, 1345—1349 (1971).

Barrett, A. M.: The effects of some autonomic blocking agents on the heart rates of anaesthtized and pithed rats. Europ. J. Pharmacol. 15, 267—273 (1971).

Barry, J., Dubois, M. P., Poulain, P., Leonardelli, J.: Caractérisation et topographie des neurones hypothalamiques immunoréactifs avec des anticorps anti-LRF de synthèse. C. R. Acad. Sci. (Paris) 276 (Série D), 3191—3193 (1973).

Björklund, A., Falck, B., Hromek, F., Owman, C., West, K. A.: Identification and terminal distribution of the tubero-hypophyseal monoamine fibre systems in the rat by means of stereotaxic and microspectrofluorimetric techniques. Brain Res. 17, 1—23 (1970).

Björklund, A., Moore, R. Y., Nobin, A., Stenevi, U.: The organization of tubero-hypophyseal and reticulo-infundibular catecholamine neuron systems in the rat brain. Brain Res. **51**, 171—191 (1973).

Blake, C. A., Sawyer, C. H.: Nicotine blocks the suckling-induced rise in circulating prolactin in rats. Science **177**, 619—621 (1972).

Collu, R., Fraschini, F., Visconti, P., Martini, L.: Adrenergic and serotoninergic control of growth hormone secretion in adult male rats. Endocrinology **90**, 1231—1237 (1972).

Cross, B. A., Dyer, R. G.: Unit activity in rat diencephalic islands — the effect of anaesthetics J. Physiol. (Lond.) **212**, 467—481 (1971).

Donoso, A. O., de Gutierrez Moyano, M.: Adrenergic activity in hypothalamus and ovulation. Proc. Soc. exp. Biol. (N. Y.) **135**, 633—635 (1970).

Donoso, A. O., Bishop, W., Fawcett, C. P., Krulich, L., McCann, S. M.: Effects of drugs that modify brain monoamine concentrations on plasma gonadotropin and prolactin levels in the rat. Endocrinology **89**, 774—784 (1971).

Ellendorff, F., Wuttke, W.: Limbic, mesencephalic and peripheral influence on preoptic neuronal activity in the rat. Pflügers Arch. ges. Physiol. **339**, Suppl. R 84 (1973).

Ellendorff, F., Colombo, J. A., Blake, C. A., Whitmoyer, D. I., Sawyer, C. H.: Effects of electrical stimulation of the amygdala on gonadotropin release and ovulation in the rat. Proc. Soc. exp. Biol. (N. Y.) **142**, 417—420 (1973).

Fuxe, K., Hökfelt, T., Nilsson, O.: Castration, sex hormones, and tubero-infundibular dopamine neurons. Neuroendocrinology **5**, 107—120 (1969).

Fuxe, K., Hökfelt, T., Sundstedt, C.-D., Ahrén, K., Hamberger, L.: Amine turnover changes in the tubero-infundibular dopamine (DA) neurons in immature rats injected with PMS. Neuroendocrinology **10**, 282—300 (1972).

Heinrich, U., Lichtensteiger, W., Langemann, H.: Effect of morphine on the catecholamine content of midbrain nerve cell groups in rat and mouse. J. Pharmacol. exp. Ther. **179**, 259—267 (1971).

Hökfelt, T., Fuxe, K.: Effects of prolactin and ergot alkaloids on the tubero-infundibular dopamine (DA) neurons. Neuroendrocrinology **9**, 100—122 (1972).

Kalra, S. P., McCann, S. M.: Modification of brain catecholamine level and LH release by preoptic stimulation. Excerpta Medica Int. Congress Series No. 256, Abstracts, IV Int. Congress of Endocrinology, Washington 1972, Abstract No. 508. Amsterdam: Excerpta Medica 1972.

Kamberi, I. A., Mical, R. S., Porter, J. C.: Effect of anterior pituitary perfusion and intraventricular injection of catecholamines and indoleamines on LH release. Endocrinology **87**, 1—12 (1970a).

Kamberi, I. A., Mical, R. S., Porter, J. C.: Prolactin-inhibiting activity in hypophysial stalk blood and elevation by dopamine. Experientia (Basel) **26**, 1150—1151 (1970b).

Keller, P. J., Lichtensteiger, W.: Stimulation of tubero-infundibular dopamine neurones and gonadotrophin secretion. J. Physiol. (Lond.) **219**, 385—401 (1971).

Kordon, C.: Effects of selective experimental changes in regional hypothalamic monoamine levels on superovulation in the immature rat. Neuroendocrinology **4**, 129—138 (1969).

Kordon, C.: Blockade of ovulation in the immature rat by local microinjection of α-methyl-dopa into the arcuate region of the hypothalamus. Neuroendocrinology **7**, 202—209 (1971).

Kordon, C.: Rôle de la sérotonine hypothalamique dans la libération de prolactine induite par succion du mamelon chez la rate lactante. Lille méd. **17**, 1406 (1972).

Lienhart, R., Lichtensteiger, W., Langemann, H.: Studies on midbrain dopamine (DA) neurons in morphine-tolerant mice. Experientia (Basel) **29**, 764—765 (1973).

Lichtensteiger, W.: Cyclic variations of catecholamine content in hypothalamic nerve cells during the estrous cycle of the rat, with a concomitant study of the substantia nigra. J. Pharmacol. exp. Ther. **165**, 204—215 (1969a).

Lichtensteiger, W.: The catecholamine content of hypothalamic nerve cells after acute exposure to cold and thyroxine administration. J. Physiol. (Lond.) **203**, 675—687 (1969b).

Lichtensteiger, W.: Katecholaminhaltige Neurone in der neuroendokrinen Steuerung. Prinzip und Anwendung der Mikrofluorimetrie. Progr. Histochem. Cytochem. 1 (No. 4), 185—276 (1970).

Lichtensteiger, W.: Effect of electrical stimulation on the fluorescence intensity of catechol-amine-containing tuberal nerve cells. J. Physiol. (Lond.) **218**, 63—84 (1971).

Lichtensteiger, W.: Changes in hypothalamic monoamines in relation to endocrine states: Functional characteristics of tubero-infundibular dopamine neurons. In: Endocrinology, Proc. of the Fourth Int. Congress, Washington 1972. Int. Congr. Ser. No. 273, pp. 131—137. Amsterdam: Excerpta Medica 1973.

Lichtensteiger, W., Keller, P. J.: Tubero-infundibular dopamine neurons and the secretion of luteinizing hormone and prolactin: extrahypothalamic influences, interaction with cholin-ergic systems and the effect of urethane anesthesia. Brain Research **74**, 279—303 (1974).

Lu, K.-H., Meites, J.: Inhibition by L-dopa and monoamine oxidase inhibitors of pituitary prolactin release; stimulation by methyldopa and amphetamine. Proc. Soc. exp. Biol. (N. Y.) **137**, 480—483 (1971).

Müller, E. E., Cocchi, D.: Brain monoamines and the control of growth hormone release. In: Neurosecretion — The Final Neuroendocrine Pathway (VI. Int. Symposium on Neuro-secretion, London 1973), (F. Knowles, L. Vollrath, Eds.). Berlin-Heidelberg-New York: Springer 1974.

Murphy, J. T., Dreifuss, J. J., Gloor, P.: Response of hypothalamic neurons to repetitive amygdaloid stimulation. Brain Res. **8**, 153—166 (1968).

Raziano, J., Cowchock, S., Ferin, M., Vande Wiele, R. L.: Estrogen-dependency of monoamine-induced ovulation. Endocrinology **88**, 1516—1518 (1971).

Reinert, H.: Urethane hyperglycaemia and hypothalamic activation. Nature (Lond.) **204**, 889—891 (1964).

Sawyer, C. H., Markee, J. E., Townsend, B. F.: Cholinergic and adrenergic components in the neurohumoral control of the release of LH in the rabbit. Endocrinology **44**, 18—37 (1949a).

Sawyer, C. H., Everett, J. W., Markee, J. E.: A neural factor in the mechanism by which estro-gen induces the release of luteinizing hormone in the rat. Endocrinology **44**, 218—233 (1949b).

Scapagnini, U., van Loon, G. R., Moberg, G. P., Preziosi, P., Ganong, W. F.: Evidence for central norepinephrine-mediated inhibition of ACTH secretion in the rat. Neuroendo-crinology **10**, 155—160 (1972).

Schneider, H. P. G., McCann, S. M.: Mono- and indolamines and control of LH secretion. Endocrinology **86**, 1127—1133 (1970).

Taleisnik, S., Tomatis, M. E., Celis, M. E.: Rôle of catecholamines in the control of melanocyte-stimulating hormone secretion in rats. Neuroendocrinology **10**, 235—245 (1972).

Valverde, R., Chieffo, V., Reichlin, S.: Prolactin-releasing factor in porcine and rat hypothala-mic tissue. Endocrinology **91**, 982—993 (1972).

Velasco, M. E., Taleisnik, S.: Release of gonadotropins induced by amygdaloid stimulation in the rat. Endocrinology **84**, 132—139 (1969).

Zarrow, M. X., Quinn, D. L.: Superovulation in the immature rat following treatment with PMS alone and inhibition of PMS-induced ovulation. J. Endocr. **26**, 181—188 (1963).

Brain Monoamines and the Control of Growth Hormone Release

E. E. Müller and D. Cocchi

Department of Pharmacology, University of Milan, Milan (Italy)

Many data on the central nervous system (CNS) control of pituitary growth hormone (GH) secretion have been accumulated in recent years following the introduction of specific and sensitive radioimmunoassay methods in plasma of man (Berson and Yalow, 1964) and laboratory animals (Schalch and Reichlin, 1966). Studies in primates have shown GH secretion to be altered by hypothalamic lesions, pituitary stalk section, infusion of microliter quantities of glucose near the median eminence and by injections of hypothalamic extracts.

Similar studies in the rat have shown that electrolytic lesions of the ventro-medial nucleus of the hypothalamus lower plasma GH, whereas electrical stimulation of this structure produces an elevation of plasma GH (see Martin, 1973; Müller, 1973). A GH-releasing factor (GRF) activity has been detected in the hypothalami of animals of different species (McCann and Porter, 1969), and, recently, it has been possible to isolate from sheep hypothalamus a tetradecapeptide, somatostatin, which possesses GH-inhibiting (GIF) activity both "*in vitro*" and "*in vivo*" (Brazeau et al., 1973).

The introduction eleven years ago (Falck et al., 1962) of a highly specific and sensitive fluorescence histochemical technique has allowed the demonstration of the cellular localization in the CNS of many animal species of primary monoamine-containing nerve fibres. Details concerning the distribution of the main mono-aminergic pathways in the CNS can be found in this book. The topographical localization of brain monoamine systems strongly indicate that they function in the neuroendocrine control of anterior pituitary secretion (McCann and Porter, 1969).

The aim of this article is to provide a brief review of the current state of knowledge regarding participation of CNS dopamine (DA), norepinephrine (NE) and serotonin (5-HT) in the control of GH secretion, especially in primates.

Monoamine Participation in GH Release

The neuropharmacological studies performed in rodents gave evidence for a role of brain monoamines in GH release (see Müller, 1973; Collu et al., 1972; Sinha et al.,

1972). Studies performed in the monkey and the human have shown this to be the case also in primates. In the monkey, α-adrenergic blockade resulting from intra-venous infusion of phentolamine, significantly depressed GH secretion, while β-adrenergic blockade with propranolol was associated with a prompt rise in plasma GH levels (Werrbach et al., 1970). In addition, the direct infusion of systematically ineffective doses of pentholamine into the anterior hypothalamus or third ventricle of the brain of baboons significantly lowered serum GH without concomitant changes in glucose and non-esterified fatty acid levels (Toivola et al., 1972). These data suggested the existence in the CNS of the monkey of α-adrenergic receptors regulating GH secretion. In fact, NE injected directly into the ventro-medial nucleus (VMN) of the hypothalamus consistently elevated GH in the conscious monkey. Microinjections of 5-HT in the same area did not elevate GH. In contrast to central administration of NE, intrahypothalamic infusion or direct microinjection of DA into the VMN resulted in an inhibition of GH secretion (Toivola and Gale, 1972, 1973). In the human, the administration of L-Dopa, the immediate precursor of DA which readily crosses the blood brain barrier, caused a significant rise in plasma GH levels in patients with parkinsonism (Boyd et al., 1970) as well as in normal subjects (Cavagnini et al., 1972). The stimulatory effect on GH secretion by L-Dopa was not blocked by either oral or intravenous glucose (Boyd et al., 1970), but was reduced or potentiated respectively by the concomitant infusion of phentolamine (Kansal et al., 1972) or propranolol (Massara and Ca-manni, unpublished results), stressing the involvement of adrenergic α- and β-receptors in the regulation of GH secretion. Consistent with these findings, earlier studies have shown that blockade of α-adrenergic receptors by phentolamine prevented the increase in plasma GH that follows insulin-induced hypoglycemia. In contrast, β-adrenergic receptor blockade by propranolol augmented the levels of GH in hypoglycemic subjects (Blackard and Heidingsfelder, 1968). Catechol-amines (CA) were also shown to be implicated in the vasopressin-induced growth hormone release since phentolamine was effective also in suppressing the increased GH secretion which follows vasopressin administration in the human (Heidings-felder and Blackard, 1968). These findings demonstrated that central α- and β-adrenergic mechanism(s) have respectively a stimulatory and an inhibitory effect on GH secretion, opposite to that described for regulation of insulin secretion by the pancreas (Porte, 1967). In addition to L-Dopa, apomorphine, a direct stimulant of DA receptors (Andén et al., 1967), induced a rise of GH (Lal et al., 1972; Brown et al., 1973), an effect which is compatible with a dopaminergic mechanism. Con-cerning the role of serotonin, recently increased GH levels have been found in plasma of patients with excessive 5-HT secretion due to the carcinoid syndrome (Feldman and Lebovitz, 1972) and impaired GH response to insulin hypoglycemia has been reported following methysergide and cyproheptadine, two 5-HT receptor blockers (Bivens et al., 1973). In addition, rises in plasma GH levels have been reported in Japanese subjects following oral administration of 5-hydroxytryptophan (Imura et al., 1973). However, in our hands, administration of L-tryptophan, the amino acid precursor of 5-HT evoked at much higher doses, only small and erratic GH rises in normal subjects (Müller et al., unpublished data).

Identity of the Monoamine and Sites of Action

Although a wealth of investigations has pointed to the participation of brain CA in the neurohumoral control of GH secretion, some aspects, however, are still unclear and worthy of further studies. One of the problems is whether NE or DA acts as the true neurotransmitter for the GRF-secreting structures. Dopamine and NE seem to have an antagonistic role in rodents (Müller, 1973) and possibly in the monkey (Toivola and Gale, 1973), while the available evidence would indicate that both amines facilitate GH release in man. The plasma GH rise elicited by L-Dopa might be due to activation of the NE system in the hypothalamus or limbic structures. Quite interestingly in fact, both phentolamine and propranolol interact with the effect of L-Dopa. However, suggestions for a direct stimulation of DA receptors in the release of GH come from the reported stimulant action of apomorphine and the suppressive effects on GH release of anti-dopaminergic drugs (Kim et al., 1971). It appears rather surprising, therefore, that 2-Br-α-ergocriptine (CB 154, Sandoz), a drug which like apomorphine possesses a direct DA-like activity in the neostriatum (Corrodi et al., 1973) does not influence GH release in normal subjects (Del Pozo et al., 1973).

Strictly connected with and dependent upon the nature of the neurotransmitter is that of the possible site(s) at which CA act to regulate GH secretion. Figure 1 shows schematically the possible sites of catecholamine action. Assuming that the most probable area at which these neurotransmitters could operate to modulate GRF release is the hypothalamus (Toivola and Gale, 1972), the more likely mechanism in man is either (1) through a direct axo-dendritic or axo-somatic contact with the "transducer neurons" of the ventromedial-arcuate nucleus complex responsible for GRF production or (2) through neurons distant to the transducer

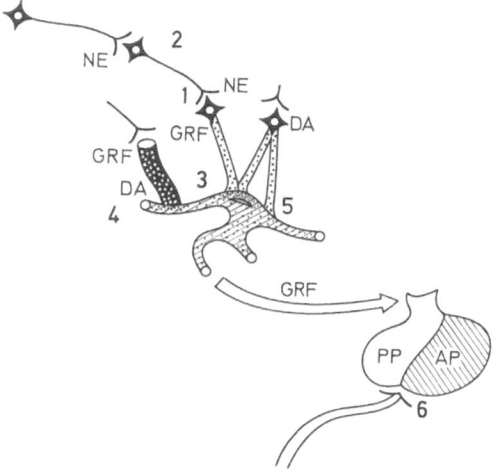

Fig. 1. Possible sites at which catecholamines might participate in the neuroendocrine control of GH release. See text for explanation. NE = indicates norepinephrinergic neurons. DA = dopaminergic neurons. GRF = hypophysiotrophic neurons. PP = posterior pituitary. AP = anterior pituitary

neurons or (3) axo-axonic synapses at the level of the median eminence between peptidergic nerve terminals and neurotransmitter nerve terminals, or both. Another alternative might be that (4) GRF secreting neurons also contain neurotransmitter granules and that the intracellular release of the neurotransmitter may trigger release of GRF. Two final possibilities include that (5) neurotransmitters could be released into the portal circulation to directly stimulate GH release (McLeod, 1969) or (6) delivered to the pituitary by the general circulation.

It seems essential to bear in mind that the demonstration of neuroendocrine influences inhibiting the secretion of GH (Vale et al., 1972; Brazeau et al., 1973) requires the existence in the CNS of neurotransmitter(s) providing the critical intermediate link between brain and GIF-secretory structure(s).

Until now, with the exception of the decrease of GH in the plasma of acromegalic subjects following L-Dopa administration (Liuzzi et al., 1972), an effect which on the ground of the present knowledge has to be considered paradoxical, no clear-cut evidence has been presented in man for a neurotransmitter function inhibitory to GH release.

In summary, the bulk of these data are without doubt compatible with the view that brain CA intervene in the process of GH secretion; information is still scanty for definitely assessing the role of 5-HT. Further studies are needed for a better knowledge of brain loci shown diagrammatically in Fig. 1 and for the recognition of the (multi)synaptic pathways mediating the neuroendocrine reflex responsible for GH release. Clarification of these points may also help understand contradictions in the literature.

References

Andén, N. E., Rubenson, A. A., Fuxe, K., Hökfelt, T.: Evidence for dopamine receptor stimulation by apomorphine. J. Pharm. Pharmacol. 19, 627—629 (1967).

Berson, S. A., Yalow, R. S.: In: Pincus, G., Thiman, K. V., Astwood, E. B. (Eds.): The Hormones, Vol. IV, pp. 557—630. New York: Academic Press 1964.

Bivens, C. M., Lebovitz, H. E., Feldman, J. M.: Inhibition of hypoglycemia induced growth hormone secretion by the serotonin antagonists cyproheptadine and methysergide. New Engl. J. Med. 289, 236—239 (1973).

Blackard, W. G., Heidingsfelder, S. A.: Adrenergic receptor control mechanism for growth hormone secretion. J. clin. Invest. 47, 1400—1414 (1968).

Boyd, A. E., Lebovitz, H. E., Pfeiffer, J. B.: Stimulation of human growth hormone by L-dopa. New Engl. J. Med. 238, 1425—1429 (1970).

Brazeau, P., Vale, W., Burgus, R., Ling, N., Butcher, M., Rivier, J., Guillemin, R.: Hypothalamic polypeptide that inhibits the secretion of immunoreactive pituitary growth hormone. Science 179, 77—79 (1973).

Brown, W. A., van Voert, M. H., Ambani, L. M.: Effect of apomorphine on growth hormone release. J. clin. Endocr. 37, 463—465 (1973).

Cavagnini, F., Peracchi, M., Scotti, G., Raggi, U., Pontiroli, A. E., Bana, R.: Effect of L-Dopa administration on growth hormone secretion in normal subjects and parkinsonian patients. J. Endocr. 54, 425—433 (1972).

Collu, R., Fraschini, F., Visconti, P., Martini, L.: Adrenergic and serotoninergic control of growth hormone secretion in adult male rats. Endocrinology 90, 1231—1237 (1972).

Corrodi, H., Fuxe, K., Hökfelt, T., Lidbrink, P., Ungerstedt, U.: Effect of ergot drugs on central catecholamine neurons: evidence for a stimulation of central dopamine neurons. J. Pharm. Pharmacol. 25, 409—412 (1973).

Del Pozo, E., Friesen, H., Burmeister, P.: Endocrine profile of a specific prolactin inhibitor: Br-ergocryptine (CB I54). Schweiz. med. Wschr. **103**, 847—848 (1973).

Falck, B., Hillarp, N.A., Thieme, G., Torp, A.: Fluorescence of catecholamines and related compounds condensed with formaldehyde. J. Histochem. Cytochem. **10**, 348—354 (1962).

Feldman, J.M., Lebovitz, H.E.: Control of insulin and growth hormone secretion by serotonin and dopamine. Abstracts, 4th Int. Congr. Endocr. Washington. Excerpta Med. Int. Congr. Series, No. 256, p. 35 (1972).

Heidingsfelder, S.A., Blackard, W.G.: Adrenergic control mechanism for vasopressin induced plasma growth hormone response. Metabolism **17**, 1019—1024 (1968).

Imura, H., Nakai, I., Yoshimi, T.: Effect of 5-hydroxytryptophan (5-HTP) on growth hormone and ACTH release in man. J. clin. Endocr. **36**, 204—206 (1973).

Kansal, P.C., Buse, J., Talbert, O.R., Buse, M.: The effect of L-Dopa on plasma growth hormone, insulin and thyroxine. J. clin. Endocr. **34**, 99—105 (1972).

Lal, S., de la Vega, C.E., Sourkes, T.L., Friesen, H.G.: Effect of apomorphine on human-growth-hormone secretion. Lancet **1972 I**, 661.

Liuzzi, A., Chiodini, P.G., Botalla, L., Cremascoli, G., Silvestrini, F.: Inhibitory effect of L-Dopa on GH release in acromegalic patients. J. clin. Endocr. **35**, 941—943 (1972).

Martin, J.B.: Neural regulation of growth hormone secretion. New Engl. J. Med. **288**, 1384—1393 (1973).

McCann, S.M., Porter, J.C.: Hypothalamic pituitary stimulating and inhibiting hormones. Physiol. Rev. **49**, 240—284 (1969).

McLeod, R.: Influence of norepinephrine and catecholamine-depleting agents on the synthesis and release of prolactin and growth hormone. Endocrinology **85**, 916—923 (1969).

Müller, E.E.: Nervous control of growth hormone secretion. Neuroendocrinology **11**, 338—369 (1973).

Porte, D., Jr.: Beta adrenergic stimulation of insulin release in man. Diabetes **16**, 150—155 (1967).

Schalch, D.S., Reichlin, S.: Plasma growth hormone concentration in the rat determined by radioimmunoassay. Influence of sex, pregnancy, lactation, anesthesia, hypophysectomy and extrasellar pituitary transplants. Endocrinology **79**, 275—280 (1966).

Sinha, Y., Selby, F.W., Lewis, U.Y., Vanderlaan, W.P.: Studies of GH secretion in mice by a homologous radioimmunoassay for mouse GH. Endocrinology **91**, 784—792 (1972).

Toivola, P.T.K., Gale, C.C.: Norepinephrine and dopamine microinjection into hypothalamus of baboons: effects on growth hormone secretion. Fed. Proc. **32**, 265 Abs. (1973).

Toivola, P.T.K., Gale, C.C.: Stimulation of growth hormone release by microinjection of norepinephrine into hypothalamus of baboons. Endocrinology **90**, 895—902 (1972).

Toivola, P.T.K., Gale, C.C., Goodner, C.J., Werrbach, J.H.: Central α-adrenergic regulation of growth hormone and insulin. Hormones **3**, 193—213 (1972).

Vale, W., Brazeau, P., Grant, G., Nussey, A., Burgus, R., Rivier, J., Ling, N., Guillemin, R.: Premières observations sur le mode d'action de la somatostatine, un facteur hypothalamique qui inhibe la sécrétion de l'hormone de croissance. C. R. Acad. Sci. (Paris) **275**, 2913—2916 (1972).

Werrbach, J.H., Gale, C.C., Goodner, C.J., Conway, M.J.: Effect of autonomic blocking agents on growth hormone, insulin, free fatty acids and glucose in baboons. Endocrinology **86**, 77—82 (1970).

The Characterization of Monoaminergic Nerve Terminals in the Brain by Fine Structural Cytochemistry

J. G. RICHARDS and J. P. TRANZER †

Department of Experimental Medicine, F. Hoffmann-La Roche & Co. Ltd., Basle (Switzerland)

It is now accepted that noradrenaline (NA) acts as the transmitter of the post-ganglionic adrenergic neuron (Euler, 1971) while in the brain the monoamines NA, dopamine (DA) and 5-hydroxytryptamine (5-HT) are putative transmitters (Vogt, 1971). Fluorescence microscopy has shown that the amines are distributed through-out the neuron (Eränkö and Härkönen, 1963; Falck, 1962) although they are to be found in their greatest concentration in highly fluorescent varicosities or termi-nals which are noticeable in the course of the terminal axon and it is there that the transmitter appears to be released in close proximity to the effector cell e.g. smooth muscle or adjacent neuron.

Ultrastructural studies of peripheral adrenergic nerve terminals after various pharmacological manipulations (Pellegrino de Iraldi and De Robertis, 1961; Tranzer and Thoenen, 1968) have identified the small dense core (sdc) and large dense core (ldc) vesicles, measuring approximately 50 nm and 100 nm in diameter respectively, as among the storage sites of NA. Moreover, it appears that the pro-portion of vesicles with a dense core depends on the tissue and the type of fixative used (Bloom, 1972; Hökfelt, 1971; Tranzer et al., 1969). Thus, with osmium tetroxide alone, or in combination with aldehydes, the proportion with dense cores is lower than with potassium permanganate, although the general morphological appearance of the tissue is better preserved. The storage sites for monoamines in the brain are more difficult to demonstrate than NA in peripheral adrenergic nerve terminals (see review by Bloom, 1970) and up to now only the permanganate technique (Richardson, 1966) employed by Hökfelt (1967, 1968) has been suc-cessful in revealing endogenous amines.

A more sensitive and specific cytochemical method, based on the chromaffin reaction, for the ultrastructural localization of biogenic monoamines has recently been developed in our laboratory (Tranzer and Richards, in preparation) whereby it has been possible to detect sites of monoamine storage in the whole adrenergic neuron and in selective regions of the central nervous system which have been implied in the neural control of endocrine function. Since this cytochemical pro-cedure was first tried and tested on the peripheral nervous system where it was found to be consistent, a brief mention of the localization and distribution of the amine storage sites in these nerves will be made.

† deceased on January 15th, 1974

NA Storage Sites in the Peripheral Adrenergic Neuron

When sympathetically-innervated organs of the rat e.g. iris, vas deferens, mesenteric artery or heart are fixed for electron microscopy using the conventional cacodylate-buffered glutaraldehyde and osmium procedure, examination of their terminal adrenergic axons reveals the presence of some ldc and many small vesicles mostly empty-looking but occasionally with a dense core (Fig. 1a). However, tissues fixed in chromate-dichromate buffered aldehydes and osmium contain nerve terminals with sdc vesicles filled with a highly electron dense material and ldc vesicles of an enhanced electron density (Fig. 1b). In addition to these vesicles a fine reticulum containing electron dense material was observed in most terminals. In tissues from animals pretreated with reserpine (Fig. 1c) all the small vesicles appeared empty and the large had a dense core of reduced electron opacity. Moreover, when the osmium post-fixation was omitted in control animals both small and large electron dense cores, of a similar size and distribution to those found in the vesicles of osmium-treated tissues, could be detected (Fig. 1d). These observations indicate that the electron dense material represents the neurotransmitter NA (Tranzer et al., 1969). The tubular reticulum storing amine (trsa) was first described in the adrenergic nerve axons supplying arteries of the mesentery (Tranzer, 1972) where it was found in abundance, as in the iris although in other organs, e.g. rat vas deferens, it is only occasionally observed. The precise function of these amine storing compartments is at present unknown.

The post-ganglionic adrenergic axons innervating the iris originate from some cell bodies found in the superior cervical ganglion. After the improved fixation technique described above, similar storage sites for amines to those found in nerve terminals of the iris could be observed (Richards and Tranzer, in preparation). In addition, however, the storage sites revealed a characteristic distribution in the cell body and its processes, namely: many sdc and the occasional ldc vesicles which were isolated and dispersed; sdc and ldc vesicles and sometimes trsa associated with the Golgi apparatus; and finally, groups of amine storage organelles (sdc and trsa) usually found at the cell perimeter and in dendritic processes. These observations confirm and extend similar results of Hökfelt (1969) in studies of potassium permanganate-fixed sympathetic ganglia.

The presence of numerous sdc vesicles in the perikaryon is not surprising in view of recent fine structural observations on non-terminal adrenergic axons (Tranzer, 1973) which revealed that a large proportion of the amine storage vesicles in the nerve trunk were of the sdc type. The presence of trsa also in cell bodies and dendrites raises the question of whether all three types of amine storage organelles have different functions in the transport, storage or release of the neurotransmitter NA.

From these investigations on the peripheral adrenergic neuron it became clear that the success of the cytochemical reaction as well as the preservation of tissue ultrastructure depend on the precise control of various parameters, e.g. the nature and concentration of the fixative components, and the temperature and duration of fixation (Tranzer and Richards, in preparation).

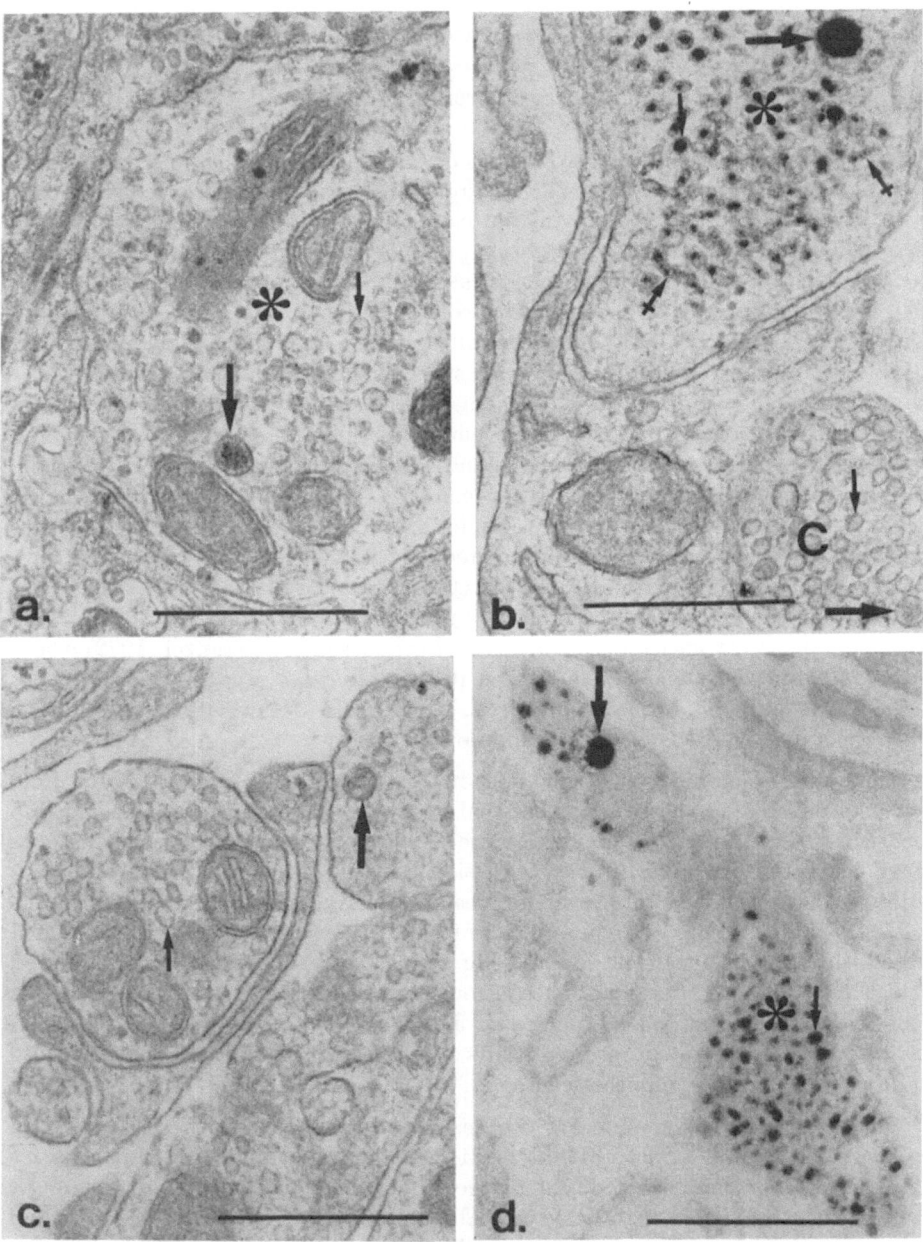

Fig. 1a—d. Ultrastructural aspect of sympathetic nerve terminals (*) in the rat iris under various experimental conditions. a Control. Fixation with glutaraldehyde buffered with cacodylate and followed by osmium tetroxide. Note the presence of many small vesicles, only a few of which contain a dense core (→), and a single ldc vesicle (⟶). b Control. Fixation with chromate-dichromate buffered aldehydes followed by osmium results in the appearance in some nerve terminals of sdc (→) and ldc (⟶) vesicles and also a tubular reticulum (+→) with a highly electron dense content. C, cholinergic nerve terminal. c Reserpine pretreatment. Fixation as in Fig. 1b. The electron density of the small vesicles (→) has been lost and that of the large vesicles (⟶) greatly reduced. d Control. Fixation as in Fig. 1b except that the osmium post-fixation was omitted. Note the presence of small (→) and large (⟶) electron dense cores in profiles resembling, in size and distribution, the nerve terminals in Fig. 1b. 0.5 μm; × 56000

Monoamine Storage Sites in the Central Nervous System

Although biochemical (Vogt, 1971) and fluorescence microscopical (Dahlström and Fuxe, 1964; Fuxe, 1965) investigations have provided for some time a vast amount of information concerning the identification of various monoamines in different parts of the brain and their localization in specific neuronal systems, little was known of their precise ultrastructural storage sites until the permanganate fixation method was employed by Hökfelt (1967) in electron microscope investigations. From these studies it was confirmed that, as in the peripheral sympathetic nervous system, sdc and ldc vesicles are among the storage sites for amines in the brain. While this technique has provided a great deal of information on the identification of monoaminergic nerve terminals and their distribution in the brain (Hökfelt, 1968, 1970) it is readily acknowledged (Bloom, 1972; Hökfelt, 1971) that an amine-specific cytochemical reaction, e.g. based on an aldehyde fixation, is desirable.

Two main approaches have thus been used to investigate the sites of monoamine storage in the brain at the ultrastructural level, namely, a) the replacement of the physiological transmitter, i.e. endogenous amine by large amounts of exogenous amines, e.g. 5-hydroxydopamine (Richards and Tranzer, 1970; Tranzer and Thoenen, 1967) which are known to be more readily localized with conventional fixation methods and b) the application of cytochemically-reactive fixatives which selectively and perhaps quantitatively localize different endogenous biogenic monoamines, e.g. the improved chromaffin-based reaction described here.

a) Localization of Exogenous Amines

This rather indirect approach stems from the finding of an active re-uptake mechanism in peripheral and central nerve terminals storing monoamines. The use of this phenomenon in morphological studies was first demonstrated by Wolffe et al. (1962) when the selective uptake of tritium-labelled NA was shown in sympathetic nerve terminals of the pineal organ by electron microscopic radio-autography. Subsequent investigations (Hökfelt, 1968) combining permanganate fixation with the loading of central nerve terminals with near physiological concentrations of NA, DA or 5-HT have helped in the identification of specific monoamine nerve terminals in the brain.

The fixation of rat brain tissue by the conventional cacodylate-buffered aldehydes and osmium procedure reveals the presence of nerve terminals containing small empty-looking vesicles and the occasional ldc vesicle (Fig. 2a).

Although it was long debated whether the ldc vesicles are storage sites for amines in the central nervous system and has indeed now been affirmed, the mere presence of ldc vesicles in a nerve process is not sufficient in itself to allow their identification as monoaminergic since other nerve terminals, such as those storing acetylcholine, also exhibit the presence of ldc vesicles.

When various brain regions are exposed to 5-OH-DA-containing solutions, either *in vitro* or *in vivo* after incubation of brain slices or intraventricular administration, nerve terminals containing sdc and ldc vesicles of a marked electron density could be observed (Fig. 2b). The proportion of nerve terminals labelled

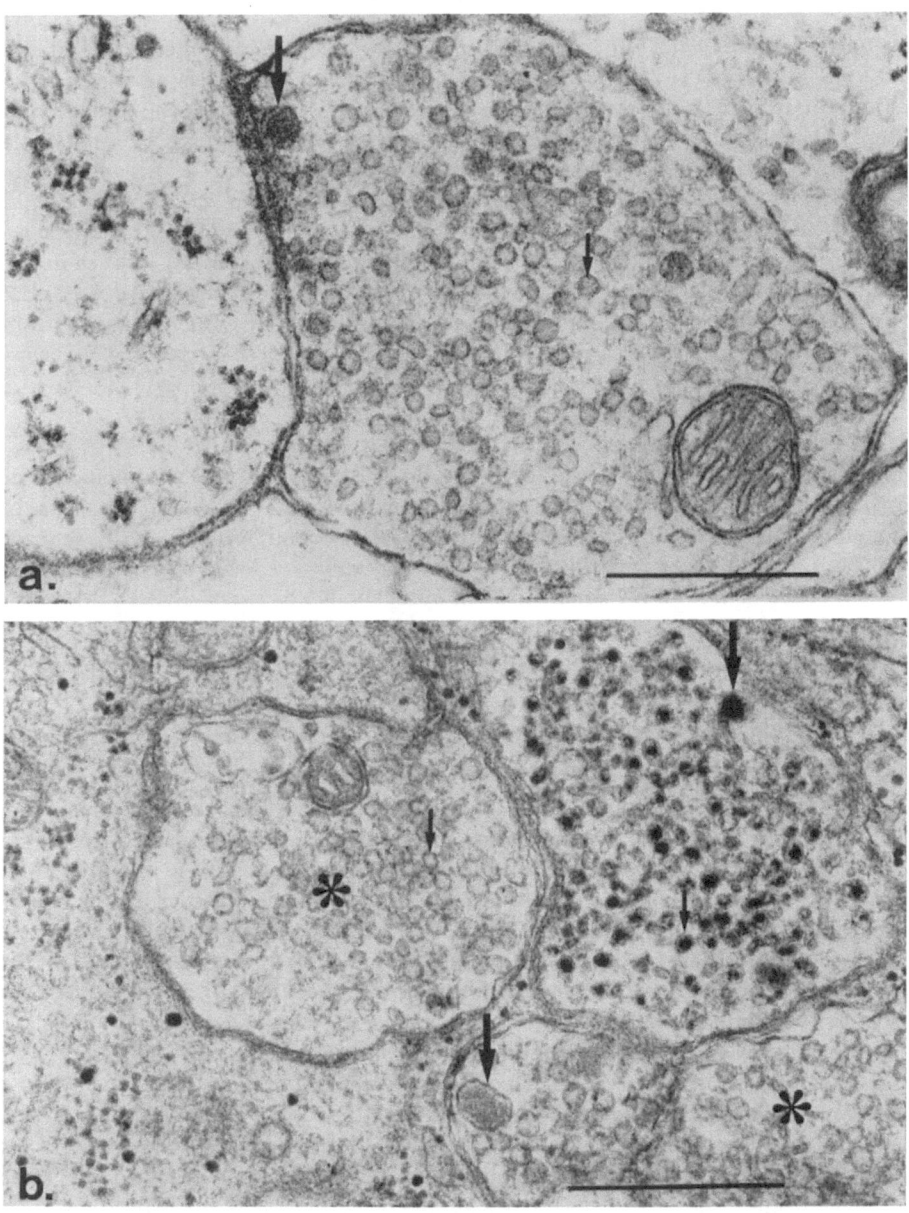

Fig. 2a and b. Ultrastructural aspect of nerve terminals in the periventricular region of the anterior hypothalamus in the rat after fixation with cacodylate-buffered glutaraldehyde and osmium. a Control. The nerve terminal contains many small empty-looking vesicles (→) and the occasional ldc vesicles (→). b 5-OH-DA pretreatment (intraventricular injection). One terminal profile contains sdc (→) and ldc (→) vesicles with a marked electron density while others (*) retain a similar ultrastructural aspect to that illustrated in a. 0.5 μm; × 56000

with this technique was usually small and varied from 3–5 % in the periventricular region of the anterior hypothalamus to up to approximately 25–30 % in the lateral part of the median eminence (for a comparison with the permanganate method see Hökfelt, 1968; Ajika and Hökfelt, 1973). In all regions investigated no accumulation was observed in reserpine-pretreated animals.

Other possibilities of identifying central monoaminergic nerve terminals by electron microscopy include degeneration studies with 6-hydroxydopamine (Bloom et al., 1969; Richards, 1971) and radioautography with various tritium-labelled amines (Aghajanian and Bloom, 1966; Descarries and Droz, 1970).

There were, however, certain disadvantages in using the approach of labelling with exogenous amines when studying the accumulation of tritium-labelled amines by radioautography of substances such as 5-OH-DA and α-methyl-noradrenaline. Both techniques have inherent problems associated with the poor penetration and/or uptake of the administered amine into deeper brain regions and the non-specific nature of the accumulation at other than physiological concentrations. Moreover, as clearly discussed by Bloom (1970) in a review on the fine structural localization of biogenic monoamines in nervous tissue, the use of radioautography in the precise localization of amines is seriously hindered by limits in the resolution which, at approximately 150–200 nm, "under the best of circumstances would only be able to distinguish certain types of axons and structures of the size of chromaffin granules, while completely unable to distinguish among adjacent synaptic vesicles". Consequently, the second and a more direct approach, namely the localization of endogenous amines by fine structural cytochemistry is preferred.

b) Localization of Endogenous Amines

This has been achieved by the vascular perfusion of rat brain with chromate-dichromate buffered aldehydes followed by immersion fixation of selected brain regions in similarly-buffered osmium tetroxide (see Tranzer and Richards, in preparation). The results reported here are preliminary in the sense that the cytochemical technique has not been applied with success in all parts of the central nervous system. However, endogenous monoamines have been localized in at least three different brain regions which have been implied in the control of endocrine function, namely the hypothalamus, median eminence and cerebral ventricles of which only the last will be described in detail here.

The ultrastructural aspect of these brain regions changed markedly upon fixation with the improved cytochemical technique. Thus, monoamine-specific sdc and ldc vesicles could be detected in nerve terminals in both the periventricular region of the anterior hypothalamus and in the lateral part of the median eminence (Fig. 3a and b). Moreover, the dense cores persisted in tissues not post-fixed in osmium but were sensitive to reserpine treatment. The latter observations allow the conclusion that the terminals so identified are monoaminergic in nature. The above described terminals in the hypothalamus sometimes showed the presence of a tubular reticulum containing an amine-specific electron dense material (trsa).

The third brain region in which we were able to localize an endogenous amine was that bordering the cerebral ventricles. Although previous electron microscope studies had described the presence of vesiculated nerve fibres (i.e. varicosities or ter-

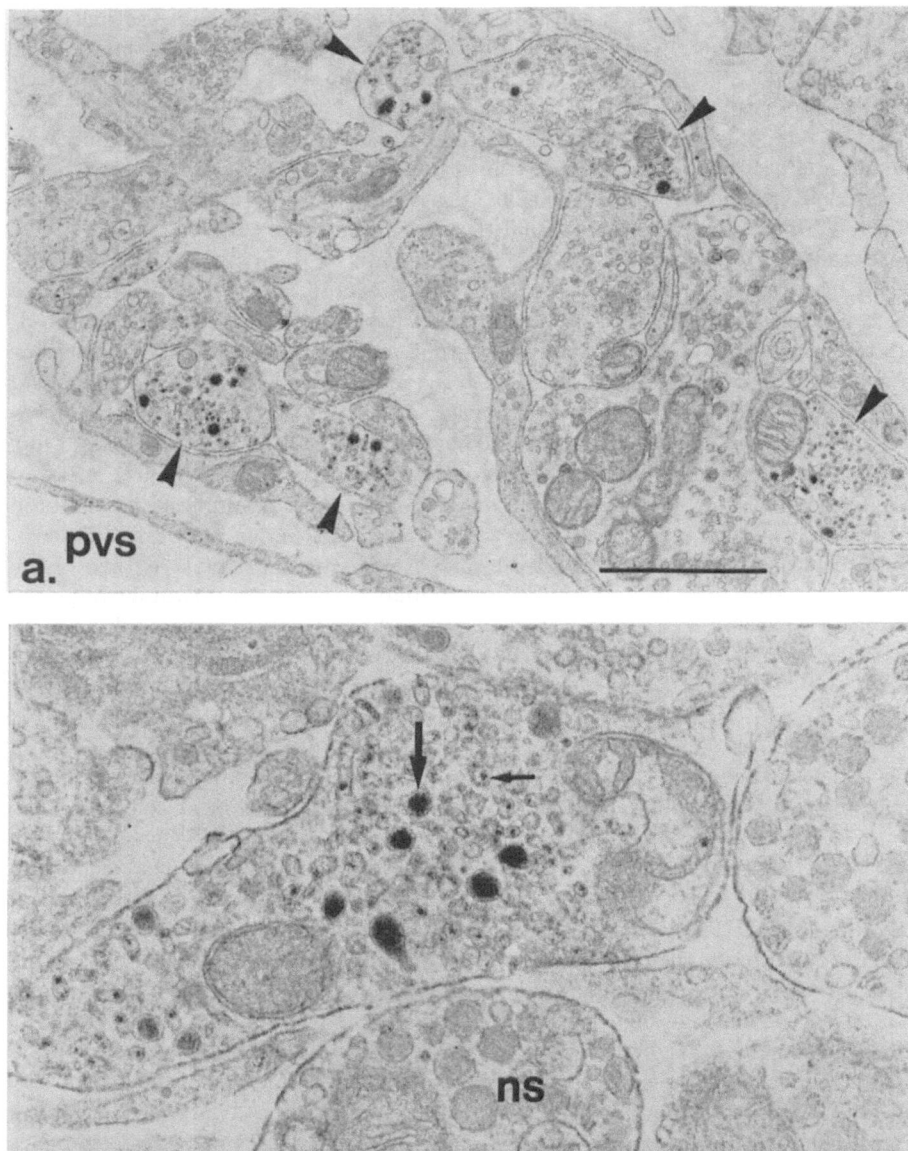

Fig. 3a and b. Rat median eminence after fixation with chromate-dichromate buffered aldehydes and osmium. Note that several nerve terminal profiles (▶) contain sdc (→) and ldc (→) vesicles with a marked electron density while others, presumably neurosecretory neurones (ns), remain unreactive with this fixation method. pvs, perivascular space. a: 1 μm; × 22000. b: 0.5 μm; × 56000

minals) within the ventricles of the central nervous system in various species of mammals (Brightman and Palay, 1963; Le Beux, 1972; Leonhardt, 1968; Leonhardt and Backus-Roth, 1969; Leonhardt and Lindner, 1967; Leonhardt and Prien, 1968; Lindemann and Leonhardt, 1973; Noack et al., 1972; Noack and Wolff, 1970, 1971; Rinne, 1966; Rohrschneider et al., 1972; Westergaard, 1970, 1972), the nature of the transmitter employed by these nerves was completely unknown. As in other brain regions after conventional fixation, terminals contained many small empty-looking vesicles and a few ldc vesicles from which the type of nerve could not be determined (Fig. 4a). However, recent fine structural investigations combined with fluorescence microscopy (Lorez and Richards, 1973; Richards et al., 1973) have enabled this to be clarified.

The following observations allow these nerves (above the striatum and in the interventricular foramen) to be identified as of the indolealkylamine type, probably storing 5-HT:

1) 5-OH-DA is taken up and stored in these nerves after intraventricular administration (Fig. 4b). Both sdc and ldc vesicles appear in virtually all supra-ependymal nerve terminals, the dense cores being reserpine-sensitive.

2) The presence of endogenous amines could be demonstrated using the specific cytochemical technique (Fig. 4c and d).

3) The fluorescence histochemical findings revealing an amine-specific fluorescence on the ventricular surface of the ependyma, of a similar size and distribution to the axon profiles observed by electron microscopy.

That the fluorescence represents an indolealkylamine, most probably 5-HT, rather than a catecholamine is suggested by the following observations: a) the fluorescence was yellow and faded rapidly upon irradiation with violet-blue light; b) when tissues were not exposed to formaldehyde gas, no fluorescence appeared; c) its colour and reaction to drugs interfering with the sythesis, storage and/or metabolism of monoamines, e.g. reserpine, nialamide, reserpine + nialamide, p-chlorophenylalanine (p-CPA) and α-methyl-p-tyrosine (α-MPT), corresponded to those of the specifically yellow fluorescing 5-HT terminal axons in e.g. the suprachiasmatic nucleus or just beneath the subcommissural organ and not to those of the specifically blue-green fluorescing catecholamine axons in e.g. the neostriatum or the periventricular nucleus of the hypothalamus (see Richards et al., 1973).

Furthermore, conclusive evidence for the storage of an indolealkylamine in these nerve terminals came from combined cytochemistry and pharmacology at the ultrastructural level (Richards and Tranzer, 1974). Thus, after blocking either the synthesis of NA [α-MPT (Hanson, 1965)] or 5-HT [p-CPA (Koe and Weissmann, 1966, Bloom and Giarman, 1970)] the precise nature of these supra-ependymal nerves could be determined. The following observations strongly suggest, in confirmation of the fluorescence histochemical findings, that the endogenous amine is an indolealkylamine, probably 5-HT:

The amine-specific sdc and ldc vesicles in these nerve terminals were consistantly observed in virtually all terminals of control and α-MPT treated animals whereas, after treatment with reserpine or p-CPA, the amine-specific electron dense cores disappeared (Fig. 5a—d).

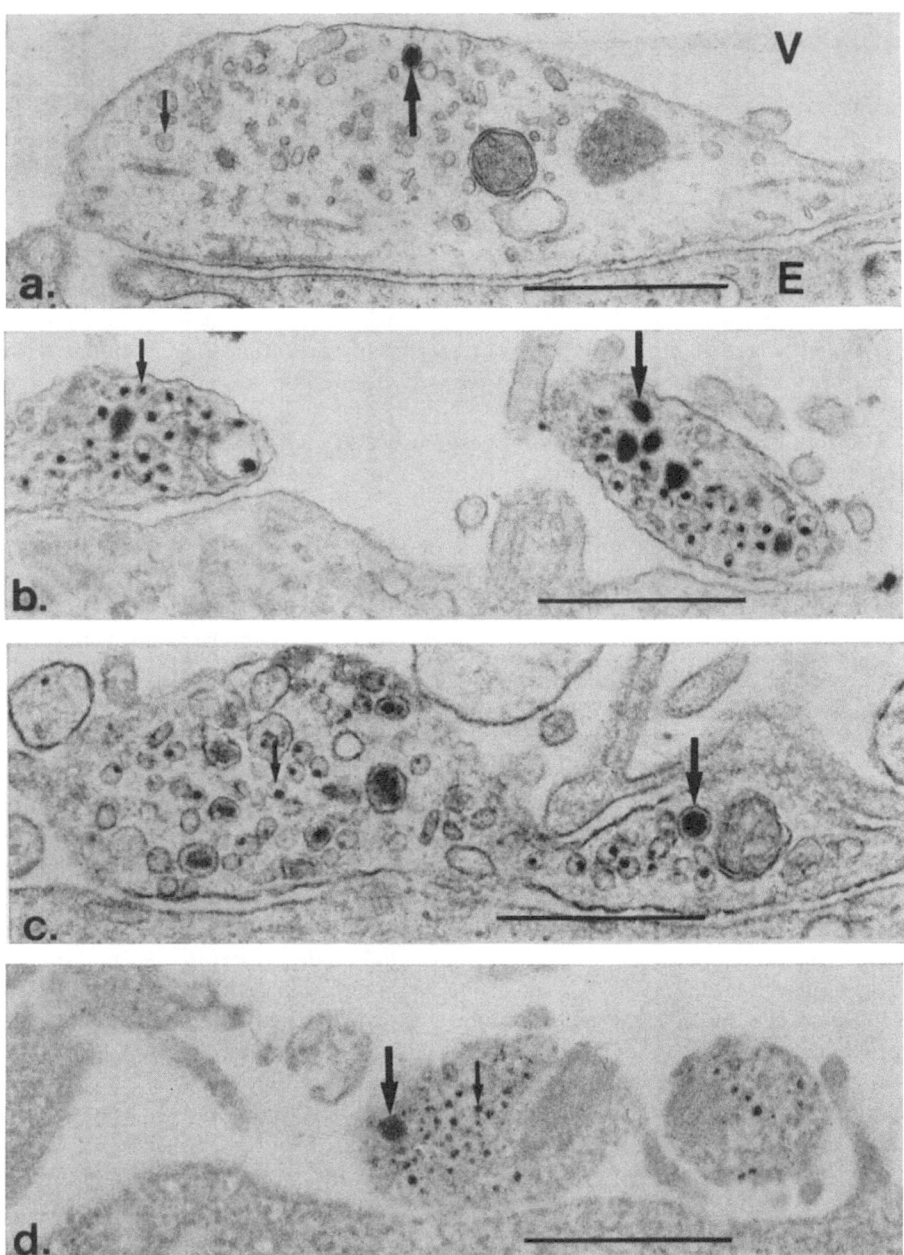

Fig. 4a—d. Ultrastructural aspect of supra-ependymal nerve terminals at the ventricle-ependyma interface under various experimental conditions. Nucleus caudatus of the rat. a Control. Fixation with cacodylate-buffered glutaraldehyde and osmium. The varicose region of the nerve fibre contains many small empty-looking vesicles (→) and a few ldc vesicles (➔). E, ependyma: V, ventricle. b 5-OH-DA pretreated rat. Similar fixation to that in a. Virtually all the nerve terminals contained sdc (→) and ldc (➔) vesicles with a highly electron dense material. c Control, after chromate-dichromate buffered aldehydes and osmium fixation. Note that compared with a, the small vesicles (→) now contain an electron dense core and the density of the large vesicles (➔) is somewhat enhanced. d Control, after a similar fixation to that in c except that the osmium post-fixation was omitted. Many small (→) and large (➔) electron dense cores can be observed in supra-ependymal profiles resembling in size and distribution the nerve terminals illustrated in c. 0.5 μm; × 56000

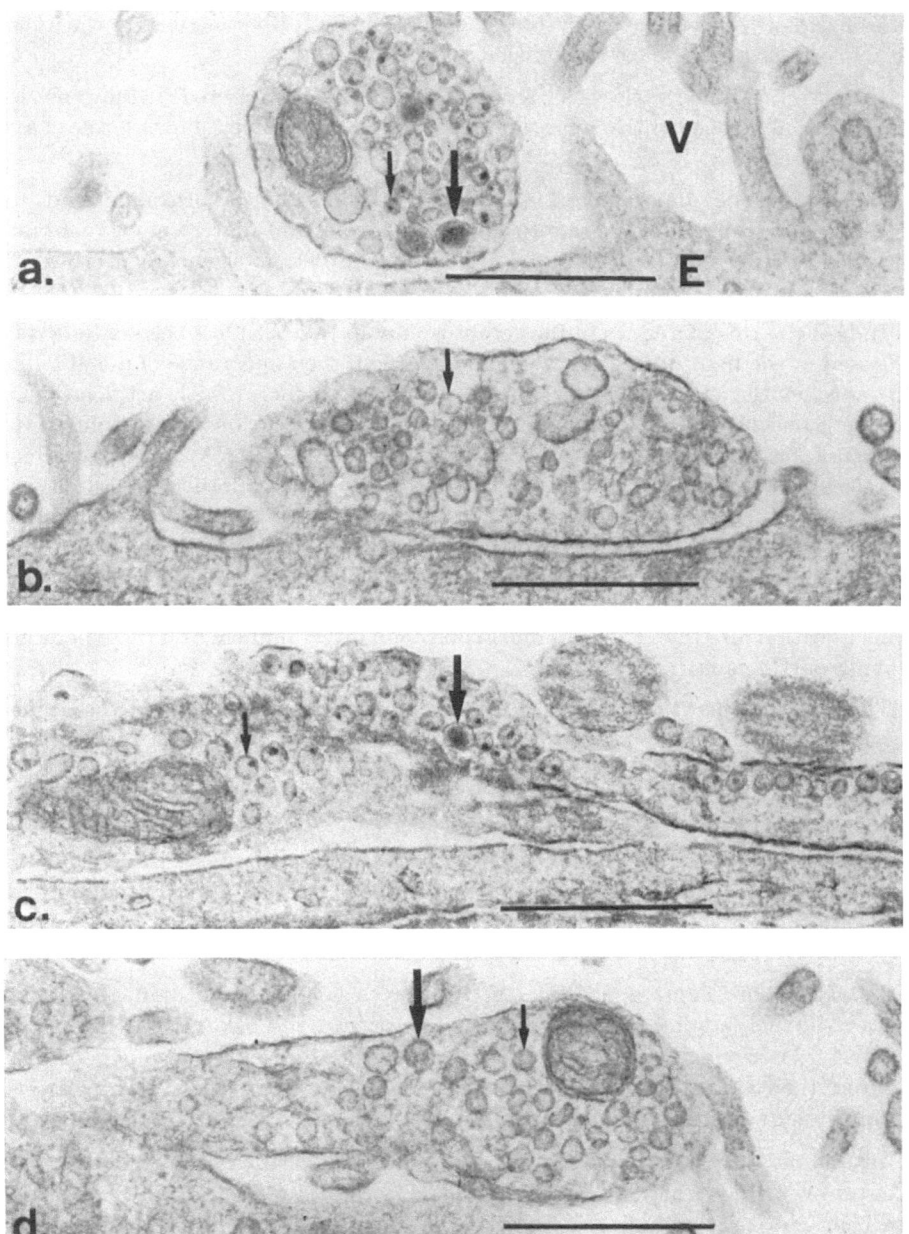

Fig. 5a—d. Effect of various pharmacological manipulations on the ultrastructural aspect of supra-ependymal nerve terminals after fixation with the cytochemical procedure. Stria medullaris thalami of the rat. a Control, b Reserpine, c α-MPT, and d p-CPA. Note the presence of sdc vesicles (-→) in a and c and small empty-looking vesicles (→) in b and d. 0.5 μm; × 56000

Preliminary investigations suggest that similar nerve fibres occur throughout many parts of the ventricular system, e.g. roof of the third ventricle, in the aqueduct, and floor of the fourth ventricle.

Because until now little was known of the transmitter stored in these nerves their function has been little more than speculated upon. The following roles have been proposed:

As receptors possibly registering the composition of the cerebrospinal fluid; by releasing their transmitter content to act locally through intimate synaptic contacts with ependymal cells or that they may influence some distant organs, e.g. the median eminence and neurohypophysis via the infundibular recess.

Indeed the role of amines in the cerebrospinal fluid (c.s.f.) has been extensively discussed in the light of findings which have shown the appearance of a 5-HT-like substance in the effluent from cerebral ventricles perfused with artificial c.s.f. (Feldberg and Myers, 1966) and the effects of injecting various monoamines into the ventricles. Thus, it has been found that injection of DA, NA, and 5-HT affect the release of the hormones LH, FSH, and prolactin, some stimulating and others suppressing it (Porter et al., 1972). Furthermore, intraventricular injection of amines has also been shown to affect body temperature regulation (Feldberg and Myers, 1964). While these observed effects may only partially reflect the physiological role of these amines in the c.s.f., nevertheless any study of the effects of amine injection into the ventricles must consider a direct influence on these neurons as being partly causal.

The fact that previous electron microscopic studies have described the occurrence of similar supra-ependymal nerve fibres in the third and fourth ventricles of other mammals may indicate that indolealkylamine nerves are a common feature to the ventricular system of mammals and perhaps even man. In the latter event their wide distribution in the cerebral ventricles may suggest that they could play some role in the brain affecting behaviour. Indeed, changes in c.s.f. levels of 5-hydroxyindoleacetic acid, the major acid metabolite of 5-HT, have been recorded in patients with psychiatric disorders although the results are conflicting (Barchas and Usdin, 1973).

Clearly, before supra-ependymal 5-HT nerves can be implied in any brain function further studies are required to investigate the behavioural effects of selectively destroying these nerves, e.g. by the intraventricular injection of 5,6-dihydroxytryptamine a 5-HT derivative which somewhat selectively destroys serotonin neurons in the central nervous system (Baumgarten et al., 1972).

In summary, the possibilities for the fine structural localization of monoamines in neurons is briefly reviewed. Nerve terminals in certain regions of the brain have been characterized by fine structural cytochemistry. Endogenous monoamines have been localized in small and large dense core vesicles in the anterior hypothalamus, median eminence and certain supra-ependymal nerve fibres in the cerebral ventricles. Moreover, in the last region the type of monoamine could be further characterized and was found to be an indolealkylamine. The possible function of this heretofore unidentified neuronal system is discussed.

References

Aghajanian, G. K., Bloom, F. E.: Electron-microscopic autoradiography of rat hypothalamus after intraventricular H³-norepinephrine. Science **153**, 308—310 (1966).

Ajika, K., Hökfelt, T.: Ultrastructural identification of catecholamine neurones in the hypothalamic periventricular-arcuate nucleus—median eminence complex with special reference to quantitative aspects. Brain Res. **57**, 97—118 (1973).

Barchas, J., Usdin, E. (Eds.): Serotonin and behaviour. New York: Academic Press 1973.

Baumgarten, H. G., Björklund, A., Holstein, A. F., Nobin, A.: Chemical degeneration of indolealamine axons in rat brain by 5,6-dihydroxytryptamine. An ultrastructural study. Z. Zellforsch. **129**, 256—271 (1972).

Bloom, F. E.: The fine structural localization of biogenic monoamines in nervous tissue. Int. Rev. Neurobiol. **13**, 27—66 (1970).

Bloom, F. E.: Localization of neurotransmitters by electron microscopy. Assoc. Res. nerv. Dis. Proc. **50**, 25—57 (1972).

Bloom, F. E., Algeri, S., Groppetti, A., Revuelta, A., Costa, E.: Lesions of central norepinephrine terminals with 6-OH-dopamine: biochemistry and fine structure. Science **166**, 1284—1286 (1969).

Bloom, F. E., Giarman, N. J.: The effects of p-Cl-phenylalanine on the content and cellular distribution of 5-HT in the rat pineal gland: combined biochemical and electron miscroscopic analyses. Biochem. Pharmacol. **19**, 1213—1219 (1970).

Brightman, M. W., Palay, S. L.: The fine structure of ependyma in the brain of the rat. J. Cell Biol. **19**, 415—439 (1963).

Dahlström, A., Fuxe, K.: Evidence for the existence of monoamine-containing neurons in the central nervous system. I. Demonstration of monoamines in the cell bodies of brain stem neurons. Acta physiol. scand. **62**, 1—55 (1964).

Descarries, L., Droz, B.: Intraneural distribution of exogenous norepinephrine in the central nervous system of the rat. J. Cell Biol. **44**, 385—399 (1970).

Eränkö, O., Härkönen, M.: Histochemical demonstration of fluorogenic amines in the cytoplasm of sympathetic ganglion cells of the rat. Acta physiol. scand. **58**, 285—286 (1963).

von Euler, U. S.: Adrenergic neurotransmitter functions. Science **173**, 202—206 (1971).

Falck, B.: Observations on the possibilities of the cellular localization of monoamines by a fluorescence method. Acta physiol. scand. **56**, Suppl. **197**, 1—25 (1962).

Feldberg, W., Myers, R. D.: Effects on temperature of amines injected into the cerebral ventricles. A new concept of temperature regulation. J. Physiol. (Lond.) **173**, 226—237 (1964).

Feldberg, W., Myers, R. D.: Appearance of 5-hydroxytryptamine and an unidentified pharmacologically active lipid acid in effluent from perfused cerebral ventricles. J. Physiol. (Lond.) **184**, 837—855 (1966).

Fuxe, K.: Evidence for the existence of monoamine neurons in the central nervous system. IV. The distribution of monoamine terminals in the central nervous system. Acta physiol. scand. **64**, Suppl. **247**, 37—85 (1965).

Hanson, L. C. F.: The disruption of conditioned avoidance response following selective depletion of brain catecholamines. Psychopharmacologia (Berl.) **8**, 100—110 (1965).

Hökfelt, T.: On the ultrastructural localization of noradrenaline in the central nervous system of the rat. Z. Zellforsch. **79**, 110—117 (1967).

Hökfelt, T.: *In vitro* studies on central and peripheral monoamine neurons at the ultrastructural level. Z. Zellforsch. **91**, 1—74 (1968).

Hökfelt, T.: Distribution of noradrenaline storing particles in peripheral adrenergic neurons as revealed by electron microscopy. Acta physiol. scand. **76**, 427—444 (1969).

Hökfelt, T.: Electron microscopic studies on peripheral and central monoamine neurons. In: Bargmann, W., Scharrer, B. (Eds.): Aspects of Neuroendocrinology, V. Int. Symp. on Neurosecretion. Berlin-Heidelberg-New York: Springer 1970.

Hökfelt, T.: Ultrastructural localization of intraneuronal monoamines. Some aspects on methodology. In: Eränkö, O. (Ed.): Histochemistry of nervous transmission. Prog. Brain Res. **34**, 213—222 (1971).

Koe, B. K., Weissman, A.: p-Chlorophenylalanine: a specific depletor of brain serotonin. J. Pharmacol. exp. Ther. **154**, 499—516 (1966).

Le Beux, Y. J.: An ultrastructural study of the neurosecretory cells of the medial vascular prechiasmatic gland. II. Nerve endings. Z. Zellforsch. **127**, 439—461 (1972).

Leonhardt, H.: Ependym. In: Sterba, G. (Ed.): Zirkumventrikuläre Organe und Liquor, pp. 177—190. Jena: Fischer 1968.

Leonhardt, G., Backus-Roth, A.: Synapsenartige Kontakte zwischen intraventrikulären Axonendigungen und freien Oberflächen von Ependymzellen des Kaninchengehirns. Z. Zellforsch. **97**, 369—376 (1969).

Leonhardt, H., Lindner, E.: Marklose Nervenfasern im III. und IV. Ventrikel des Kaninchen- und Katzengehirns. Z. Zellforsch. **78**, 1—18 (1967).

Leonhardt, H., Prien, H.: Eine weitere Art intraventrikulärer kolbenförmiger Axonendigungen aus dem IV. Ventrikel des Kaninchengehirns. Z. Zellforsch. **92**, 394—399 (1968).

Lindemann, B., Leonhardt, H.: Supraependymale Neuriten, Gliazellen und Mitochondrienkolben im caudalen Abschnitt des Bodens der Rautengrube. Z. Zellforsch. **140**, 401—412 (1973).

Lorez, H. P., Richards, J. G.: Distribution of indolealkylamine nerve terminals in the ventricles of the rat brain. Z. Zellforsch. **144**, 511—522 (1973).

Noack, W., Dumitrescu, L., Schweichel, J. V.: Scanning and electron microscopical investigations of the surface structures of the lateral ventricles in the cat. Brain Res. **46**, 121—129 (1972).

Noack, W., Wolff, J. R.: Über neuritenähnliche intraventrikuläre Fortsätze und ihre Kontakte mit dem Ependym der Seitenventrikel der Katze. Corpus callosum und Nucleus caudatus. Z. Zellforsch. **111**, 572—585 (1970).

Noack, W., Wolff, J. R.: Axon-like processes within the lateral ventricles of cat (corpus callosum and nucleus caudatus). Experientia (Basel) **27**, 172 (1971).

Pellegrino De Iraldi, A., De Robertis, E.: Action of reserpine on the submicroscopic morphology of the pineal gland. Experientia (Basel) **17**, 122—124 (1961).

Porter, J. C., Kamberi, I. A., Ondo, J. G.: Role of biogenic amines and cerebrospinal fluid in neurovascular transmittal of hyperphysiotrophic substances. In: Knigge, K. M., Scott, D. E., Weidl, A. (Eds.): Brain-endocrine interaction. Median eminence: Structure and function. Int. Symp. Munich 1972, pp. 245—253. Basel: Karger 1972.

Richards, J. G.: Ultrastructural effects of 6-hydroxydopamine on catecholamine containing neurones in the rat brain. In: Malmfors, T., Thoenen, H. (Eds.): 6-hydroxydopamine and catecholamine neurons, pp. 151—161. Amsterdam-London: North-Holland 1971.

Richards, J. G., Lorez, H. P., Tranzer, J. P.: Indolealkylamine nerve terminals in cerebral ventricles: Identification by electron microscopy and fluorescence histochemistry. Brain Res. **57**, 277—288 (1973).

Richards, J. G., Tranzer, J. P.: The ultrastructural localization of amine storage sites in the central nervous system with the aid of a specific marker, 5-hydroxydopamine. Brain Res. **17**, 463—469 (1970).

Richards, J. G., Tranzer, J. P.: Ultrastructural evidence for the localization of an indolealkylamine in supra-ependymal nerves from combined cytochemistry and pharmacology. Experienta (Basel) **30**, 287—289 (1974).

Richardson, K. C.: Electron microscopic identification of autonomic nerve endings. Nature (Lond.) New Biol. **210**, 756 (1966).

Rinne, U. K.: Ultrastructure of the median eminence of the rat. Z. Zellforsch. **74**, 98—122 (1966).

Rohrschneider, I., Schinko, I., Wetzstein, R.: Der Feinbau der Area postrema der Maus. Z. Zellforsch. **123**, 251—276 (1972).

Tranzer, J. P.: A new amine storing compartment in adrenergic axons. Nature (Lond.) **237**, 57—58 (1972).

Tranzer, J. P.: New aspects of the localization of catecholamines in adrenergic neurons. Proceedings of III. Int. Catecholamine Symp. J. Neurochem. In press (1973).

Tranzer, J. P., Thoenen, H.: Electron microscopic localization of 5-hydroxydopamine (3,4,5-trihydroxy-phenyl-ethylamine), a new "false" sympathetic transmitter. Experientia (Basel) **23**, 743—745 (1967).

Tranzer, J. P., Thoenen, H.: Various types of amine-storing vesicles in peripheral adrenergic nerve terminals. Experientia (Basel) **24**, 484—486 (1968).

Tranzer, J. P., Thoenen, H., Snipes, R. L., Richards, J. G.: Recent developments on the ultrastructural aspect of adrenergic nerve endings in various experimental conditions. In: Akert, K., Waser, P. G. (Eds.): Mechanisms of synaptic transmission. Progr. Brain Res. **31**, 33—46 (1969).

Vogt, M.: Functional aspects of the localization of transmitter substances. Progr. Brain Res. **34**, 1—8 (1971).

Westergaard, E.: The lateral cerebral ventricles and the ventricular walls. An anatomical, histological and electron microscopic investigation on mice, rats, hamster, guinea pigs and rabbits. Thesis. Odense: Andelsbogtrykkeriet 1970.

Westergaard, E.: The fine structure of nerve fibres and endings in the lateral cerebral ventricles of the rat. J. comp. Neurol. **144**, 345—354 (1972).

Wolffe, D. E., Potter, L. T., Richardson, K. C., Axelrod, J.: Localizing tritiated norepinephrine in sympathetic axons by electron microscopic autoradiography. Science **138**, 440—442 (1962).

Sensory and Secretory Catecholamine-Containing Cells Bordering the Third Ventricle of the Toad Brain

Olivia C. McKenna and Jack Rosenbluth

Departments of Physiology and Rehabilitation Medicine, New York University, School of Medicine, New York (USA)

Recent studies in this laboratory have demonstrated the presence of two discrete populations of unusual catecholamine-containing cells, one bordering the infundibular recess and the other bordering the preoptic recess, in the hypothalamus of the toad *Bufo marinus* (McKenna and Rosenbluth, 1971, 1974; McKenna et al., 1973). The cytological characteristics of the two cell types revealed by fluorescence histochemical, electron microscopic and Golgi impregnation methods indicate that neither cell can be categorized as a typical central adrenergic neuron. Instead one appears to be a receptor cell while the other may serve a secretory role.

Cytology

When the two cell types are compared to one another, it becomes apparent that they share some characteristics but are dissimilar in other respects (Fig. 1). The cells are similar in that both lie beneath the ependymal cells of their respective recesses and send apical processes between the overlying cells to border on the cerebrospinal fluid. Within the perikarya and apical processes of both, catecholamines can be demonstrated by fluorescence histochemistry and dense cored vesicles are found in electron micrographs. Neither cell type is stained by the paraldehyde fuchsin or chrome alum-hematoxylin phloxin methods for neurosecretory material, and both have basal processes extending away from the cell bodies into the underlying neuropil. Finally, axons filled with either clear vesicles or a mixture of clear and dense cored vesicles form synapses with the cell bodies of both types.

The cells differ in several important respects, however. First, the apical processes of the cells bordering the infundibular recess balloon out into the ventricle while those of the preoptic recess cells usually terminate flush with the adjacent ependymal cells, although these may occasionally protrude slightly into the ventricle. Second, the catecholamine of the preoptic recess cells is principally epinephrine while that of the infundibular subependymal cells is a primary catecholamine, either norepinephrine or dopamine. The fluorescence intensity of the former does not vary appreciably between males and females while the fluorescence intensity of the infundibular recess cells is considerably greater in males than in

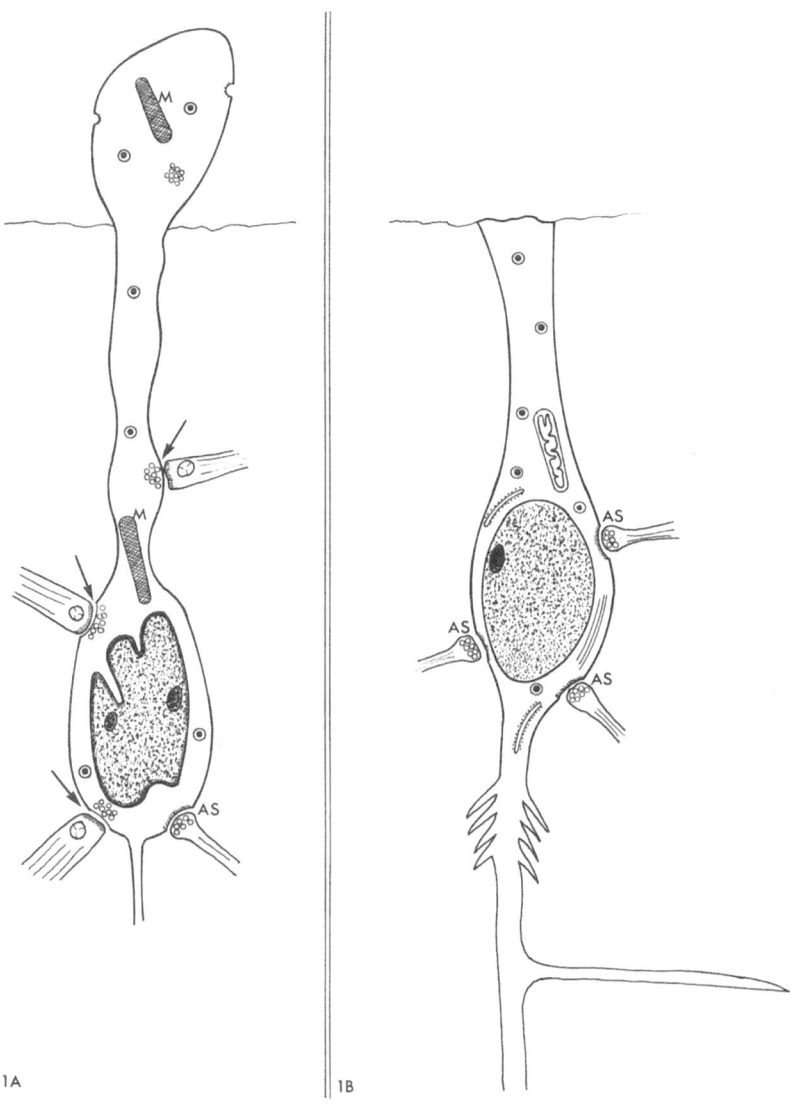

Fig. 1. A) Diagram of a subependymal cell bordering the infundibular recess. Its apical process balloons out into the ventricular cavity. The cell characteristically contains mitochondria with crystalline inclusions (M), dense cored vesicles and clusters of clear vesicles. It receives a sparse axosomatic innervation (AS) but forms numerous somatodendritic synapses (arrows). B) Diagram of a subependymal cell bordering the preoptic recess. The cells sends an apical process to the ventricle and a basal process into the underlying neuropil. The latter, in regard both to its diameter and to the type of projections found on it, is indistinguishable from ependymal processes seen in Golgi impregnation studies. The cell contains dense cored vesicles and is innervated (AS) but does not form somatodendritic synapses

females except when ovulation is induced. At this time the intensity becomes equivalent to that found in males.

The basal processes of these cells also exhibit differences. In electron micrographs the initial portion of the basal processes of the preoptic recess cells contains elements of the granular endoplasmic reticulum indicating that they are not axons. This impression is substantiated by Golgi impregnation studies which discloses that the basal processes, which extend laterally toward the surface of the hypothalamus, are thick and covered with projections unlike the thin smooth axons of neighboring neurons. In fact, were it not for the presence of an apical process the contour of this cell type would be indistinguishable from that of the adjacent ependymal cells. In contrast the basal processes of the infundibular recess cells are considerably narrower than those of the preoptic recess cells ($\sim 0.3\,\mu$ versus $\sim 2.5\,\mu$), and their initial segments lack elements of the granular endoplasmic reticulum. Although Golgi impregnation studies have not yet been extended to this second cell type, the present evidence suggests that their basal processes bear little resemblance to ependymal tails.

Although both cells are innervated by axons, only the infundibular recess cells are presynaptic to adjacent dendrites. The somatodendritic synapses formed by them are numerous and represent a pathway for the transmission of information from the cell body to surrounding dendrites. There is no evidence that preoptic recess cells have an equivalent function.

Finally, fluorescence histochemical studies indicate that the ontogenetic development of the two cell types differs. Those of the infundibular recess develop their fluorescence at stages equivalent to 23—24 (Shumway, 1940) while those bordering the preoptic recess do not appear until metamorphic climax. Such a wide difference in the time of appearance of the two cell types further supports the conclusion that they have dissimilar functions.

Functions

The cytological features of the subependymal cells bordering the infundibular recess plus the fact that they form numerous somatodendritic synapses point to a sensory function for these cells. Presumably they relay information obtained from the CSF to surrounding neurons. The resemblance of their basal processes to certain axons suggests the additional possibility that signals may also be conducted along these processes to more distant locations. These cells are able to pick up materials from the ventricle as shown by a study in which ferritin was injected directly into the infundibular recess and the cells examined at varying time intervals after the injection (Fig. 2). Initially ferritin particles were seen within coated invaginations of the cell surface exposed to the ventricle. At later times the particles were found concentrated within multivesicular bodies. Although ferritin is not a normal constituent of the CSF and its uptake may be nonspecific (Rosenbluth and Wissig, 1964), this experiment demonstrates that the cells have the capacity to pick up at least one protein from the CSF.

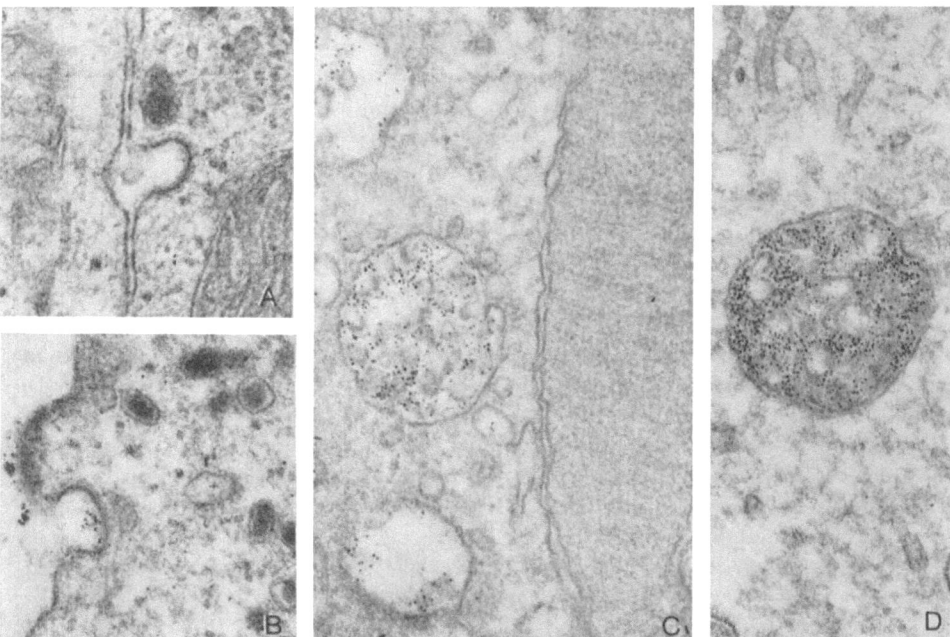

Figs. 2 A—D. Profiles of infundibular recess cells found within the ventricle (cf. Fig. 1 A) after injection of 2% ferritin in amphibian Ringer directly into the recess. A) Untreated control tissue showing coated invaginations of cell membrane. × 81000. B) Thirty minutes after injection ferritin particles are found within a coated invagination of the cell membrane. × 68000. C) Four hours after ferritin injection particles are found in multivesicular bodies. No ferritin particles are seen free in the cyctoplasm. × 68000. D) In the same tissue as C a multivesicular body contains heavier concentrations of ferritin particles. × 68000

The dramatic increase in cellular fluorescence seen in ovulating female toads suggests further that these cells play a role in reproductive function. Thus, one possibility is that regulatory substances derived from cells within the brain are released into the CSF and that the cells bordering the infundibular recess detect changes in their concentration and in this manner play a role in the regulation of reproduction.

In contrast the cells bordering the preoptic recess do not form somatodendritic synapses and their basal processes have none of the characteristics of axons. Instead, their high concentration of catecholamines in the apical processes bordering the ventricle and their innervation by axons suggest that these are chromaffin-like secretory cells which release their amines directly into the CSF and for which we have coined the term "encephalochromaffin cells". Their appearance at metamorphic climax suggest that they may be involved in a system used by a terrestrial rather than an aquatic animal.

Relation to other Cell Types

In recent years it has become increasingly apparent that the cerebral ventricles are not bordered exclusively by typical ependymal cells but also by other cell types that have special functions.

Evidence for secretory ependymal cells in the hypothalamus has been reviewed by Knowles (1969). More recently secretory cells have been described in the paraventricular organ (Braak, 1968; Peute, 1969, 1971) and the nucleus infundibularis dorsalis in nonmammalian vertebrates (Peute, 1973). In mammals secretory activity in ependymal cells in the preoptic recess of the rat (Leveque, 1972), in the anterior hypothalamus (Knowles and Anand Kumar, 1969) and the habenula (Anand Kumar, this volume, p. 294) of the rhesus monkey has been reported and correlated with reproductive activity. The tanycytes of the median eminence which are innervated may also have a secretory role. In addition reports of axon terminals of neurosecretory cells (Leonhardt, 1970; Rodriguez, 1970; Weindl and Schinko, this volume, p. 327) and of serotoninergic neurons (Richards and Tranzer, this volume, p. 246) extending into the ventricle suggest these two cell types may also secrete directly into the CSF.

Cells that may serve a sensory role have been described both in reptiles and amphibia in the paraventricular organ and the nucleus infundibularis dorsalis (Braak, 1968; Peute, 1969, 1973; Vigh-Teichmann et al., 1970). It is not yet clear, however, whether these cells should be considered sensory epithelial cells or sensory neurons. In addition dendrites of hypothalamic neurosecretory cells extend through the ependyma to the ventricular surface, and it has been suggested that they perform an osmoreceptor function within the CSF (Dierickx, 1962; Rodriguez, 1970). One other cell type in fish which may perform a sensory role contacts the central canal of the spinal cord at its apical surface and contacts underlying neurosecretory cells with its basal processes (Baumgarten et al., 1970; Vigh et al., 1971).

Conclusions

We have characterized two unusual catecholamine-containing cells which are in contact with the CSF in the amphibian hypothalamus. Reasons have been given for proposing that one of these, located in the infundibular recess, is sensory and that the other, located in the preoptic recess, is a chromaffin-like secretory cell. A review of the literature indicates that CSF-contacting sensory and secretory cells are probably widely distributed phylogenetically.

The existence of such cells supports the view that the CSF acts as a pathway for the distribution of biologically important materials within the brain. Thus the brain may employ not only synaptic transmission, but also a form of long distance humoral transmission analogous to that used by endocrine glands in the periphery. In the latter case the blood serves to distribute hormones to a variety of target cells; in the brain the equivalent role may be carried out by the CSF. Such a ventricular humoral system could serve to co-ordinate the activities of parts of the brain not otherwise interconnected.

References

Anand Kumar, T. C.: The habenulo-epiphysial system and the neuroendocrine regulation of menstrual cycles in the rhesus monkey. In: F. Knowles and L. Vollrath (Eds.): Neurosecretion — the final neuroendocrine pathway. VI. International Symposium on Neurosecretion, London, 1973. p. 294 Berlin-Heidelberg-New York: Springer 1974.

Baumgarten, H., Falck, B., Wartenberg, H.: Adrenergic neurons in the spinal cord of the pike *(Esox lucius)* and their relation to the caudal neurosecretory system. Z. Zellforsch. **107,** 479 (1970).

Braak, H.: Zur Ultrastruktur des Organon vasculosum hypothalami der Smaragdeidechse *(Lacerta viridis).* Z. Zellforsch. **84,** 285 (1968).

Dierickx, K.: The dendrites of the preoptic neurosecretory nucleus of *Rana temporaria* and the osmoreceptors. Arch. int. Pharmacodyn. **140,** 708 (1962).

Knowles, F.: Ependymal secretion especially in the hypothalamic region. J. Neuro-Visc. Rel. Suppl. **9,** 97 (1969).

Knowles, F., Anand Kumar, T. C.: Structural changes related to reproduction in the hypothalamus and in the pars tuberalis of the rhesus monkey. Phil. Trans. B **256,** 357 (1969).

Leonhardt, H.: Zur Frage der ventrikulären „gomoripositiven" Neurosekretion. In: Bargmann, W., Scharrer, B. (Eds.): Aspects of neuroendocrinology. V. International Symposium on Neurosecretion, p. 339. Berlin-Heidelberg-New York: Springer 1970.

Leveque, T. F.: The medial prechiasmatic area in the rat and LH secretion. In: Knigge, K. M., Scott, D. E., Weindl, D. (Eds.): Proc. Symp. Median Eminence: Structure and Function, p. 298. Basel: Karger 1972.

McKenna, O. C., Pinner-Poole, B., Rosenbluth, J.: Golgi impregnation study of a new catecholamine-containing cell type in the toad hypothalamus. Anat. Rec. **177,** 1 (1973).

McKenna, O. C., Rosenbluth, J.: Characterization of an unusual catecholamine-containing cell type in the toad hypothalamus. A correlated ultrastructural and histochemical study. J. Cell Biol. **48,** 650 (1971).

McKenna, O. C., Rosenbluth, J.: Cytological evidence for catecholamine-containing sensory cells bordering the ventricle of the toad hypothalamus. J. comp. Neurol. **154,** 133 (1974).

Peute, J.: Fine structure of the paraventricular organ of *Xenopis laevis* tadpoles. Z. Zellforsch. **97,** 564 (1969).

Peute, J.: Somatodendritic synapses in the paraventricular organ of two anuran species. Z. Zellforsch. **112,** 31 (1971).

Peute, J.: Ultrastructural aspects of the nucleus infundibularis dorsalis in the caudal hypothalamus of *Xenopus laevis.* Z. Zellforsch. **137,** 513 (1973).

Richards, J. G., Tranzer, J. P.: The characterization of monoaminergic nerve terminals in the brain by fine sreuctural cyctochemistry. In: F. Knowles and L. Vollrath (Eds.): Neurosecretion — the final neuroendocrine pathway. VI. International Symposium on Neurosecretion, London 1973. p. 246 Berlin-Heidelberg-New York: Springer 1974.

Rodriguez, E. M.: Morphological and functional relationships between the hypothalamoneurohypophysial system and cerebrospinal fluid. In: Bargmann, W., Scharrer, B. (Eds.): Aspects of Neuroendocrinology. V. International Symposium on Neurosecretion, p. 352. Berlin-Heidelberg-New York: Springer 1970.

Rosenbluth, J., Wissig, S.: The distribution of exogenous ferritin in toad spinal ganglia and the mechanism of its uptake by neurons. J. Cell Biol. **23,** 307 (1964).

Shumway, W.: Stages in the normal development of *Rana pipiens.* Anat. Rec. **78,** 139 (1940).

Vigh, B., Vigh-Teichmann, I., Aros, B.: Ultrastruktur der Liquorkontaktneurone des Zentralkanals des Rückenmarkes vom Karpfen *(Cyprinus carpio).* Z. Zellforsch. **122,** 301 (1971).

Vigh-Teichmann, I., Vigh, B., Koritsansky, S.: Liquorkontaktneurone im Nucleus paraventricularis. Z. Zellforsch. **103,** 483 (1970).

Weindl, A., Schinko, I.: Neuroendocrine activity in the organum vasculosum of the lamina terminalis. In: F. Knowles and L. Vollrath (Eds.) Neurosecretion — the final neuroendocrine pathway. VI. International Symposium on Neurosecretion, London, 1973. p. 327 Berlin-Heidelberg-New York: Springer 1974.

IV. Summaries

Aminergic Mechanisms in Neuroendocrine Control

Kjell Fuxe, Tomas Hökfelt, Gösta Jonsson, and Anders Löfström

Department of Histology, Karolinska Institutet, Stockholm (Sweden)

During the last few years the role of monoamines in neuroendocrine control has been vividly discussed especially in relation to gonadotrophin secretion (see e.g. the proceedings of last neurosecretion symposium in Kiel, Bargmann and Scharrer, 1970). In view of the extensive catecholamine (CA) and 5-hydroxytryptamine (5-HT) innervation of the median eminence, the hypothalamus and the limbic system, monoaminergic mechanisms probably operate at many levels of the CNS to control neuroendocrine function (see Fuxe et al., this volume, p. 223). Furthermore, in addition there is a CA innervation of the intermediate lobe and the neural lobe (see Björklund et al., this volume, p. 209). Various approaches have been undertaken to elucidate the role of the monoamines as is well-illustrated by the papers at the present symposium. Some workers (see Wuttke et al., and Ruf and Holmes, this volume, pp. 328 and 320) lesion the monoamine pathways or perform intraventricular injections of monoamines (see Kamberi et al., 1970; Schneider and McCann, 1970a) and measure the serum levels of luteinizing hormone (LH), follicle stimulating hormone (FSH) and prolactin or other parameters. Others (see Lichtensteiger, this volume, p. 229) study the amine turnover in terminals or cell bodies of monoamine neurons, especially of the tubero-infundibular dopamine (TIDA) neurons under various endocrine states. Due to the fact that the various approaches have given more or less contradictory results, the situation has grown very complex. The present article will summarize some of our own findings on the functional role of the monoamine neurons especially of the TIDA neurons and their role in the control of gonadotrophin secretion. From the work of Schally's group (see review by Schally et al., 1972) it is clear that LRF also can release FSH and therefore the term "FSH releasing hormone-LH releasing hormone" may be more appropriate. Thus, the dopamine (DA) system would also be inhibitory with regard to FSH secretion. At this symposium Martini (this volume, p. 135) raised the possibility that there may also be a factor selectively controlling FSH secretion and provided some evidence for this view. It was postulated that the paraventricular area could be involved in the synthesis of this "FSH releasing factor". In view of this it should be mentioned that there exists a dense noradrenaline (NA) innervation of the parvocellular part of the paraventricular nucleus and consequently a noradrenergic mechanism can control the activity of this area and of the hypothetical "FSH releasing factor".

The Tubero-Infundibular DA Neurons

As reported at this symposium by Löfström et al., using fluorescence histochemistry in combination with microfluorimetry in order to quantitate CA in the median eminence at various time-intervals following tyrosine hydroxylase inhibition, the DA turnover in the medial external layer is significantly higher than that in the lateral external layer (see Fig. 1). This difference may reflect a subdivision of the TIDA neurons. The NA terminals in the subependymal layer appear to have the lowest turnover of the CA terminal systems studied in the median eminence (Fig. 1).

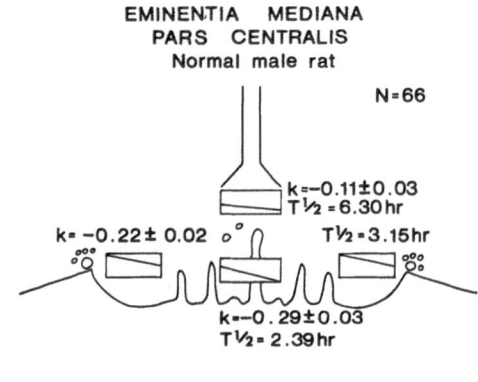

Fig. 1. Schematic representation of results from CA turnover measurements in nerve terminals in the central part of the median eminence in normal male rat, based on microfluorimetric quantitation of changes in the formaldehyde induced CA fluorescence following tyrosine hydroxylase inhibition produced by α-methyl-p-tyrosine methylester (250 mg/kg $i.\,p.$). The disappearance of the fluorescence was exponential and the calculated Tl/2 for the external layer was 2.39 h (medial part) and 3.15 h (lateral part) while Tl/2 for the subependymal layer was 6.30 h. The k-values $\pm$ S.D. for the slope are also given

It is known from previous work (see review by Fuxe and Hökfelt, 1969) that the TIDA neurons are markedly activated in lactation and pregnancy. Recent work by Löfström et al. (1974) suggest that the turnover of DA in certain parts of the external layer may be considerably increased up to ten times. These results have been interpreted to suggest that the TIDA neurons may contribute to the maintenance of the low LH and FSH secretion found in pregnancy and lactation and thus that the TIDA neurons may inhibit the luteinizing hormone releasing factor (LRF) secretion. Further support for this view was obtained, when 17-β-estradiolbenzoate was found markedly to increase DA turnover in this system (Fuxe et al., 1967, 1969, 1972) when administered repeatedly to castrated rats, exerting an inhibitory feedback on LRF secretion. It has also been found that in rats antifertility steroids (estrogen derivatives, 19-nortestosterone derivatives) and clomiphene in high doses, known to inhibit LH secretion, activate the TIDA neurons (Fuxe et al., 1971). In agreement new types of DA receptor stimulating agents have been found to cause blockage of PMS-induced ovulation in immature rats (see Fuxe and Hökfelt, 1973).

Of the hypophysial hormones prolactin but neither FSH nor LH markedly increases turnover in the TIDA neurons of hypophysectomized rats (Hökfelt and Fuxe, 1972b). This finding was interpreted to suggest that the inhibitory feedback of prolactin on its own secretion may partly be mediated via release of DA which enhance PIF secretion. Other authors have reached similar conclusions based on intraventricular CA injections (Kamberi et al., 1970) or treatment with monoamine drugs (Meites and Clemens, 1972). It is not known whether there are two types of TIDA neurons, one controlling PIF and one LRF secretion, or whether the same neuron system coordinates the secretion of LRF and PIF. Under all conditions prolactin has been found to increase DA turnover in the lateral external layer (see Fuxe et al., 1973a). Thus, conditions with hypersecretion of prolactin may result in the activation of dopaminergic mechanisms in the median eminence inhibiting LRF secretion. This could be part of the basis for the inverse interrelationship found between prolactin and LH secretion and could explain the blockage of ovulation found in relation to states with hypersecretion of prolactin (e.g. Chiari-Frommels syndrom). At the present symposium Lichtensteiger presented evidence for the existence of a cholinergic mechanism probably controlling the activity of the TIDA neurons, since anticholinergic drugs such as atropine blocked the increase in fluorescence intensity obtained in the DA cell bodies following electrical stimulation of various parts of the limbic system.

At this meeting Müller and Cocchi provided pharmacological evidence that in rat growth hormone (GH) secretion may be under an inhibitory dopaminergic control. It is therefore of interest that GH although in high doses increases amine turnover in the TIDA neurons of hypophysectomized rat. It should be realized, however, (see Fuxe et al., this symposium) that there exists a massive DA innervation of the limbic system which also can participate in the control of hormone secretion from the anterior pituitary.

Ascending NA Neurons

As pointed out in the introduction there are a number of observations starting already with the pioneering work of Sawyer, Everett and coworkers (see reviews by Wurtman, 1971; Coppola, 1971) that NA neurons may enhance the release of LH. Recent work in our laboratory (Löfström et al., 1974) seem to support this view, since after ovariectomy there occurs an increase of amine turnover in probable NA terminals in the subependymal layer and in the medial external layer, an effect which is counteracted by estrogen-priming. These findings are in good agreement with the results of Bapna et al. (1971) demonstrating a decrease of NA turnover in the anterior but not in the posterior hypothalamus following combined treatment with 17-β-estradiol benzoate and progesterone of ovariectomized rats. In the experiments mentioned above the gonadal steroids can be expected to exert a negative feedback on gonadotrophin secretion. The reduction of NA neuron activity observed would therefore be in agreement with the hypothesis that some NA pathways facilitate LH secretion. The high turnover of NA found in the anterior hypothalamus and the median eminence after castration may partly be mediated via the increases in FSH secretion (see Anton-Tay et al., 1969). However, different results have been obtained when progesterone is given to estrogen-primed castrated female rats under conditions of which progesterone probably causes a rise in LH and FSH levels (Kalra et al., 1971) similar to that found in proestrus. Thus, in this case progesterone has been found to increase NA turnover as assessed by whole brain analysis (Fuxe et al., 1973a) which gives further support for the view mentioned above.

Previous work has failed to reveal any marked effects of estrogen on CA uptake and release. *In vitro*, 17-β-estradiol benzoate has been found to cause a clear-cut inhibition of ³H-NA uptake into synaptosomes of the hypothalamus only in concentrations of 10^{-5} M, whereas in brain slices the uptake was not affected (see Janowsky and Davis, 1970; Fuxe et al., 1971; and Fig. 2). It has therefore been assumed that the changes in amine turnover observed mainly have been due to changes in nervous impulse flow.

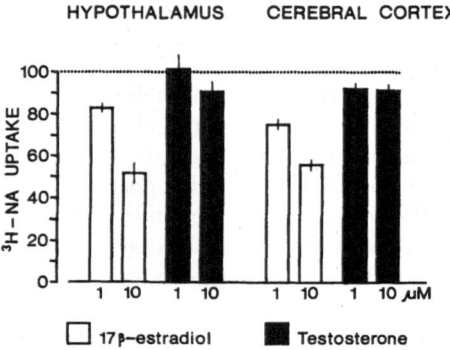

Fig. 2. Effect of 17-β-estradiol and testosterone on the *in vitro* uptake of ³H-NA at $+37°$ C in homogenates (synaptosomes) from hypothalamus and cerebral cortex of castrated female rat. The synaptosomes were preincubated with 1 or 10 μM hormone in Krebs-Ringer bicarbonate buffer for 10 min after which ³H-NA was added to give a final concentration of 0.05 μM and the incubation was continued for another 5 min. Each column represents the mean $\pm$ S.E.M. of 6 determinations and is expressed as a percentage of control

At the present symposium Ruf and Holmes presented some evidence based on intraventricular injections of the neurotoxic compound 6-OH-DA that the NA neurons may be involved in the control of puberty, since puberty was postponed in the 6-OH-DA treated animals. — It has been speculated that NA neurons could also be involved in control of prolactin secretion (Fuxe and Hökfelt, 1970; Fuxe et al., 1970; Donoso et al., 1971; Ajika et al., 1972). It may be of interest to mention that Wuttke and coworkers (this volume, p. 328) found initial increases in prolactin secretion following intraventricular injections of 6-OH-DA which mainly lesion the NA tracts but not the TIDA neurons.

It is the opinion of the present authors that the existence of a NA mechanism at the level of the median eminence enhancing LRF secretion, can be one of the explanations for the findings of an increase in LRF secretion following DA injection into the third ventricle (Schneider and McCann, 1970b; Kamberi et al., 1970). The DA injected can release NA from their stores, and increases in NA receptor activity may occur (see Andén and Fuxe, 1971) which could overcome the inhibitory DA mechanism in the external layer on LRF secretion (see above). A corresponding situation does not exist with regard to control of PIF secretion in which case both DA and NA mechanism may act to enhance PIF secretion, and consequently the results obtained in DA turnover studies (see above) or studies involving intraventricular DA injections (Kamberi et al., 1970) agree; thus injected DA enhances PIF secretion.

For the possible involvement of NA neurons in the control of ACTH and GH secretion the reader is referred to other review articles (see Fuxe et al., 1973b; Van Loon, 1973; Müller and Cocchi, this volume, p. 241). The possibility has to be stressed that the physiological role of the NA neurons could partly be to coordinate hormonal secretion from the pituitary gland and to favour certain patterns of hormonal secretions.

Ascending 5-HT Neurons

Previous findings have mainly revealed the existence of 5-HT terminals in the suprachiasmatic area and certain other areas of the hypothalamus (review by Fuxe et al., 1968). At the present symposium, however, autoradiographic results indicated that 5-HT nerve terminals may exist also at the level of the external layer of the median eminence (see Calas, this volume, p. 299). From the pharmacological studies of Kordon (see review article by Kordon et al., 1971/72) activation of 5-HT receptors appears to result in inhibition of the cyclic surge of LH secretion. In agreement with this view it has been found (Fuxe et al., 1973a) that estrogen increases 5-HT turnover in castrated female rats, an effect which seems to be related to the inhibitory feedback action of estrogen on LH secretion. When progesterone is administered to these estrogen primed rats probably resulting in peak secretion of LH and FSH (Kalra et al., 1971), the 5-HT turnover is again restored to normal. The situation is, however, still complex, since a tryptophane hydroxylase inhibitor, parachlorophenylalanine, given 24 h before the critical period will inhibit PMS-induced ovulation (see Kordon et al., 1971/72) as will intraventricularly injected 5.7-HT also given 24 h before the critical period (unpublished data). The possibility may be considered that 5-HT neurons may control FSH secretion also via a LRF independent mechanism. The role of 5-HT in control of prolactin secretion is also complex, but the pharmacological evidence for a facilitating action of 5-HT on suckling induced increases in prolactin secretion is convincing (Kordon et al., 1971/72).

The role of 5-HT neurons in regulation of other anterior pituitary hormones is not dealt with in the present article (see Ganong, 1972; Fuxe et al., 1973a; Van Loon, 1973). Here also the possibility has to be mentioned that the 5-HT neurons, like the NA neurons, may be coordinators of hormonal secretion from the pituitary gland.

Conclusions

The hypothesis is favoured that there exist a dopamine mechanism in the median eminence *inhibiting luteinizing hormone releasing factor secretion* and *enhancing prolactin inhibitory factor secretion* and in the anterior pituitary *inhibiting prolactin release* (see Fuxe and Hökfelt, 1969; Hökfelt and Fuxe, 1972a) and a noradrenaline mechanism in the hypothalamus *facilitating luteinizing hormone releasing factor secretion* (see Sawyer et al., 1949; Kalra et al., 1971; Ojeda and McCann, 1973). Furthermore, the hypothesis is advanced that the amenorrhea found in relation to hyperprolactinemia in man (e.g. Chiari-Frommels syndrom) can be partly caused by the selective activation by prolactin of certain tubero-infundibular dopamine neurons resulting in inhibition of luteinizing hormone releasing factor secretion. – The role of 5-hydroxytryptamine neurons in gonadotrophin secretion is also discussed.

Acknowledgements. This work was supported by grants from the Swedish Medical Research Council (04X—715, 04X—2887, 04X—2295) and by grants from the Population Council (M73.73) and from Svenska Livförsäkringsbolags Nämnd för Medicinsk Forskning.

References

Ajika, K., Krulich, L., McCann, S. M.: The effect of pentobarbital (nembutal) on prolactin release in the rat (36742). Proc. Soc. exp. Biol. (N. Y.) **141**, 203 (1972).

Andén, N.-E., Fuxe, K.: A new dopamine-β-hydroxylase inhibitor: Effects on the noradrenaline concentration and on the action of L-dopa in the spinal cord. Brit. J. Pharmacol. **43**, 747 (1971).

Anton-Tay, F., Pelham, R. W., Wurtman, R. J.: Increased turnover of ^{3}H-norepinephrine in rat brain following castration or treatment with ovine follicle-stimulating hormone. Endocrinology **84**, 1489 (1969).

Bapna, J., Neff, N. H., Costa, E.: A method for studying norepinephrine and serotonin metabolism in small regions of rat brain: Effect of ovariectomy on amine metabolism in anterior and posterior hypothalamus. Endocrinology **89**, 1345 (1971).

Bargmann, W., Scharrer, B. (Eds.): Aspects of neuroendocrinology. Berlin-Heidelberg-New York: Springer 1970.

Coppola, J. A.: Brain catecholamines and gonadotropin secretion. In: Martini, L., Ganong, W. F. (Eds.): Frontiers in neuroendocrinology, p. 129. New York: Oxford University Press 1971.

Donoso, A. P., Bishop, W., Fawcett, C. P., Krulich, L., McCann, S. M.: Effects of drugs that modify brain monoamine concentrations on plasma gonadotropin and prolactin in the rat. Endocrinology **89**, 774 (1971).

Fuxe, K., Hökfelt, T.: Catecholamines in the hypothalamus and the pituitary gland. In: Ganong, W. F., Martini, L. (Eds.): Frontiers in neuroendocrinology, p. 47. New York: Oxford University Press 1969.

Fuxe, K., Hökfelt, T.: Participation of central monoamine neurons in the regulation of anterior pituitary function with special regard to the neuro-endocrine role of tubero-infundibular dopamine neurons. In: Bargmann, W., Scharrer, B. (Eds.): Aspects of neuroendocrinology, p. 192. Berlin-Heidelberg-New York: Springer 1970.

Fuxe, K., Hökfelt, T.: The effects of hormones and psychoactive drugs on the tubero-infundibular neurons. Paper presented at a symposium on "Some aspects of hypothalamic regulation of endocrine functions". Vienna, June 1973.

Fuxe, K., Hökfelt, T., Jonsson, G.: Participation of central monoaminergic neurons in the regulation of anterior pituitary secretion. In: Martini, L., Meites, J. (Eds.): Neurochemical aspects of hypothalamic function, p. 61. New York-London: Academic Press 1970.

Fuxe, K., Hökfelt, T., Jonsson, G.: The effect of gonadal steroids on the tubero-infundibular dopamine neurons. In: Hormonal steroids. Excerpta Med. Intern. Congr. Ser., No. **219**, 806 (1971).

Fuxe, K., Hökfelt, T., Jonsson, G., Levine, S., Lidbrink, P, Löfström, A.: Brain and pituitary-adrenal interactions. Studies on central monoamine neurons. In: Brain-pituitary-adrenal interrelationships, p. 239. Basel: Karger 1973 b.

Fuxe, K., Hökfelt, T., Jonsson, G., Löfström, A.: Recent morphological and functional studies on hypothalamic dopaminergic and noradrenergic mechanisms. In: Usdin, E., Snyder, S. (Eds.): Frontiers in cetacholamine research, p. 787. New York: Pergamon Press 1973 a.

Fuxe, K., Hökfelt, T., Nilsson, O.: Activity changes in the tubero-infundibular DA neurons of the rat during various states of the reproductive cycle. Life Sci. **6**, 2057 (1967).

Fuxe, K., Hökfelt, T., Nilsson, O.: Castration, sex hormones and tubero-infundibular dopamine neurons. Neuroendocrinology **5**, 107 (1969).

Fuxe, K., Hökfelt, T., Nilsson, O.: Effect of constant light and androgen-sterilization on the amine turnover of the tubero-infundibular dopamine neurons: Blockade of cyclic activity and induction of a persistent high dopamine turnover in the median eminence. Acta Endocr. (Kbh.) **69**, 625 (1972).

Fuxe, K., Hökfelt, T., Ungerstedt, U.: Localization of indolealkylamines in CNS- Advances Pharmacol. **6**, A, 235 (1968).

Ganong, W. F.: Evidence for a central noradrenergic system that inhibits ACTH secretion. In: Knigge, K. M., Scott, D. E., Weindl, A. (Eds.): Brain-endocrine interaction. Median eminence: Structure and function, p. 254. Basel: Karger 1972.

Hökfelt, T., Fuxe, K.: On the morphology and the neuroendocrine role of the hypothalamic catecholamine neurons. In: Brain-endocrine interaction. Median eminence: Structure and function, p. 181. Basel: Karger 1972 a.

Hökfelt, T., Fuxe, K.: Effects of prolactin and ergot alkaloids on the tubero-infundibular dopamine (DA) neurons. Neuroendocrinology **9**, 100 (1972 b).

Janowsky, D. S., Davis, J. M.: Progesterone-estrogen effects on uptake and release of nor-epinephrine by synaptosomes. Life Sci. **9**, 525 (1970).

Kalra, P. S., Krulich, L., Quijada, M., Kalra, S. P., C. P. McCann, S. M.: Feedback of gonadal steroids on gonadotropins and prolactin in the rat. In: James, V. H. T., Martini, L. (Eds.): Hormonal steroids, p. 708. Amsterdam: Excerpta Medica 1971.

Kamberi, I. A., Mical, R. S., Porter, J. C.: Prolactin-inhibiting activity in hypophysial stalk blood and elevation of dopamine. Experientia (Basel) **26**, 1150 (1970).

Kordon, C., Gogan, F., Hery, M., Rotsztejn, W. H.: Interference of serotonin-containing neurons with pituitary gonadotropins release-regulation. Hormones and Antagonists. Gynec. Invest. **2**, 116 (1971/72).

Löfström, A., Jonsson, G., Fuxe, K.: A quantitative fluorescence analysis of catecholamine terminals of the median eminence. To be published (1974).

Loon, G. R. van: Brain catecholamines and ACTH secretion. In: Martini, L., Ganong, W. F. (Eds.): Frontiers in neuroendocrinology, p. 209, New York: Oxford University Press 1973.

Meites, J., Clemens, J. A.: Hypothalamic control of prolactin secretion. Vitamines and Hormones. **30**, 165 (1972).

Ojeda, S. R., McCann, S. M.: Evidence for participation of a catecholaminergic mechanism in the post-castration rise in plasma gonadotropins. Neuroendocrinology **12**, 295 (1973).

Sawyer, C. H., Markee, J. E., Townsend, B. F.: Cholinergic and adrenergic components in the neurohumoral control of the release of LH in the rabbit. Endocrinology **44**, 18 (1949).

Schally, A. V., Kastin, A. J., Arimura, A.: FSH-Releasing hormone and LH-releasing hormone. Vitamines and Hormones **30**, 83 (1972).

Schneider, H. P. G., McCann, S. M.: Mono- and indolamines and control of LH secretion. Endocrinology **86**, 1127 (1970 a).

Schneider, H. P. G., McCann, S. M.: Dopaminergic pathways and gonadotropin releasing factors. In: Bargmann, W., Scharrer, B. (Eds.): Aspects of Neuroendocrinology, p. 177. Berlin-Heidelberg-New York: Springer 1970 b.

Wurtman, R. J.: Brain monoamines and endocrine function. Neurosci. Res. Prog. Bull. **9**, 172 (1971).

New Trends in Vertebrate Neurosecretion

LUTZ VOLLRATH

Department of Anatomy, King's College, London (Great Britain)

In a review dealing with the physiology of the neurohypophysis published in 1968 (Farrell et al.) the authors felt that in the preceding four years little new of fundamental nature had appeared. I am not sure whether the present audience will agree with this view. I feel however that, had this really been the case, it could only have meant that those years represented a phase of seeming quiescence in which the foundation was laid for the enormous progress to take place in the last quinquennium. The papers delivered at the present symposium have reflected this progress very clearly and have left no doubt that progress in the field of vertebrate neurosecretion will continue to be rapid.

In the introductory paper Sir Francis Knowles (Knowles, this volume) expressed the hope that, by the end of this symposium, we might be in a position to formulate a clearer picture of a neurosecretory neuron than has hitherto been possible. I believe that we are indeed in such a position. Particularly helpful in this respect has been the application of new techniques. Landmarks have been the increased application of electrophysiological techniques with and without iontophoresis, the use of immunochemistry and immunohistochemistry, freeze-etching, freeze-fracture and scanning electron microscopy as well as conventional electron microscopy combined with morphometric techniques, not to mention all the sophisticated biochemical refining methods.

Classical Neurosecretory System

Looking back, it is most satisfying to see that the nature of the neurosecretory neuron has become much clearer and that a number of important, yet controversial, issues have been solved.

To begin with, it is now clearer than ever that the neurosecretory neuron is a cell which combines both secretory *and* neuronal properties. As regards its *secretory* nature, evidence has been produced, a while ago (Pilgrim, 1969), that neurosecretory cells, like e.g. the exocrine cells of the pancreas, undergo a characteristic secretory cycle and that individual cells oscillate between phases of high activity and restitution respectively. The observation that the secretory cycles of individual cells are not synchronized, even after prolonged osmotic stimulation, appears of special importance because the lack of synchronization could enable the system as a whole to sustain a state of high activity without fatigue over a long period of

time (Pilgrim, 1969), a functional aspect earlier ascribed to individual neurosecretory cells (Knowles, 1967).

The *neuronal* nature of neurosecretory cells has perhaps been best illustrated
by the electrophysiological studies. Particularly noteworthy is that – speaking in
the terminology of electrophysiologists – a successful antidromic invasion of the
neurosecretory neuron has taken place. As we have heard, the development and
the application of the antidromic technique have greatly helped to provide the
basic information about the electrical properties of neurosecretory cells both under
normal and experimental conditions (Cross, this volume). Information of this kind
was hardly, if at all, available at previous symposia (Heller and Clark, 1962;
Stutinsky, 1967; Bargmann and Scharrer, 1970). At the present symposium it was
provided in such an amount and with such a high quality that even a straight-
forward morphologist cannot overlook the fact any longer that a neurosecretory
neuron possesses distinct electrical properties. With respect to the high degree of
specialization of the neurosecretory cells it is particularly astounding that,
electrically, neurosecretory neurons do not seem to differ from non-secretory
neurons (Cross, this volume). Thanks to electrophysiologists we are also beginning
to realize the functional significance of the neuronal input of neurosecretory cells
(Cross, this volume; Barker et al., 1971a), demonstrated many years ago, and we
now know what happens, both morphologically and electrically, if neurosecretory
neurons are deprived of their neuronal input by deafferentation (Dyball and Dyer,
1971; Dyer et al., 1973). Moreover, direct iontophoretic administration of drugs
has greatly helped our understanding of the function of neurosecretory cells (Cross,
this volume; Barker et al., 1971b), though we were reminded that the same drug
may produce different effects depending on whether it is administered iontophoretically or systemically (Stutinsky, this volume). Particularly interesting
also was the observation that oxytocin, directly applied to paraventricular neurons,
proved disastrous for the cells and, I presume, one would readily agree with the
interpretation that this fact could explain why such elaborate binding and packaging mechanisms for the posterior lobe hormones are required (Moss et al., 1972).

Now, which controversial issues appear to have been solved? As regards the
question of a differential function of the paraventricular and supraoptic nuclei we
seem to have an extremely clear picture. The evidence obtained by different
approaches that each nucleus is involved in the production of vasopressin *and*
oxytocin, though in varying proportions, is indeed overwhelming (Cross, this
volume; Stutinsky, this volume). One technical approach which, in my opinion,
needs special mention is the immunohistochemical demonstration of vasopressin
in both nuclei and in individual cells and fibres with such a clarity (Burlet,
Marchetti and Duheille, this volume) that one cannot fail to be impressed.

As regards the *transport* of neurosecretory material, Professor Bern (Bern, 1970)
raised the question at the last neurosecretion symposium as to what the neurosecretionists meant by axoplasmic flow, the slow one, the fast one or the very fast
one. From the elegant studies in which radioactive substances were injected
directly into the neurosecretory nuclei by means of chronically implanted cannulae,
one was under the impression that indeed three flow speeds of 0.5, 1.5, and 190 mm/
day respectively were operative (Norström and Sjöstrand, 1971) and that also in
this respect the neurosecretory neuron did not differ from non-neurosecretory ones.

However, at the present symposium this concept was questioned and just one speed of 24—48 mm/day was proposed instead (Pickering, this volume). Again our attention was focussed on the neurotubules as important structures for the axonal transport (Grainger and Sloper, this volume; Flament-Durand and Dustin, this volume) and everything seemed quite clear when we heard that administration of colchicine was followed by a proximal accumulation of neurosecretory material and that no material arrived in the pituitary until we heard that the neurotubules were intact and that colchicine was a "dirty drug" (Douglas, discussion remark) having perhaps no direct effect on the tubules at all.

A very clear picture was obtained regarding the *release* of neurosecretory material. The concept of stimulus-secretion-coupling, born ten years ago (Douglas and Poisner, 1964) is still going strong, in fact even stronger it would appear, (Douglas, this volume; Russell and Thorn, this volume).

Moreover, the exocytosis concept (Nagasawa et al., 1970) appears to have been established beyond doubt. Exocytotic profiles have been demonstrated by various techniques and an increase in their number was shown under conditions of increased release of neurosecretory material (Dreifuss, Nordmann, Akert, Sandri, and Moor, this volume; Dempsey, Bullivant, and Watkins, this volume; Santolaya

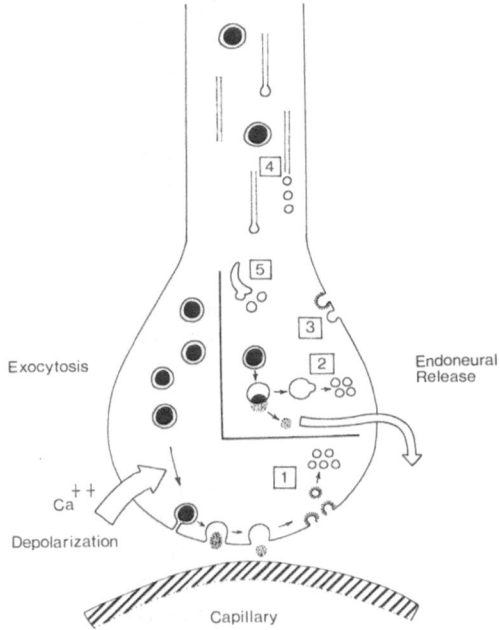

Fig. 1. Release mechanisms and formation of microvesicles in peptidergic neurosecretory axon terminals. While the concept of exocytosis of neurosecretory material appears to have been clearly established, there is some doubt as to whether an endoneural release takes place at all. 1—5 denotes different mechanisms of microvesicle formation. (1) Perhaps the majority of microvesicles originate as a result of exocytosis and the accompanying membrane vesiculation serving to restore terminal membrane area. Alternatively some microvesicles could occur resulting from (2) breakdown of large empty neurosecretory vesicles, (3) pinocytotic processes, (4) transformation of neurotubules, and (5) evaginations of endoplasmic reticulum

et al., 1972). A simultaneous release of both carrier proteins and hormones was demonstrated (Uttenthal et al., 1971) and, particularly noteworthy, in fixed ratios (Nordmann et al., 1971). Furthermore we were encouraged not to worry about the rarity of exocytotic profiles (e.g. Krisch et al., 1972) because even during increased hormone release related to milk-ejection only one in a thousand granules is released and this event takes only two seconds (Lincoln, this volume).

We also see more clearly how to interpret functionally the so-called synaptic vesicles of classical neurosecretory axon terminals, a controversial subject ever-since the introduction of electron microscopy into neurosecretory research (Holmes and Knowles, 1960; Lederis, 1964; Bargmann, 1967; Knowles et al., 1970; Vollrath, 1969, 1970). It now seems clear that they do not contain acetylcholine (Whitaker and LaBella, 1972; Bridges et al., 1973) but that they are the result of exocytosis and the accompanying membrane vesiculation serving to restore terminal membrane area and composition (Nagasawa et al., 1970, 1971; Douglas et al., 1971). However, it should be remembered that, as has been pointed out several times, the small electron-lucent vesicles probably do not represent a homogeneous population as regards their origin (Herlant, 1967; Vollrath, 1969, 1970) (Fig. 1). But apart from this reservation, it appears to me that the time has come to discontinue the use of the term synaptic vesicle for the small electron-lucent vesicles of the classical neurosecretory neuron. It would seem more appropriate to use a purely descriptive term, such as microvesicle (Douglas et al., 1971; Nagasawa et al., 1971).

With respect to the large empty-appearing elementary vesicles we now know at least that we can increase their number by using fixatives with a pH in an alkaline range (Morris and Cannata, 1973; Cannata and Morris, 1973), and this makes us have second thoughts about the concept of an endoneural release, (see Fig. 1), in particular since it has become clear at the present symposium that the question of an extragranular pool of neurosecretory material is indeed debatable (Pickering, this volume).

Hypophysiotropic Neurosecretory System

The present symposium has also clearly demonstrated that the classical neuro-secretory system has found a partner and, particularly noteworthy, of equal rank: the hypothalamic system elaborating the hypophysiotropic hormones. As we have heard, the development in this field has been breathtakingly fast (Martini, this volume). About two years ago it was felt that biochemistry and pharmacology had outpaced morphology (Knowles, 1972). At present we are witnessing that the morphologists are coming up fast.

To begin with, morphologists have been very successful in their search for morphologic correlates of releasing factors. Not only has the correlate of the CRF been found (Bock, 1972; Bock, Brinkmann, and Feldmann, this volume) but it is most interesting to see that CRF material has exactly the same staining properties as the classical neurosecretory material provided that the right fixative is used. Moreover, there have been many indications by electron microscopy in a wide range of species that Type A or peptidergic neurosecretory fibres are very likely candidates for containing hypophysiotropic hormones (Dierickx, this volume, amphibians; Oksche, Oehmke, and Hartwig, this volume, birds; Deery, this volume; and Knowles, Vollrath, and Meurling, this volume, elasmobranch fish).

Until fairly recently we were in a similar position with the releasing factor materials as with the classical neurosecretory material during the ontogenetic development: it was only demonstrable in the distal part of the system and one could already hear the view expressed that the releasing factors might be formed distally. However, at the present symposium, we have, I believe, witnessed an historic event; the clear demonstration, by immunohistochemistry, of releasing factor perikarya, namely those containing LH-RF (Barry and Dubois, this volume).

We are also beginning to understand the mechanisms regulating the function of the two neurosecretory systems. We have heard which role the aminergic systems play (Lichtensteiger, this volume; Fuxe, Hökfelt, Jonsson, and Löfström, this volume) and that amines affect pituitary pars intermedia function direct (Björklund, Falck, Nobin, and Stenevi, this volume). Moreover, we have heard that also mechanical factors may play an important role in neuroendocrine regulation: namely, that the neurohaemal contact area of the tubero-infundibular system in the external zone of the median eminence changed considerably in size due either to an active growth of nerve fibres or to changes in volume of tanycytic or glial processes (Wittkowski, 1973, and this volume).

Prospects

Looking ahead, one cannot help feeling that in the field of neurosecretion in the future the emphasis will probably lie in that of the releasing factor system. In my view, it should not take long before we have a fairly complete picture of the localization of at least a few releasing factor neuron pathways. Immunohistochemical methods, antidromic and orthodromic stimulation, lesions experiments and the application of the beautifully demonstrated cobalt-iontophoresis technique (Mason and Nishioka, this volume) represent such potent tools that progress is inevitable. In this respect we have already got a foretaste by the recent discovery of a third hypothalamo-neurohypophysial tract containing a neurophysin and terminating in the external zone of the median eminence and originating probably in the parvicellular parts of the paraventricular and supraoptic nuclei (Parry and Livett, 1973).

The search for electron microscopic correlates of releasing and inhibitory hormones will certainly continue. Since granule size has always been regarded as an important distinguishing feature of neurosecretory granules, it should be borne in mind that granule size appears to be a highly questionable distinguishing feature because it seems to be directly related to the size of the cross section of an axon (Wittkowski, 1973). Moreover it has to be taken into consideration that granule size may change under different physiological and experimental conditions, as indicated by the increase in size of the CRF granules according to the time of survival after adrenalectomy (Wittkowski, 1973).

Undoubtedly also the classical neurosecretory system will continue to attract attention. In view of the present concept that each of the classical neurosecretory nuclei is involved in the production of both vasopressin and oxytocin, attempts are likely to be made to morphologically identify the vasopressin- and the oxytocin-producing cells. Moreover, the Golgi apparatus of neurosecretory neurons, because of its functional bipolarity (Picard, Michel-Bechet, and Tasso, this volume), could turn out to be a favourite object of study in cell biology.

Perhaps one of the most challenging problems is that of finding the recurrent collaterals of neurosecretory neurons postulated by electrophysiologists (Cross, this volume) and to characterise their synapses with interneurons and to elucidate their neuronal circuits. Moreover, it would be most interesting to clearly define the areas and the mode of termination of the ascending peptidergic neurons which appear to have such a consistent distribution throughout the vertebrate species (Sterba, this volume).

As regards the distal part of the classical neurosecretory system, challenging problems have been posed with regard to the easily releasable pool of neurosecretory material. A most intriguing working hypothesis has been put forward (Pickering, this volume) that the easily releasable pool of neurosecretory material consisting of newly formed material travels, in the axon terminal, closely related to the cell membrane and if not released moves into the centre of the axon terminal and subsequently back into preterminal axonal swellings.

As to the neurophysins, we are at present witnessing the attempts to study the distribution of the carrier proteins in a wide variety of species and to determine how many different neurophysins there are (Ellis et al., 1972; Watkins and Evans, 1972), and in particular whether the minor components represent distinct neurophysins or metabolic products which arise in the neural lobe itself (Pickering, this volume). Moreover, it remains to be shown what the functional significance of the different neurophysins is.

In my view, also the pituicytes require special attention. Interesting starting points have been provided by the degeneration studies presented at the present symposium (Dellman et al., this volume) and the observation made earlier that neurosecretory neurons can regenerate only in the presence of pituicytes and that peripheral nerves are unable to do so among pituicytes (Kiernan, 1971), not forgetting the finding that rat pituicytes are innervated by dopaminergic fibres (Baumgarten et al., 1972).

Finally there is the challenging new concept that within certain hypothalamic nuclei there are cell clusters comprising specialized secretory elements and ependymal cells which together form functional units (Oksche, Oehmke, and Hartwig, this volume), challenging in particular because, so far, our view was mainly directed along and down the "neurosekretorische Bahn". Now we are challenged to regard the neurosecretory neuron not as an isolated and independent unicellular gland but as a functional unit intimately related to its neighbours, the final common pathway thus representing a small neuronal machine by itself.

In this context our attention was also focussed on the functionally enigmatic ependymal elements, the tanycytes, forming contacts with neuronal elements and the portal blood vessels (Oksche, Oehmke, and Hartwig, this volume). It appears to me that by the end of this symposium tanycytes were slightly less enigmatic than at the beginning of this conference.

In my view the concept of a preferential uptake from the CSF of certain substances by the tanycytes, as suggested by the incorporation of intraventricularly injected tritiated TRF (Scott et al., this volume) could prove most fruitful. No doubt also the innervation of the tanycytes (Güldner and Wolff, 1973), and this volume) and their changes in volume (Wittkowski, 1973) will attract attention and might give clues as to their precise function in neuroendocrine control.

Let me finish by mentioning two points which, though speculative, could, in my view, turn out to be rather important. The first point concerns the pineal gland. Those members of the present audience who took part in the Bristol Neurosecretion Symposium will recall that then the unsuccessful attempt was made to classify the pineal gland as a neurosecretory organ. At the present conference the pineal gland has made its debut at a neurosecretion symposium (Smith and Kappers, this volume), but not as a neurosecretory organ yet. In this context it is however interesting to note that recent studies have shown that the mammalian pineal gland contains polypeptides of low molecular weight, which inhibit FSH- and LH-release respectively (Benson et al., 1972; Orts and Benson, 1973; Moszkowska et al., 1971; Reiter, 1973). Since these substances appear to belong to the same category as the hypothalamic hypophysiotropic hormones, one wonders whether perhaps eventually the pineal gland will be classified as a neurosecretory organ.

The second point relates to parturition. In view of the ill-defined role of oxytocin during parturition (Farrell et al., 1968) there is the intriguing current concept that not the mother but the fetus with its hypothalamo-hypophysial-adrenocortical system is responsible for the initiation of labour (Liggins, 1968, 1969; Liggins et al., 1967; Anderson et al., 1971; Murphy, 1973; Jöchle, 1973). However, the study of the well-established neuroendocrine reflex pathways should not be neglected because recently it has been shown that, in pregnant women, mechanical breast stimulation by suction cup led to initiation of labour in 70% of cases (Jhirad and Vaga, 1973).

And so we are left with the interesting possibility that at birth both the classical and the hypophysiotropic neurosecretory systems are functionally closely interrelated: The hypophysiotropic neurosecretory CRF-system of the fetus, via the adrenal cortex, stimulating the classical neurosecretory system of the mother to release oxytocin.

References

Anderson, A. B. M., Laurence, K. M., Davies, K., Campbell, H., Turnbull, A. C.: Fetal adrenal weight and the cause of premature delivery in human pregnancy. J. Obstet. Gynaec. Brit. Cwlth. 78, 481—488 (1971).

Bargmann, W.: Conclusions-Schlußwort-Résumé. In: Stutinsky, F. (Ed.): Neurosecretion, pp. 241—247. Berlin-Heidelberg-New York: Springer 1967.

Bargmann, W., Scharrer, B.: Aspects of neuroendocrinology. Berlin-Heidelberg-New York: Springer 1970.

Barker, J. L., Crayton, J. W., Nicoll, R. A.: Supraoptic neurosecretory cells: autonomic modulation. Science 171, 206—207 (1971a).

Barker, J. L., Crayton, J. W., Nicoll, R. A.: Supraoptic neurosecretory cells: adrenergic and cholinergic sensitivity. Science 171, 208—210 (1971b).

Baumgarten, H. G., Björklund, A., Holstein, A. F., Nobin, A.: Organization and ultrastructural identification of the catecholamine nerve terminals in the neural lobe and pars intermedia of the rat pituitary. Z. Zellforsch. **126**, 483—517 (1972).

Benson, B., Matthews, M. J., Rodin, A. E.: Studies on a non-melatonin pineal antigonadotrophin. Acta endocr. (Kbh.) **69**, 257—266 (1972).

Bern, H. A.: Concluding remarks. Bargmann, W., Scharrer, B. (Eds.): Aspects of neuroendocrinology, pp. 374—377. Berlin-Heidelberg-New York: Springer 1970.

Bock, R.: Morphometrische Untersuchungen zum histologischen Nachweis des Corticotropin-releasing factor im Infundibulum der Ratte. Z. Anat. Entwickl.-Gesch. **137**, 1—29 (1972).

Bridges, T. E., Fisher, A. W., Gosbee, J. L., Lederis, K., Santolaya, R. C.: Acetylcholine and cholinesterases (assays and light- and electron microscopical histochemistry) in different parts of the pituitary of rat, rabbit and domestic pig. Z. Zellforsch. **136**, 1—18 (1973).

Cannata, M. A., Morris, J. F.: Changes of the appearance of hypothalamo-neurohypophysial neurosecretory granules associated with their maturation. J. Endocr. **57**, 531—538 (1973).

Douglas, W. W., Nagasawa, J., Schulz, R. A.: Coated microvesicles in neurosecretory terminals of posterior pituitary glands shed their coats to become smooth "synaptic" vesicles. Nature (Lond.) **232**, 340—341 (1971).

Douglas, W. W., Poisner, A. M.: Stimulus-secretion coupling in a neurosecretory organ: the role of calcium in the release of vasopressin from the neurohypophysis. J. Physiol. (Lond.) **172**, 1—18 (1964).

Dyball, R. E. J., Dyer, R. G.: Plasma oxytocin concentration and paraventricular neurone activity in rats with diencephalic islands and intact brains. J. Physiol. (Lond.) **216**, 227—235 (1971).

Dyer, R. G., Dyball, R. E. J., Morris, J. F.: The effect of hypothalamic deafferentation upon the ultrastructure and hormone contents of the paraventricular nucleus. J. Endocr. **57**, 509—615 (1973).

Ellis, H. K., Watkins, W. B., Evans, J. J.: Distribution of soluble proteins in the mammalian neurohypophysis and their cross-species reactivity with anti-neurophysin. J. Endocr. **55**, 565—575 (1972).

Farrell, G., Fabre, L. F., Rauschkolb, E. W.: The neurohypophysis. Ann. Rev. Physiol. **30**, 557—588 (1968).

Güldner, F.-H., Wolff, J. R.: Neuro-glial synaptoid contacts in the median eminence of the rat: ultrastructure, staining properties and distribution on tanycytes. Brain Res. **61**, 217—234 (1973).

Heller, H., Clark, R. B.: Neurosecretion. London, New York: Academic Press 1962.

Herlant, M.: Mode de libération des produits de neurosécrétion. In: Stutinsky, F. (Ed.): Neurosecretion, pp. 20—35. Berlin-Heidelberg-New York: Springer 1967.

Holmes, R. L., Knowles, F. G. W.: "Synaptic" vesicles in the neurohypophysis. Nature (Lond.) **185**, 710 (1964).

Jhirad, A., Vaga, T.: Induction of labor by breast stimulation. Obstet. and Gynec. **41**, 347—350 (1973).

Jöchle, W.: Corticosteroid-induced parturition in domestic animals. Ann. Rev. Pharmacol. **13**, 33—55 (1973).

Kiernan, J. A.: Pituicytes and the regenerative properties of neurosecretory and other axons in the rat. J. Anat. (Lond.) **109**, 97—114 (1971).

Knowles, F.: Neuronal properties of neurosecretory cells. In: Stutinsky, F. (Ed.): Neurosecretion, pp. 8—19. Berlin-Heidelberg-New York: Springer 1967.

Knowles, F.: Concluding remarks. In: Knigge, K. M., Scott, D. E., Weindl, A. (Eds.): Brain-endocrine interaction. Median eminence: Structure and function, pp. 364—368. Basel: Karger 1972.

Knowles, F., Weatherhead, B., Martin, R.: The ultrastructure of neurosecretory fibre terminals after zinc-iodine-osmium impregnation. In: Bargmann, W., Scharrer, B. (Eds.): Aspects of neuroendocrinology, pp. 159—165. Berlin-Heidelberg-New York: Springer 1970.

Krisch, B., Becker, K., Bargmann, W.: Exocytose im Hinterlappen der Hypophyse. Z. Zellforsch. **123**, 47—54 (1972).

Lederis, K.: Fine structure and hormone content of the hypothalamo-neurohypophysial system of the rainbow trout *(Salmo irideus)* exposed to sea-water. Gen. comp. Endocr. **4**, 638—661 (1964).

Liggins, G. C.: Premature parturition after infusion of corticotrophin or cortisol into foetal lambs. J. Endocr. 42, 323—329 (1968).

Liggins, G. C.: Premature delivery of foetal lambs infused with glucocorticoids. J. Endocr. 45, 515—523 (1969).

Liggins, G. C., Kennedy, P. C., Holm, L. W.: Failure of initiation of parturition after electro-coagulation of the pituitary of the foetal lamb. Amer. J. Obstet. Gynec. 98, 1080—1086 (1967).

Morris, J. F., Cannata, M. A.: Ultrastructural preservation of the dense core of posterior pituitary neurosecretory granules and its implications for hormone release. J. Endocr. 57, 517—529 (1973).

Moss, R. L., Dyball, R. E. J., Cross, B. A.: Excitation of antidromically identified neurosecretory cells of the paraventricular nucleus by oxytocin applied iontophoretically. Exp. Neurol. 34, 95—102 (1972).

Moszkowska, A., Kordon, C., Ebels, I.: Biochemical fractions and mechanisms involved in the pineal modulation of pituitary gonadotropin release. In: Wolstenholme, G. E. W., Knight, J. (Eds.): The pineal gland, pp. 241—258. Edinburgh, London: Churchill Livingstone 1971.

Murphy, B. E. P.: Does the human fetal adrenal play a role in parturition? Amer. J. Obstet. Gynec. 115, 521—525 (1973).

Nagasawa, J., Douglas, W. W., Schulz, R. A.: Ultrastructural evidence of secretion by exocytosis and of "synaptic vesicle" formation in posterior pituitary glands. Nature (Lond.) 227, 407—409 (1970).

Nagasawa, J., Douglas, W. W., Schulz, R. A.: Micropinocytotic origin of coated and smooth microvesicles ("synaptic vesicles") in neurosecretory terminals of posterior pituitary glands demonstrated by incorporation of horseradish peroxidase. Nature (Lond.) 232, 341—342 (1971).

Nordmann, J. J., Dreifuss, J. J., Legros, J. J.: A correlation of release of polypeptide hormones and of immunoreactive neurophysin from isolated rat neurohypophyses. Experientia (Basel) 27, 1344—1345 (1971).

Norström, A., Sjöstrand, J.: Axonal transport and turnover of neurohypophysial proteins of the rat. J. Neurochem. 18, 2007—2016 (1971).

Orts, R. J., Benson, B.: Inhibitory effects on serum and pituitary LH by a melatonin-free extract of bovine pineal glands. Life Sci. 12, Part II, 513—519 (1973).

Parry, H. B., Livett, B. G.: A new hypothalamic pathway to the median eminence containing neurophysin and its hypertrophy in sheep with natural scrapie. Nature (Lond.) 242, 63—65 (1973).

Pilgrim, C.: Morphologische und funktionelle Untersuchungen zur Neurosekretbildung. Enzymhistochemische, autoradiographische und elektronenmikroskopische Beobachtungen an Ratten unter osmotischer Belastung. Erg. Anat. Entw.-Gesch. 41, No. 4, 1—79 (1969).

Reiter, R. J.: Comparative physiology: pineal gland. Ann. Rev. Physiol. 35, 305—328 (1973).

Santolaya, R. C., Bridges, T. E., Lederis, K.: Elementary granules, small vesicles and exocytosis in the rat neurohypophysis after acute haemorrhage. Z. Zellforsch. 125, 277—288 (1972).

Stutinsky, F.: Neurosecretion. Berlin-Heidelberg-New York: Springer 1967.

Uttenthal, L. O., Livett, B. G., Hope, D. B.: Release of neurophysin together with vasopressin by a Ca²⁺ dependent mechanism. Phil. Trans. B 261, 379—380 (1971).

Vollrath, L.: Über die Herkunft „synaptischer" Bläschen in neurosekretorischen Axonen. Z. Zellforsch. 99, 146—152 (1969).

Vollrath, L.: The origin of "synaptic" vesicles in neurosecretory axons. In: Bargmann, W., Scharrer, B. (Eds.): Aspects of neuroendocrinology, pp. 173—176. Berlin-Heidelberg-New York: Springer 1970.

Watkins, W. B., Evans, J. J.: Demonstration of neurophysin in the hypothalamo-neurohypophysial system of the normal and dehydrated rat by the use of cross-species reactive anti-neurophysins. Z. Zellforsch. 131, 149—170 (1972).

Whitaker, S., LaBella, F. S.: Electron microscopic histochemistry of cholinesterase in the posterior, intermediate and anterior lobes of the rat pituitary. Z. Zellforsch. 130, 152—170 (1972).

Wittkowski, W.: Elektronenmikroskopische Untersuchungen zur funktionellen Morphologie des Tubero-hypophysären Systems der Ratte. Z. Zellforsch. 139, 101—148 (1973).

New Trends in Invertebrate Neurosecretion

Berta Scharrer

Department of Anatomy, Albert Einstein College of Medicine, New York (USA)

Four years ago, the Fifth International Symposium in Kiel featured a comprehensive overview on the state of neurosecretion in invertebrates (Scharrer and Weitzman, 1970). Therefore, in updating this report, we can confine ourselves to a few focal areas which spotlight current progress in this field. Most of these advances, conceptual as well as factual, are based largely on recent studies in insects and parallel those obtained in vertebrates. In both groups, the critical evaluation of the neurosecretory neuron, and its place within the spectrum of neurochemical mediation, continues to occupy center stage in our interest.

The new trend in this interpretive effort reflects our growing awareness of the remarkable versatility with which this special neuron operates in transmitting neurally derived information to various receptors.

There is increasing evidence that, in their bioelectric properties, neurosecretory neurons behave much like conventional neurons.

The role of axonal spike potentials in the release of neurosecretory mediators has been demonstrated in molluscs (Kandel and Kupfermann, 1970) and insects (Normann, 1973).

Considerable progress has been made in the elucidation of the precise topographic relationships between neurosecretory neurons and cells with which they interact. For example, painstaking studies carried out with conventional methods have detailed not only the existing neurosecretory pathways but also their afferent connections (Brousse-Gaury, 1971, a, b). As documented by experimental data, this synaptic input conveys sensory information intended primarily for the governance of the endocrine apparatus. Furthermore, neurons known to belong to such neurosecretory systems have been traced in their entirety with the aid of a novel procedure, axonal iontophoresis and cobalt sulfide precipitation (Mason and Nishioka, this volume, p. 48). One result of this approach is the clarification of the innervation of the corpora allata which, in the case of *Schistocerca*, has been traced to the lateral neurosecretory cells of the protocerebrum, and to a group of neurons in the subesophageal ganglion.

What other gains have been made in the elucidation of the diverse types of neurosecretory signals conveyed to this and other effector organs or cells ? Within the *neurohormonal* class, control mechanisms responsible for sequential changes in behavior are of particular interest. For example, in lepidopterans (Truman and Riddiford, 1974), an "eclosion hormone" triggers the movements necessary for emergence (preprogrammed in the abdominal ganglia), and the transition to adult behavior. The action of this factor, derived from the medial neurosecretory cells of the protocerebrum, is governed by a circadian clock which is sensitive to photoperiod. Two additional factors, both released from intrinsic cells of the corpus cardiacum under the direction of the brain, elicit subsequent reproductive events. In virgin females, the "calling hormone" causes the release of a sex pheromone. After mating, which affects the secretion of a bloodborne substance by the bursa copulatrix, the brain dictates a switchover to an "oviposition stimulating hormone" which, in turn, is responsible for an increase in the rate of oviposition.

In recent years, our special attention has been directed to *non-hormonal* activities of neurosecretory mediators, the existence of which had not been conceived before the advent of electron microscopy. The neurosecretory systems of insects provide us with instructive models for the demonstration of close range interaction between neurosecretory neurons and their effector sites. The latter include endocrine as well as non-endocrine cells. In both instances, the range of their spatial closeness to the release sites of the respective neurosecretory messengers is the same. Quite frequently, the extracellular pathway consists of a narrow zone of stromal material which may narrow down to the point where it is virtually nonexistent.

Such neuroeffector junctions resemble the more conventional types, except that the neurochemical mediator involved differs from the usual (cholinergic or aminergic) varieties in that its chemical composition appears to be the same as that of classical neurohormones.

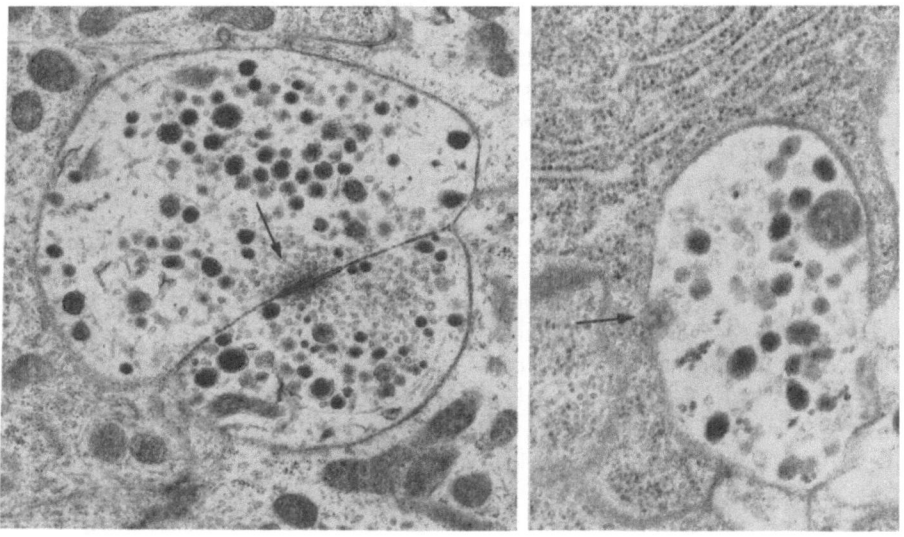

Fig. 1   Fig. 2

Fig. 1. Neurosecretory "innervation" of the corpus allatum in the orthopteran *Arphia pseudonietana*. Note release sites (arrow) between two contiguous axon profiles surrounded by parts of corpus allatum cells. (Specimen courtesy of Dr. S. N. Visscher). × 17000

Fig. 2. Synaptoid release site (arrow) of neurosecretory fiber within the salivary gland of the cockroach *Byrsotria fumigata*. × 31250

We still know very little about either the special circumstances that call for this kind of "private" peptidergic input, or the characteristics of its mode of operation. Although the frequency of such neurosecretory junctions seems to vary from one species to another, their presence is being reported in an increasing number of organs of insects.

As to endocrine receptors, synaptoid contact sites have been demonstrated in the prothoracic glands, the corpora cardiaca, and particularly the corpora allata (Fig. 1). The conclusion that, at these sites, the release of a neurosecretory mediator can be elicited upon appropriate stimulation has been substantiated by exposure of the tissue to excessive concentrations of potassium prior to fixation. The ultrastructural results are an increased number of synaptoid vesicles and an appearance of extracellular neurosecretory material.

Two examples, among the varied non-endocrine recipients of such special neural signals, are striated musculature and salivary glands (Fig. 2).

Recognition of these and other intermediate modes of neural signalling has removed the sharp boundary line originally thought to separate conventional neurons from the highly specialized elements that dispatch bloodborne chemical messengers. Thus the neurosecretory neuron with its distinctive biosynthetic and bioelectric properties has found its place within an impressively rich spectrum of possibilities available for neural communication.

References

Brousse-Gaury, P.: Influence de stimuli externes sur le comportement neuro-endocrinien de blattes. I. — Les organes sensoriels céphaliques, point de départ de réflexes neuro-endocriniens. Ann. Sci. net. Zool. Ser. 12 ^{e}, **13**, 181—332 (1971 a).

Brousse-Gaury, P.: Influence de stimuli externes sur le comportement neuro-endocrinien de blattes. II. — Histophysiologie des voies réflexes neuro-endocriniennes. Ibid 333—450 (1971 b).

Kandel, E. R., Kupfermann, I.: The functional organization of invertebrate ganglia. Ann. Rev. Physiol. **32**, 193—258 (1970).

Normann, T. C.: Membrane potential of the corpus cardiacum neurosecretory cells of the blowfly, *Calliphora erythrocephala*. J. Insect Physiol. **19**, 303—318 (1973).

Scharrer, B., Weitzman, M.: Current problems in invertebrate neurosecretion. In: Bargmann, W., Scharrer, B. (Eds.): Aspects of Neuroendocrinology, pp. 1—23. Berlin-Heidelberg-New York: Springer 1970.

Truman, J. W., Riddiford, L. M.: Hormonal mechanisms underlying behaviour. In: Treherne, J. E., Berridge, M. J., Wigglesworth, V. B. (Eds.): Advances in Insect Physiology, Vol. 10, pp. 297—352. London-New York: Academic Press 1974.

Concluding Remarks

W. BARGMANN

Department of Anatomy, University of Kiel (Federal Republic of Germany)

Mr. Chairman, Ladies, and Gentlemen!

When you read our programme you had certainly no difficulty in imagining what the item "Introductory Lecture" meant, because it was clearly explained as a historical survey dealing with 20 years of research work on neurosecretion beginning with the Naples Symposium. Incidentally, the exact birthday of our concept was earlier, on April 21st, 1952, Denver, Colorado – the obstetricians and baptizers were Ernst and Berta Scharrer, Professor Kleinholz, and my late co-worker, Ernst Horstmann. Some cups of tea were used for sprinkling the newborn.

But what means the announcement of "Concluding remarks", which Professor Knowles has asked me to give? Perhaps a further summary of the summarizing reviews presented by Professor Berta Scharrer and Professor Vollrath? Well, those papers of our colleagues already reflected brilliantly the essential features and progress presented in our research field during this symposium, progress based on the invention of new methods. Therefore it does not seem to me that it is necessary to go again into the details. Let me mention only a few points.

It has turned out once more, as was already demonstrated at our former meetings at Naples, Lund, Bristol, Strasbourg, and Kiel, that vertebrates and invertebrates should not be discussed separately in separate Symposia. The neurosecretory systems and their products are admittedly different in the different groups of the animal kingdom, but the basic phenomena of neurosecretion are processes at the cellular level and it is at this level that investigators try to understand the mechanisms of elaboration, transport and release of neurohormones and neurohumors. At this conference the number of participants made the arrangement of some separate and simultaneous sessions inevitable and this will presumably be necessary also in the future. But might I suggest that at forthcoming meetings there might be at least one or two surveys comparing the cellular events in vertebrates and invertebrates in one session for all the participants. I would hope that this proposal would have the approval of many of the symposiasts, especially Professor Douglas.

A second point deals with the sometimes passionate enjoyment one may have in creating definitions, for example a definition of neurosecretion. In background discussions I have got the impression that almost every third neurosecretionist has a concept more or less different from that of his neighbour! I do not intend to add a new one but, rather, draw attention to our use of a limited number of terms namely Peptidergic Neurosecretion, Neurohormonal Cells, Neurohaemal organs, Aminergic Control of peptidergic systems. This common application of terms is certainly the equivalent of a certain degree of mutual understanding.

Some investigators tend to adopt the aminergic neurons as neurosecretory cells. Whether this is to be recommended or not, it is clear that the non-peptidergic systems must be thoroughly considered in our symposia. I should like to stress this, because it demonstrates a process of maturation we have undergone since the first Symposium at Naples. The first circular sent round in 1952 contained the sentence, "The symposium will *not* be concerned with substances such as acetylcholine or adrenalin". "Tempora mutantur et nos mutamur cum illis."

Instead of producing further comments of this kind I prefer to conclude my remarks by saying some words of admiration, recognition and gratitude.

As you perhaps know, it was originally planned – somewhat in a mood of nostalgia – to return with the VIth Symposium on Neurosecretion to the Stazione Zoologica Napoli, where we started twenty years ago. Sir Francis Knowles was kind and brave enough to take over the burden of organization in Italy. But finally, after years of toil and difficulty, he has said as our host, "Welcome to London" and not as organizer in Italy, "Benvenuti in Napoli"! Some of the senior neurosecretionists were kept closely in touch with the long prophasic negotiations and other problems which Professor Knowles had to overcome before the switch from Naples to London seemed indicated. His final proposal to organize the Symposium in London was gratefully accepted, with strong feelings of decompression.

Professor Knowles' multilateral diplomacy finally has resulted in this meeting characterized by its atmosphere of high scientific standard, generous hospitality and friendship. Let me therefore take this opportunity of expressing the sentiments of gratitude of the participants to you, Professor Knowles, to your co-worker, Professor Vollrath, and your many helpers, more or less behind the scene, for all your efforts which created this climate. Thanks are also due to the Royal Society for having made accessible her famous institution as a framework for our meetings, to the Zoological Society and to the Warden of King's College Hall where many of us lived so comfortably. Last but not least we owe special thanks of course to Lady Knowles for psychologically assisting her husband.

Today the participants of this meeting will be "released", following different patterns of extrusion, and reach their laboratories in the near future. We shall bring with us to our various workshops new information and stimulating concepts. Let me express the hope, still using terms of Neuroendocrinology, that one of the most important principles in neurohormonal regulation, namely, feedback will once again, as it has in the past twenty years, bring our family or tribe of neurosecretionists together once more, for a VII symposium, wherever in the world its place may be.

V. Abstracts

Studies on the Medial Neurosecretory Cells in the Protocerebrum of Water Beetle, *Dytiscus Marginalis*

A. ÁBRAHÁM

Institute of Zoology, University of Szeged (Hungary)

The medial neurosecretory cells are situated at both sides of the pars intercerebralis. Each cell group consists of 15 large unipolar cells, their processes facing centrally. Neurosecretory granules leave the cells at any point on the cell membrane of the perikaryon and of the processes. The processes form pathways in the neuropil and leave it as brain nerves. In the middle of the neuropil the pathways cross over. In the vicinity of this place many granules appear which indicate three pathways of secretion, two of them ending in the neuropil and one in the corpus cardiacum.

The change of the different water ions (Na+, K+, Ca++), the quantity of light and temperature, the stimulation with UV rays or alternating current cutting of the palpes or the extirpation of the eyes resulted in differences in the production of granules. The neurosecretion consists of dense core granules originating in the Golgi complex but it is possible that the endoplasmic reticulum or the mitochondria also play a role in their production. The granules show some functional similarity with synaptic vesicles but are different in appearance. We can follow the granules from the cell body to the site of release but the synaptic vesicles are visible only at the synaptic region. The form of extrusion of granules indicates a possibility that the functional role of the granules in the neuropil is different from that in the corpus cardiacum. It is not clear whether the axons containing neurosecretory granules make true synaptic formations or not.

Ábrahám, A.: Acta anat. (Basel) **65**, 435—446 (1966).
Ábrahám, A.: Revue Roumaine de Biol., Sér. Zool. **11**, 25—33 (1966).
Ábrahám, A.: Z. mikr.-anat. Forsch. **80**, 469—484 (1969).
Bloch, B., Thomson, E., Thomson, A.: Z. Zellforsch. **70**, 185—208 (1966).

Functional Morphology of the Cephalic Neuroendocrine Complex of Two Species of Blattidae: an in Situ Study

K. G. ADIYODI

Department of Zoology, Calicut University (South India)

In *Periplaneta americana* and *Neostylopyga rhombifolia* a cardiaca-allatal commissural plexus (CACP) lies between and partly overlapping the postcommissural lobes of the corpora cardiaca (CC), the nervi corpori allati I (NCA I) and the corpora allata (CA). CACP, which is often continuous posteriorly with a complicated postallatal nerve plexus (PNP), comprises a variable number of connectives with neurosecretory processes linking the cardiac commissural organ (containing tritocerebral fibres) to NCA I, allatal commissure and the CA. Neurosecretory processes are exchanged between the two halves of the cephalic neuroendocrine apparatus (CNC) both intracerebrally and extracerebrally at different places, possibly to ensure functional synchrony of CNC components.

NCA I and CACP are drawn out with their stroma to varying extents over the CA. Histophysiological evidence suggests that part of the stainable secretion stored in, and/or in axonal transit through CA may be released through CA surface; limitedly though, NCA I, CACP, and perhaps also NCA II may function as neurohaemal areas. A „directed" neurosecretory pathway could be distinguished from PNP to the foregut and the fat body. The degree of spatial intimacy detected between neurosecretory and stomatogastric components of CNC suggests that the two systems may function in an integrated fashion. The recurrent-oesophageal nerve complex serves not only for a direct transport of neurosecretion, but also as one of the sites of its release.

Supported in part by research grants from the Indian National Science Academy.

Moult-Related Neuroendocrine Events in the Crab, *Paratelphusa Hydrodromous* (Herbst)

R. G. ADIYODI and K. G. ADIYODI

Department of Zoology, Calicut University (South India)

The complete picture of the neurosecretory system and the cyclic changes temporally related to ecdysis have been investigated in the crab, *P. hydrodromous*. All types of neurosecretory cells located in the eyestalk (except the e-cells), brain and thoracic ganglia show two peaks of release of neurosecretion (NSM) axonally and or extraneuronally: Release I during C_4—D_0 and Release II during D_2—D_3. Each release is preceded by periods of NSM accumulation in the perikarya of the neurosecretory cells. Release of NSM is either absent or very low in postmoult, and practically absent in D_1 and D_4. X-organ cells, conventionally implicated in the production of the moult-inhibiting hormone (MIH) also show, like other neurosecretory cells, only two peaks of release of NSM, Release I in C_4—D_0 and Release II in D_2—D_3. Surprisingly no notable release of NSM from the a-cells (which form most of the X-organ) is visible during postmoult, when moult is inhibited and a high titre of MIH may be expected in the blood. NSM released from other cell types of the eyestalk, brain and thoracic ganglia, simultaneously with that from the X-organ cells, may be mostly metabolic hormones concerned with the controls of moult-related phenomena like calcium deposition, oxygen consumption and water metabolism. Some problems in causally relating activities of X-organ and other neurosecretory cells with the control of moult are discussed. Light microscopically detectable changes occur in the NSM (1) very near the axon hillock; (2) at a somewhat distal end of the axon; (3) in the preterminal part of the axon located within the sinus gland and (4) on reaching the axon terminals.

The Habenulo-Epiphysial System and the Neuroendocrine Regulation of Menstrual Cycles in the Rhesus Monkey

T. C. ANAND KUMAR

Department of Anatomy, All-India Institute of Medical Sciences, New Delhi (India)

Light and electron microscopic studies, in rhesus monkeys, on the ventricular lining in the habenular region indicate that this is a site at which both ependymosecretory and neurosecretory substances are discharged into the cerebrospinal fluid. A correlation exists between the habenular ependymosecretion and the stages of the menstrual cycle: the ependymo-secretion occurs maximally only during menstruation. The pineal concentrates radioactivity maximally in contrast to all other known target organs of the body in monkeys injected with tritium-labelled oestradiol. An oestrogen receptor has been identified in the pineal. The activity of adenyl cyclase, an enzyme whose role in increasing the output of the antigonadal pineal principle, melatonin, is well-known, is enhanced in response to oestrogen administration.

An antigonadotropic function has been attributed to the habenula (Faure et al., 1966; Motta et al., 1968) and the pineal (Wurtman et al., 1968). The demonstration of a habenular innervation of the pineal (David and Herbert, 1973) indicates that these two components are functionally linked. The results of our studies, when viewed against this background, suggest that the habenulo-epiphysial system may constitute an important neuroendocrine component in the regulation of menstrual cycles in response to circulating levels of gonadal hormones. The effects of this system are presumably effected *via* the hypothalamo-hypophysial system through substances secreted by the habenular ependyma and the pineal into the cerebrospinal fluid.

David, G. F. X., Herbert, J.: Brain Res. **64**, 327—343 (1973).
Faure, J., Vincent, D., Bensch, C.: C. R. Soc. Biol. (Paris) **160**, 1557 (1966).
Motta, M., Fraschini, F., Giuliani, G., Martini, L.: Endocrinology **83**, 1101 (1968).
Wurtman, R. J., Axelrod, J., Kelly, D. E.: The pineal. New York: Academic Press 1968.

ADH as a Transmitter of Recurrent Inhibition in the Supraoptic Neuro-secretory System?

E. Arnauld and J. D. Vincent

Laboratoire de Neurophysiologie, Bordeaux (France)

Five unanaesthetized rhesus monkeys fitted for single cell recording were subjected to water deprivation up to 8 days, followed by a 4 days rehydration period. Four to 8 supraoptic neu-rones identified by antidromic invasion following stimulation of the posterior pituitary were recorded daily. Frequency and pattern of firing, as well as the presence or absence of recurrent inhibition (RI) were studied. RI was defined by a period of reduced firing following antidromic invasion of the cells. Blood samples were collected from a chronic intracardiac cannula, allow-ing for plasma electrolyte, osmotic pressure and haematocrit determinations.

The mean firing frequency of supraoptic neurones increased in relation with the observed rise in plasma osmotic pressure. Initially, an increasing proportion of cells displayed a phasic pattern of discharge with alternances of bursts followed by silent periods. In a majority of cells, clear-cut RI was observed. After the 5th day of water deprivation, most of the cells discharged continuously at a high rate, and RI was no longer present. The mean firing fre-quency returned to control values after 2 days of rehydration. On the 4th day, the cells were either silent or firing very slowly. RI could again be demonstrated when a sufficient level of spontaneous firing existed.

On the basis of iontophoretic administration and of intracarotid injection of ADH, it has been proposed that the neurosecretory product may act as a neurotransmitter and could mediate RI. Since it has been shown that the hormonal content of the neurohypophysis decreases progressively during dehydration, the disappearance of RI and of the phasic pattern of discharge after prolonged dehydration is not inconsistent with this view, provided that the general increase in firing does not as such reduce the silent period which follows the antidromic spike.

Synapses in the Neurosecretory System of the Earthworm

B. Aros

2nd Department of Anatomy, Semmelweis University Medical School, Budapest (Hungary)

In earlier studies we found that the neurosecretory cells of the circumpharyngeal ring of *Lumbricidae* send their nerve processes into the fibrous zone situated below the cellular layer of the ganglia. It is possible that secretory material of these nerve fibers passes to the capillaries present in this zone. In a recent electron microscopic study of this fibrous zone we observed numerous synapses mainly axo-dendritic, containing granulated vesicles of different types, one of them resembling neurosecretory elementary granules.

Under the light microscope, we observed nerve fibers coming from the receptor area of the prostomium and terminating in the above-mentioned fibrous zone. We postulate that there may be synaptic connections between these fibers and the nerve processes of the neurosecretory cells, and that the neurosecretory system may receive information from the prostomium which modifies the neurosecretory activity, but up to now we have not been able to demonstrate any neurohormonal synapses in the ganglia. Further investigations are needed to determine the site of hormonal release by the neurosecretory cells.

Aros,B., Röhlich,P., Vigh,B.: Acta biol. Acad. Sci. hung. **22**, 141—153 (1971a).
Aros,B., Röhlich,P., Vigh,B.: Acta biol. Acad. Sci. hung. **22**, 443—456 (1971b).
Röhlich,P., Aros,B., Vigh,B.: Z. Zellforsch. **58**, 524—545 (1962).

Histological Observations on the Problem of Hyperfunction and Exhaustion in the Magnocellular Nuclei of the Rat

D. Bara

Institutum Anatomiae Pathologicae, Szeged (Hungary)

As is known, in case of stress induced by chronic dehydration, in the supraoptic and paraventricular nuclei one can observe virtually only hypertrophied ganglion cells in which the Nissl substance [ribonucleicproteides] and neurosecretory material of the cytoplasm are extensively decreased. Various histological methods were used in attempts to clarify whether these are neurons in protracted hyperfunction or functionally exhausted. A light microscopically demonstrable increase of the ribonucleic acid content of the nucleolar substance and the intensification of the corresponding enzyme histochemical reactions of the cytoplasm, and ultrastructurally the preservation of the supramolecular organisation of the elementary secretion granules in the Golgi-complex, point to a prolonged neuronal activity.

Bachrach,D.: Z. Zellforsch. **47**, 147—157 (1957).
Bara,D., Bartók,I., Csapó,Zs.: Endokrinologie **53**, 385—396 (1968).
Bara,D., Skaliczki,J.: Acta morph. Acad. Sci. hung. **16** (4), 439—453 (1968).

Influence of Corticoids on the Amount of CRF Granules in the Median Eminence of Adrenalectomized Rats

R. Bock, H. Brinkmann, and M. Feldmann

Anatomisches Institut der Rheinischen Friedrich-Wilhelms Universität, Bonn (Federal Republic of Germany)

In the outer layer of the median eminence of the rat "Gomori-positive" granules occur which probably represent the morphological equivalent of the corticotropin-releasing factor (CRF). After bilateral adrenalectomy their amount increases depending on the length of the postoperative survival period. This increase parallels the rise in CRF activity which is observed in pharmacological investigations under the same experimental conditions. The quantitative changes of the granules following adrenalectomy can be influenced by application of corticoids. Substitution with corticoids, which is begun immediately after the operation, inhibits the augmentation of the granules. This inhibitory effect of a corticoid is closely related to its ACTH-suppressive activity and its antiphlogistic potency.

Application of corticoids from the 15th to 21st day p.o. causes an enhanced augmentation of the granules. This enhancement is more pronounced following administration of DOCA than after dexamethason.

The findings suggest:

(a) That corticoids inhibit the production of the granules (of the CRF) as well as their (its) release,

(b) that inhibition of the release takes place earlier than that of production.

Bock, R.: Z. Anat. Entwickl.-Gesch. **137**, 1—29 (1972).

Studies on the Hypothalamic Control of the Pituitary Gland of the Toad, *Bufo Bufo*

P. E. Budtz

Zoophysiological Laboratory A., Copenhagen (Denmark)

In studies of the central nervous control of the function of the toad pars distalis, the effect of ectopic transplantation and transection of the hypothalamus behind the optic chiasma were compared.

Transection of the hypothalamus results in degeneration of all nerve terminals in the median eminence except for a few Type 3 neurons (1000—1300 Å granules) (Budtz, 1970). Therefore the *release* of hormones in transected and transplanted toads was expected to be similar, but in fact the TSH release as revealed by studies on iodine uptake and GTH release as revealed by studies of the thumb pads were higher in denervated than in grafted toads (see Jørgensen, 1968). As also the *storage* of granules in the glycoproteinaceous cell Types 1 and 2 (Doerr-Schott, 1971), assumed to secrete gonadotropin and TSH, was higher in denervated than in transplants—as shown by quantitative measurements, using a Zeiss TGZ 3 particle analyzer—it is concluded, that also the rate of *synthesis* is higher in thyrotrophs and gonadotrophs of hypothalamus-transected toads than in those of transplants. This conclusion was supported by the finding of a well developed Golgi apparatus with frequent observations of granule formation in denervated toads, whereas in transplants the Golgi apparatus is less developed and granule formation less frequent.

This means that cells of the pars distalis in toads with hypothalamic transection immediately behind the optic chiasma are more active with regard to synthesis and release of gonadotropin and TSH than those of the transplanted pars distalis. From the present findings it seems justified to assume that the very few fibres left intact after denervation in fact are able to exert some control of the activity of the gonadotrophs and thyrotrophs.

It may therefore be concluded that one nerve type in the median eminence, namely the Type 3 fibres, must be the morphological equivalent of two hypophysiotrophic functions, namely the release of GRF and TRF.

Budtz, P. E.: Z. Zellforsch. **107**, 210—233 (1970).
Doerr-Schott, J.: Ann. Endocr. (Paris) **32**, 371—379 (1971).
Jørgensen, C. B.: In: Barrington, E. J. W., Jørgensen, C. B. (Eds.): Perspectives in endocrinology, pp. 469—541. New York: Academic Press 1968.

Double Tag Study (Cesium 131, Cr⁵¹-Tagged Red Blood Cells) of Capillary Exchanges in the Neurohypophysis of a Lerot (*Eliomys Quercinus* L.) during His Awakening from Hibernation

C. BURLET, J. ROBERT, and E. LEGAIT

U.E.R. Sciences Médicales A., Laboratoire d'Histologie, Nancy (France)

In the active anaesthetized lerot (basal temperature 35.5° C), the neurohypophysial vascular space, estimated through the use of radioactive erythrocytes, represents 12% of the glandular tissue; it is less developed than that of the adenohypophysis or the thyroid (16%), or of pulmonary tissue (40%) whereas it is greater than that of the kidney (10%) or liver (8%). Seventeen minutes after the awakening process begins (basal temperature 10° C), vascular space is increased in all endocrine glands: +25% in the adenohypophysis, +75% in the neurohypophysis, +80% in the thyroid. After 35 min (basal temperature 20° C), the variations are still greater: +75% in the adenohypophysis, +225% in the neurohypophysis, +280% in the thyroid.

The neurohypophysis is a veritable target-organ for cesium: its tissue concentration is 400 times that of blood. However, the study—in the neurohypophysis and the adenohypophysis—of the ratio: intra-tissue cesium activity/vascular space activity using Cr⁵¹ shows that in the course of the awakening, there is no particular metabolic process in the neurohypophysis; the intensity of the trans-capillary passage of cesium being conditioned chiefly by the evolution of tissue temperature. One observes, on the other hand, a very great hypervascularization of the neurohypophysis, especially after 35 min, at which period one can detect a high concentration of vasopressin in peripheral plasma.

Boer, G. J.: J. Histochem. Cytochem. **20**, 621—626 (1972).
Bullard, R. W., Funkhouser, G. E.: Amer. J. Physiol. **203**, 266—270 (1962).
Sooriyamoorthy, T., Livingston, A.: J. Endocr. **54**, 407—415 (1972).

Identification of Axon Terminals in Some Neuroendocrine Organs with Special Reference to Monoaminergic Neurons

ANDRÉ CALAS

Laboratory of Neuroendocrinology, E.R.A. 85 C.N.R.S., Department of Physiology, University of Montpellier II, Montpellier Cédex (France)

Radioautographic studies on the uptake of tritiated monoamines have been performed on the hypothalamic neurosecretory systems leading to the neural lobe (NL) and to the median eminence (ME) of the neurohypophysis in the duck and in the rat. Catecholaminergic (CA) axons have been found to innervate neurosecretory neurons of the anterior hypothalamus in both species (Alonso, in prep.). CA fibers are also present:

(1) in perivascular spaces of ME and NL in both species;

(2) in the internal and external zones of ME as well as within the parenchyma of NL in the rat;

(3) in the inner zone of ME in the duck. In this region they form synaptic contacts upon infundibular neurosecretory neurons (Calas, 1973).

Microspectrofluorimetry on formaldehyde-treated material has revealed that these CA fibers of the duck contain noradrenaline. They are specifically destroyed by 6-OH-Dopamine (Calas et al., 1974).

Indolaminergic (IA) axons may also be found by radioautography, after administration of 5-HT-^{3}H, within the anterior hypothalamus in both species. In the ME of ducks, they are restricted to the external zone. They are destroyed by 5,6-HT. At the ultrastructural level, CA and IA fibers differ with respect to their granular and vesicular contents (Calas, 1972, and in preparation).

Using the same techniques, axons that retain labelled monoamines could be evidenced within the corpora cardiaca of *Locusta migratoria* although their ultrastructure exhibits peculiar patterns (Lafon-Cazal et al., 1973).

Calas, A.: C. R. Acad. Sci. (Paris) **274**, 925—927 (1972).
Calas, A.: Z. Zellforsch. **138**, 503—522 (1973).
Calas, A., Hartwig, H. G., Collin, J. P.: Z. Zellforsch. **147**, 491—504 (1974).
Lafon-Cazal, M., Calas, A., Bosc, S.: J. Microsc. **17**, 197—200 (1973).

Hypothalamic Regulation of the Dogfish Pituitary

D. J. DEERY

Department of Anatomy, King's College, London (Great Britain)

Neutralised acid extracts of the anterior and posterior median eminence were prepared from the hypothalamus of the dogfish *Scyliorhinus canicula*. The effects of these extracts, and of similar extracts of other brain regions, on the adenyl cyclase system of particulate preparations of each of the four lobes of the dogfish pituitary were studied. While the hypothalamic extracts were found to promote a dose-related activation of the enzyme in each lobe, the control extracts failed to stimulate the enzyme activity. The putative neurotransmitters dopamine, melatonin, acetylcholine, serotonin, epinephrine and norepinephrine were tested at 10^{-4} M and failed to promote activation of the enzyme in any of the four pituitary preparations.

The synthetic mammalian hypophysiotropic hormones TRH and LHRH were found to activate specifically the enzyme in the ventral lobe preparation, being without effect on the enzyme of the rostral, median or neuro-intermediate lobes. These results suggest that the hypothalamus of the dogfish may elaborate substances capable of stimulation of the pituitary gland and that these substances are unlikely to correspond to any of the neurotransmitters tested. This view is supported by the observed sensitivity of the ventral lobe enzyme to the peptide releasing-hormones.

Ultrastructural Changes in the Rat Neural Lobe Following Stalk Transection and Heterotopic Transplantation, and in Organ Culture

H.-D. DELLMANN, M. E. STOECKEL, A. PORTE, F. STUTINSKY, N. CHANG, and H. K. ADLDINGER
Department of Veterinary Anatomy, University of Missouri, Columbia (USA)
Laboratoire de Physiologie générale, Strasbourg (France)

Between the first and fifth day following stalk transection, the peptidergic neurosecretory axons in the vicinity of the lesion were characterized by nonspecific reactive changes, such as proliferation of the axoplasmic reticulum, and accumulation of granulated vesicles, mitochondria and multilamellar bodies. In the nerve terminals an increase in small non-granulated vesicles, some of which are possibly derived from the granulated vesicles was observed. Subsequently the fibres degenerated and became surrounded by pituicyte processes; then they lost their proper membrane and were obviously disposed of through the action of lytic enzymes secreted by the pituicytes. During degeneration neurosecretory granules were frequently found to be condensed into crystal-like structures. The changes observed during involutionary processes in normal peptidergic neurosecretory axons and especially in Herring-bodies are similar to those found in degenerating neurosecretory axons prior to necrosis. From the seventh day on the neural lobe was composed of clusters of pituicytes which progressively reacquired embryonic characteristics (absence of lipid inclusions, extensive endoplasmic reticulum, active Golgi apparatus), and sinusoidal capillaries surrounded by wide connective tissue spaces. A pronounced connective tissue reaction as well as macrophages did not occur. The pituicyte reactions resemble those of oligodendroglial (and Schwann) cells. Following heterotopic transplantation, the same reactive and degenerative events were observed. However, the pituicytes did not eliminate their lipid droplets and lysosomes. In organ culture the early reactive and degenerative phases were also identical, but many pituicytes subsequently became necrotic.

Immunofluorescence Localization of Bovine Neurophysin II

J. DE MEY and F. VANDESANDE
Department of Embryology and Histology, State University, Gent (Belgium)

Rabbits (5) were immunized with bovine neurophysin II. The specificity of the antisera was assessed by micro-immuno diffusion. From two rabbits, antibodies to bovine neurophysin II were obtained. The two sera reacted also with neurophysin C, but not with neurophysin I. Polyacrylamide gel electrophoresis and gel electrofocusing showed that the purified antigen contained some traces of neurophysin C, but from the pattern of precipitation lines, obtained by micro-immuno diffusion, it was concluded that this was not the cause of the cross-reaction of our serum with neurophysin C.

Cryostat-sections of the bovine hypothalamic-hypophysial region were fixed in 94% ethanol and immunofluorescence staining was carried out with diluted rabbit anti-neurophysin II sera, as the middle layer in the "sandwich technique" followed by an appropriate dilution of goat anti-rabbit IgG, conjugated with FITC.

Fluorescence microscopy showed an intense granular fluorescence in apparently all the cell bodies of the supraoptic nucleus, in a large number of cells of the paraventricular nucleus, in the pituitary stalk and the neural lobe.

These results suggest that in the cow, the nucleus supraopticus is specialized in the elaboration of neurophysin II, while the paraventricular region elaborates both neurophysin I and II, but in separate neurons. They also show that neurophysin C and II are immunologically related, which is in accordance with their similar amino acid composition.

Up to now, the minor products found in neurophysin preparations have been neglected.

Our results indicate the importance to work with very pure neurophysin preparations in the near future before it will be possible to draw positively definite conclusions.

Rauch, R., Hollenberg, H. D., Hope, D. B.: Biochem. J. **115**, 473 (1969).

Exocytosis in the Rat Neurohypophysis—A Freeze-Fracture Study*

G. P. DEMPSEY, S. BULLIVANT, and W. B. WATKINS

Dept. of Cell Biology and the Postgraduate School of Obstetrics and Gynaecology, University of Auckland, Auckland (New Zealand)

The technique of freeze-fracturing demonstrates large areas of cell membranes as well as many of those ultrastructural features seen by conventional thin sections. Since the mechanism of hormone release by exocytosis initially involves the attachment of the neurosecretory granule (NSG) membrane to the membrane of the nerve cell followed by fusion of the two membranes, a freeze-fracture study of the neurohypophysis is considered appropriate. During fusion of the NSG's we would expect to see "holes" in the A face of the nerve cell membrane and broken-off "necks" on the B face of the nerve cell membrane. The presence of "holes" and "necks" in the nerve fibres of the neurohypophyses of normal rats was demonstrated and after a period of 1—2 days dehydration the number of "holes" and "necks" appeared to be at a maximum. There was a significant decrease in the number of these structures after 7 days dehydration. Loss of the small (8.5 nm) membrane-associated particles from the bulges on the nerve cell membrane overlying the NSG's is considered to represent a change in membrane structure to a state which is more favourable for fusion.

Bullivant, S.: Micron **1**, 45—51 (1969).

Bullivant, S., Ames, A.: J. Cell Biol. **29**, 435—447 (1966).

Douglas, W. W., Nagasawa, J., Schultz, R.: In: Heller, H., Lederis, K. (Eds.): Subcellular organisation and function in endocrine tissues, pp. 353—378. Cambridge University Press 1971.

---

* Published in detail in Z. Zellforsch. **143**, 465—484 (1973).

The Calcium-Influx Hypothesis and the Exocytosis-Vesiculation Sequence: An Interpretation of the Mode of Secretion of Neurohypophysial Hormones and Significance of Microvesicles ("Synaptic" Vesicles)

W. W. DOUGLAS

Department of Pharmacology, Yale University School of Medicine (USA)

Ten years ago it was suggested that the release of neurohypophysial hormones is effected by the arrival of impulses in the neurosecretory terminals which, by depolarizing, promote calcium influx and that the appearance of free calcium ions somewhere in the endings then causes the release of stored hormone. At the Fourth International Symposium on Neurosecretion held in 1966 it was argued, by analogy with other secretory systems, that the role of calcium in the neurohypophysis was likely to be concerned with "reverse micropinocytosis" (exocytosis) despite the fact that exocytosis had not been observed in neurohypophysial terminals, and it was proposed that if neurophysin were found to escape with the octapeptide hormones this would provide strong grounds for supposing secretion to involve exocytosis since this bulky molecule should not traverse intact membranes.

Neurophysin has since been found to escape and electron microscopic evidence of exocytosis in mammalian neurohypophyses obtained. Moreover, there are indications that the long-enigmatic microvesicles ("synaptic vesicles") arise in consequence of exocytosis by membrane vesiculation serving to restore terminal membrane area and composition.

The present paper will discuss the concept of a "Ca-activated exocytosis-vesiculation sequence" from morphological, biochemical, pharmacological and comparative stand points.

Ultrastructural and Electrical Changes in Neurosecretory Neurones Associated with Prolonged Stimulation of Hormone Release

R. E. J. DYBALL and J. F. MORRIS

Department of Anatomy, The Medical School, Bristol (Great Britain)

Substitution of 2% NaCl for drinking water for 3 days increased electrical activity of neuro-secretory neurones in the supraoptic and paraventricular nuclei (SON, PVN) of rats and decreased pituitary stores of oxytocin and ADH.

Examination of a series of micrographs of SON and PVN in a blind trial revealed that, under these conditions, an increased proportion of neurosecretory cells have dilated endoplasmic reticulum ($p < 0.01$) and there is an increase in the number of multivesicular lysosomal bodies per cell profile ($p < 0.02$). An increase ($p < 0.05$) in the proportion of "dense" neurosecretory granules indicates that the granule population is less mature (Cannata, Morris, 1973, J. Endocr. 57, 531—538).

If after NaCl treatment rats were allowed tap water for 2 days, neurohypophysial hormone stores increased ($p < 0.01$) but were still reduced ($p < 0.01$) below normal. The increased electrical activity had subsided and the proportion of cells showing dilated endoplasmic reticulum, the number of multivesicular bodies and the proportion of "dense" granules returned towards normal. There was, however, an increase in dense lysosomal bodies ($p < 0.01$).

Thus the changes in both ultrastructure and electrical activity appear to be related rather more to the application of the hormone-depleting stimulus than to the hormone content of the posterior pituitary.

The Electrical Characteristics and Synaptic Connexions of Neurones in the Rostral Hypothalamus

R. G. DYER and P. F. HEAP

Department of Anatomy, The Medical School, Bristol (Great Britain)

A causal relationship between hypothalamic electrical activity and the secretion of anterior pituitary hormones has been difficult to establish, partly because recording procedures interfere with the neuroendocrine reflex under investigation but also because the functions and connexions of the neurones recorded were unknown. The present experiments were undertaken to define the projections of some cells in the trigger zone (i.e. preoptic/anterior hypothalamic area — PO/AH) for the pre-ovulatory secretion of LH in rats.

Two hundred and ninety-nine single units were recorded from PO/AH and of these 41% had axons terminating in the ventromedial/arcuate region (VMH/ARC). They were identified by antidromic activation from this region. Most of these cells showed little spontaneous electrical activity and were only detected by antidromic stimulation. Their impulse conduction rate was low (< 0.4 m/sec) and, unlike the adjacent population of neurones, did not fire faster at prooestrus.

Small lesions (0.5 mm diameter) in dorsal PO/AH, where many of the cells were located, caused synaptic degeneration in VMH/ARC but no evidence of degeneration was found in the median eminence. More rostral lesions did not affect the ultrastructure of VMH/ARC. These data are consistent with the hypothesis that some of the antidromically identified PO/AH cells may be interneurones regulating adenohypophysial secretion.

A Golgi and Golgi-Cox Study on the Hypothalamus of the Crested Newt

A. FASOLO, M. F. FRANZONI, and V. MAZZI

Institute of Comparative Anatomy, University of Turin, Turin (Italy)

The cell types occurring within the periventricular grey matter of the caudal hypothalamus in the crested newt have been studied by the rapid Golgi and the Golgi-Cox methods. The following cell types were observed:

1) A majority of neurons each bearing a ventrally directed dendritic shaft.

2) Abundant liquor-contacting cells with an ovoid body more or less deeply embedded in the grey matter. These cells exhibit a process of moderate caliber, generally smooth, passing between the ependymal cells to reach the infundibular lumen. Next to the ependymal layer this process frequently displays a spindle-shaped swelling and gives off a collateral beaded branch of smaller caliber which runs subependymally a long distance. In many cases it was observed that these cells also show a short stump directed ventrally, from which some coarse and scarsely spiny dendrites arise together with a thinner beaded process, presumably axonic in nature. Liquor-contacting cells are visible at various levels of the caudal hypothalamus. They might correspond, partly at least, to the CSF-contacting neurons which were demonstrated by different techniques within the vertebrate hypothalamus (see survey by Vigh, 1971). These CSF-contacting neurons might be involved, although in a way so far not fully understood, in the mechanisms controlling hypophysial activity.

After Golgi and Golgi-Cox methods, a population of specialized ependymal cells (tanycytes) is prominent along the infundibular walls and in the neurohypophysis. Tanycytes exhibit a few spiny or barbed processes passing to the blood vessels, which they contact by means of endfeet. The wide distribution of these cells may suggest, particularly in the lower vertebrates, that they play a primary role by transporting substances from the CSF to the blood vessels or vice-versa (Knowles, 1972).

Knowles, F.: In: Kappers, J. A., Schadé, J. P. (Eds.): Topics in neuroendocrinology, p. 256. Amsterdam, London: Elsevier 1972.
Vigh, B.: Studia biol. hung. **10** (1971).

Action of Colchicine on the Neurosecretory Paraventricular Neurons in the Rat

J. FLAMENT-DURAND and P. DUSTIN
Department of Neuropathology, Free University of Brussels (Belgium)

The ultrastructural aspects of the paraventricular nucleus and its neuropil in the normal rat is presented. Two types of neurons can be distinguished. The first one contains numerous dense-core vesicles of about 140 nm of mean diameter, mainly located in the juxtanuclear region. The cisternae of the endoplasmic reticulum are arranged parallel to the surface of the cell body.

The second type of neuron contains only a few dense-core vesicles of about 75 nm in mean diameter. The endoplasmic reticulum is randomly distributed in the cytoplasm.

Colchicine treatment produced an accumulation of neurosecretory granules in the first type of neurons and in their axons. Abnormal elongated structures surrounded by a unit membrane are observed mainly in the axons. Their various morphological aspects are illustrated.

Further Observations on the Action of Colchicine on the Neurosecretory Paraventricular Neurons in the Rat

J. FLAMENT-DURAND and P. DUSTIN
Department of Neuropathology, Free University of Brussels (Belgium)

In a previous work, by using autoradiography and electron microscopy, we have shown that colchicine injected intracisternally in the rat at the dose of 200 µg in 0.05 ml of distilled water interrupts the flow of elementary neurosecretory granules in the paraventricular neurons. This was proved by the stagnation of the elementary granules in the neuronal cytoplasm and by the presence of numerous axonal swellings loaded with neurosecretory granules in the neuropil. Synthesis of protein in the neurosecretory neurons was not impaired as demonstrated by autoradiography and by electron microscopy.

In this presentation, we would like to emphasize a peculiar aspect observed in the neurosecretory cells of the colchicine-treated rats: elongated structures surrounded by a unit membrane are observed in the axons emerging from the paraventricular neurons. These structures are mainly oriented parallel to the long axis of the axons in the direction of the axonal flow. They are surrounded by a unit membrane similar to that enveloping the elementary neurosecretory granules, and sometimes connected with the membrane of neighbouring granules.

The content of these elongated structures is variable. In some instances it has the same appearance, morphology and electron density as that of the neurosecretory granules. In other instances, it has a fibrillar appearance containing bundles of longitudinally arranged fibrils of approximately 2 nm in diameter. The two types of inclusions may be found in the same axon.

The endoplasmic reticulum is often closely apposed to the membrane of the inclusions in the same way as to that of neurosecretory granules. These structures are sometimes in close relation with tubules. Their length is variable, the longest one observed measuring 4.5μ. The nature of these structures remains uncertain: they may represent a fusion of elementary neurosecretory granules or an alteration of microtubules. The fibrillar appearance seems to be in favour of the second hypothesis, but the axonal microtubules are still visible. The aspect of the enveloping membrane speaks in favour of a secretory origin.

The problem still awaits further investigations.

Autoradiographic Study of the Distribution of NA$^+$, DA$^+$, and GABA$^+$ in the Neurohypophysis of the Teleost Fish, *Gasterosteus Aculeatus* L.

E. FOLLENIUS

Laboratoire de Cytologie Animale, Institut de Zoologie, Strasbourg (France)

Among the techniques used in the study of neurosecretions and neurotransmitters, the autoradiographic ones may be especially useful for those substances having a high uptake rate by the nerve fibres. This is the case, as several studies have shown, for three of them: Noradrenaline (NA), Dopamine (DA) and γ-aminobutyric acid (GABA).

These three potential neurotransmitters have been administered to *Gasterosteus aculeatus* and their localization in the neurohypophysis has been studied at the light and electron microscope levels.

Results obtained after administration of labelled NA and DA will be briefly summarized. NA and DA are taken up by fibres abutting on cells of the meta-adenohypophysis where an aminergic innervation is therefore present. It is however not clear whether the neurotransmitter is NA or DA. Some fibres in the meso-adenohypophysis are also able to take up NA and to store it, but near the pro-adenohypophysis only a very few fibres are labelled.

Recently an attempt has been made to study the potential intervention of GABA in the hypothalamo-hypophysial regulatory system. Autoradiography after administration of 2.5μg/g of GABA-H^3 shows that the whole neurohypophysis binds strongly this amino acid. 30 min and 1 h after injection the labels were found on the nerve fibres, as well on their terminal region as on their path to the hypothalamus. The fibres which reach the different hypophysial lobes are heavily labelled. This is clear for those which abut on the corticotropic cells of the pro-adenohypophysis as well as for those distributed in the meso-adenohypophysis. In several cases even the fibres of the preoptic origin are labelled in the posterior neurohypophysis.

These results demonstrate that GABA is metabolized by different types of fibres which are not typical GABA fibres. It appears that the detection of GABA fibres by autoradiography is not as easy as for the aminergic fibres. Further improvements are needed to enhance the selectivity of the labelling for those fibres which use GABA as their neurotransmitter.

Cerebral Neurohemal Area of Crickets, *Acheta Domesticus* L., *Melanogryllus Desertus* Pall.: A Correlated Light and Electron Microscope Study

S. GELDIAY (Turkey) and J. S. EDWARDS (USA)

Cerebral neurohemal regions are found in invertebrates and vertebrates but have never previously been observed in insects. For the first time a cerebral neurohemal region is investigated and reported in *Acheta domesticus* L. and *Melanogryllus desertus* Pall..

On the ventral and medial surfaces of the protocerebrum, close to the anterior end of the dorsal aorta, axons characteristic of Types II and IV cells of the pars intercerebralis, and containing neurosecretory material, terminate on the neurilemma. Distinct because of their beaded form in whole mounts, two or three large axons, after leaving the neurohemal area, pass over the posterior surface of the brain beneath the perineurium. In whole mounts and serial sections looped axons are observed which may be reservoir regions proximal to neurohemal terminals.

No success was achieved in distinguishing between axons of Types II and IV cells with the light microscope as well as in electron micrographs. It can be presumed that axons of both types are intermingled in the tracts mentioned above. However by the size of granules and by their location they show marked difference from those of the nervus corporis cardiacum internus.

Fibres of these types are located within and on the outer surface of the perineurial sheath; a neurohemal area is formed at the surface of the brain by the numerous fibres. Synaptoid figures are observed occurring in most axons passing over the neurilemma in the neurohemal area, especially at the location where they are separated by a very thin layer from the hemocoel. Synaptoids were lacking in more proximal reservoir regions of axons associated with the cerebral neurohemal area.

Effect of Social Stimulation on the Adrenal Medulla of the Bandicoot Rat

A. GHOSH and B. R. MAITI
Department of Zoology, University of Calcutta (India)

Adult healthy male bandicoot rats *(Bandicota bengalensis)* were introduced in the cages having $10'' \times 6'' \times 6''$ size for a fighting experiment after keeping them in isolation for 15 days. Rats were allowed to fight for 6 h. Twelve sets of fights were performed using 24 animals. During the course of fighting, out of two rats one was found to establish dominance (winner) over the other (defeated). The latter was identified by injuries usually in the lips which the dominant rarely showed. Twelve nonfighting isolated rats served as control. In some of the fights the subordinate rats died even before the termination of the experiment.

Fighting in the bandicoot rat increased both adrenaline and noradrenaline concentration in the medulla in animals of the defeated group. Rats which were winners showed a slight decline in the adrenaline level accompanied by a moderate rise in noradrenaline titre. Cytochemical studies of the medullary acetyl cholinesterase revealed that the activity of this enzyme was enhanced in the winning and defeated rats. Depletion of ascorbic acid was noted in both the groups. Thus, fighting stress stimulated the production of adrenaline and noradrenaline in the adrenal medulla of the defeated bandicoot rats. Winner group on the contrary showed hormonal titre almost parallel to that of the non-fighting rats. The role of acetyl cholinesterase in release and ascorbic acid in methylation mechanism of catecholamines has also been indicated.

Regulation of the MSH Secretion in *Xenopus Laevis*. An *in vitro* Study

H. J. GOOS, R. SANGSTER, and P. VAN OORDT
Zoologisch Lab., Utrecht (The Netherlands)

As argued by Terlou (see p. 323 of this volume) catecholamines (CA's), especially dopamine, produced in hypothalamic nuclei, are involved in the inhibition of the MSH secretion in *Xenopus laevis* tadpoles. His arguments are confirmed by the data from our *in vitro* experiments. Fresh intermediate lobes from adult *Xenopus laevis* were incubated for six hours in Dickstein-Ringer with 0.05% glucose. Adrenaline, noradrenaline and dopamine (10^{-3} M) respectively were added to test their inhibitory capacity on the MSH secretion. All of them strongly inhibited the MSH release into the incubation medium whereas Prol-Leuc-Glyc-NH$_2$ did not have such action. From these results it became not clear whether CA's inhibit the synthesis or the release of MSH or both. Therefore we compared the amount of MSH in the glands before and after incubations with and without CA's and also the ultrastructure. Incubation with CA's caused remarkable higher MSH contents, suggesting an inhibitory action of CA's on the MSH *release*.

Electron micrographs showed that CA's inhibited the change of dense granules into fibrillar granules, a process which might be considered as a link in hormone *release*. This does, however, not exclude the possibility of an effect of CA's on the synthesis of MSH.

Goos, H. J. Th.: Z. Zellforsch. **97**, 449—458 (1969).
Notenboom, C. D.: Z. Zellforsch. **134**, 383—402 (1972).

Overactivity of the Hypothalamo-Neurohypophysial Neurosecretory System and the Problem of the Mechanisms of Transporting Neurosecretory Material

F. GRAINGER and J. C. SLOPER
Department of Experimental Pathology, West London Hospital, London (Great Britain)

The present study is concerned with the mechanisms by which cystine-rich polypeptides are transported down the unmyelinated secretory nerve fibres of the tractus hypophyseus in the rat. Many of these fibres contain vesicles, 100—200 nm in diameter, with electron-dense contents.

In animals given 3% saline for three days, measurements made on electron micrographs across the infundibular stem revealed a conspicuous increase in the number of microtubules in these nerve fibres, as compared with the number of microtubules seen in normal animals. A greater increase was found in animals with congenital diabetes insipidus, and in these animals there was an overall increase in nerve-fibre diameter.

If it is accepted that in saline-stressed rats and in rats suffering from diabetes insipidus, increased amounts of secretory material are transported down the tractus hypophyseus to the posterior pituitary, then these preliminary findings are consistent with the participation of microtubules in this process.

(Work supported by M. R. C. Grant No. G 972/462/B.)

Fine Structure and Staining Properties of the Neurono-Glial Synaptoid Contacts in the Median Eminence (Rat)

F. H. GÜLDNER and J. R. WOLFF
Max-Planck-Institut, Göttingen-Nikolausberg (Federal Republic of Germany)

In the median eminence the existence of synaptoid contacts between neurons and glial cells (tanycytes and astrocytes) was confirmed by three-dimensional reconstructions of electron micrographs. In the presynaptic element (PE) an aggregation of about 200—600 clear vesicles (500 Å) near 5—9 dense projections, several dense-core-vesicles (1000 Å), 2—4 mitochondria and profiles of the smooth endoplasmic reticulum occur. In one part of the PE only the clear vesicles are zinc-iodide-osmium (ZIO) positive, in the other part of PE the intervesicular space, the plasma membrane and the membrane of the dense-core vesicles are also impregnated. The dense projections are stained by ethanolic-phosphotungstic-acid (E-PTA) and bismuth-iodide-uranylacetate (BIUL). The synaptic cleft (100 Å width) is only slightly stained by E-PTA, but strongly stained by E-PTAUL and BIUL. The PE seems to adhere rather strongly to the glial surface. The postsynaptic membrane does not show any densifications. A reconstruction of a part of a tanycyte demonstrated that the PE are randomly distributed from the basal parts of the perikaryon to the vascular endfoot. The number of synaptoid contacts on the whole tanycyte was calculated as about ≥ 100.

Güldner,F.-H., Wolff,J.R.: Brain Res. **61**, 217—234 (1973).
Knowles,F., Vollrath,L.: Phil. Trans. B **250**, 311—342 (1966).
Wittkowski,W.: Z. Zellforsch. **139**, 101—148 (1973).

The Control of CRF Release at the Hypothalamic Level

E. W. HILLHOUSE, JANET BURDEN, and M. T. JONES
Sherrington School of Physiology, St. Thomas's Hospital Medical School, London, SE 1 7 EH (Great Britain)

The preparation used contains the dendrites, cell bodies and axons of the neurones secreting the hypothalamic releasing hormones. The viability of the tissue was assessed by histological examination and the ability to maintain a reasonable electrolyte balance and a high degree of oxidative metabolism. CRF was assayed by a modified version of the *in vivo-in vitro* system of de Weid et al. (1969).

Hypothalami taken from rats adrenalectomised 7—14 days previously secreted considerably greater quantities of CRF in response to electrical stimulation (100 Hz, 100 µA, 1mS; 5 min on, 5 min off, for 1 h) than hypothalami taken from intact rats although the content of both tissues was not significantly different. This hypersecretion of CRF was abolished by pretreatment with 5 mg/100 g s.c. corticosterone 24 h prior to removal of the hypothalamus and the content of the tissue remained the same. It is suggested that the negative feedback action of corticosterone is exerted at the hypothalamic level on the synthesis of CRF.

A dose dependent release of CRF was obtained upon incubation of the tissue with either acetyl-choline (5.5×10^{-15} — 5.5×10^{-14} M) or 5 HT (5.7×10^{-13} — 5.7×10^{-11} M) and both these effects were significantly reduced by noradrenaline (5.9×10^{-11} M). The effect of acetyl-choline was antagonised by hexamethonium (4.9×10^{-9} — 4.9×10^{-8} M).

It is proposed that there is both a cholinergic and a serotoninergic excitatory pathway to CRF release. The neuroinhibitory pathway is probably noradrenergic.

de Weid,D., Witter,A., Versteeg,D.H.G., Mulder,A.H.: Endocrinology **85**, 561 (1969).

Interacting Controls of Crustacean Molting and Regeneration

C. A. HOLLAND and D. M. SKINNER

Biology Division, Oak Ridge National Laboratory, Tennessee (USA)

The processes of limb regeneration and molting are intimately interrelated in Crustacea. In the land crab, *Gecarcinus*, loss of >5 limbs initiates preparations for ecdysis including re-generation of missing limbs. Conversely, during the early growth phase of the regenerates, their loss is an effective inhibitor to preparations for ecdysis (e.g. synthesis of new exoskeleton; further growth of remaining regenerates) until re-regeneration of the lost limbs restores the coordinated developmental premolt phases (Skinner and Graham, 1970, 1972). This inhibition, or premolt pause, may result in an ecdysis prolonged to as much as double the usual time. These morphological observations have been extended to the molecular level, initially, to studies on DNA synthesis (i.e. rates of incorporation of ^{3}H-T into autotomized limb buds cultured *in vitro*). We find:

(a) during a normal uninterrupted premolt period, the rate of DNA synthesis in a regenerate is initially high and falls as the limb approaches its final dimensions;

(b) in early phases of regeneration, 4 buds taken for assay show the characteristic rate of DNA synthesis; the remaining 4 assayed 48 h later show a near-complete inhibition of DNA synthesis;

(c) later in the premolt period the inhibition subsequent to the loss of the first 4 limbs is not observed and, in parallel observations on the whole animal, there is no premolt pause (Skinner and Graham, 1972).

These results extend our earlier conclusions that the preparations for ecdysis are not simply a chain of events triggered by a single stimulus. Rather the complex of interrelated events suggests multiple interlocking controls.

Skinner, Graham: Science 1970.
Skinner, Graham: Biol. Bull. 1972.

Research sponsored by the USAEC under contract with the Union Carbide Corp.

Development of Neuroendocrine Regulation in Man and Rat: Morphological and Biochemical Studies on Hypothalamic Monoaminergic Systems

M. T. HYYPPÄ and U. K. RINNE

Department of Neurology, University of Turku, Turku 52 (Finland)

In the rat hypothalamus primary catecholamines were demonstrated at the 20th day of gestation, and vesicle-containing nerve endings were also seen before birth. Chemical estimations of monoamine concentrations in the hypothalamus showed low levels of DA, NE, and 5-HT at birth, but a relatively rapid increase of the contents occurred between the 4th and 10th day after birth. Hypothalamic neurons accumulated C^{14}-L-dopa in 4-day-old rat. However, no sexual differences were seen in these studies. — In human foetuses the catecholamine fluorescence in the hypothalamus appeared during the 10th fetal week, and in the median eminence during the 13th week. A very high DA concentration was found in the fetal hypothalamus.

Biochemical studies, when correlated to experimentally induced alterations in sexual differentiation, showed that during the first ten postnatal days hypothalamic monoaminergic neurons are sensitive to hormonal or neuropharmacological manipulations: Firstly, neonatally injected reserpine caused a permanent alteration of gonadotrophin secretion as well as a small depletion of hypothalamic monoamine levels. Secondly, neonatal injections of p-chlorophenyl-alanine or reserpine altered sexual activity measured 200 days later. However, 10 days after the PCPA injection hypothalamic 5-HT and 5-HIAA levels were already normal. Thirdly, neonatal intraventricular injection of a small dose of 6-hydroxydopamine acted in a sexually selective manner upon catecholamine-containing neurons within the hypothalamus, and this observation suggests that androgens act on these neurons early in life to cause permanent changes in the neuroendocrine regulation. Lastly, our observations about the 5-HT synthesis rates in brains of masculinized and male or feminized and female rats showed differences.

All these observations suggest that the role of hypothalamic monoamines is of great importance for the development of sexual functions. The possible controversial roles of hypo-thalamic monoamines (indol versus catechol) in the development of the neuroendocrine regulation needs further studies to relate their metabolism to sex hormone secretion.

Hyyppä, M.: Thesis 1969.
Hyyppä, M.: Neuroendocrinology 9, 257 (1972).
Hyyppä, M., Cardinali, D., Wurtman, R. J.: Neuroendocrinology 11, 274 (1973).
Hyyppä, M., Cardinali, D., Baumgarten, H., Wurtman, R. J.: J. Neural Transm. 34, 111 (1973).
Grant to M.T.H.: The Population Council, M 73—30.

Intercellular Connection between Corpus Cardiacum Neurosecretory Cells of *Galleria Mellonella* (L.) (Lepidoptera)

S. KARACALI

Department of General Zoology, Ege University (Turkey)

Large neurosecretory cells in the corpus cardiacum, having several processes, are mostly surrounded by glial cells. In some places, however, they are facing directly the perikaryon or process of other similar cells, and in several places the intercellular space is obliterated. Two opposing plasma membranes appear as a "five-layered" structure, having two dense and two lucent laminae on both sides of a single median lamina. The median lamina is denser and wider than a single inner cytoplasmic membrane of either side, but has more or less the same density and width as an outer lamina of a cell membrane. These junctional complexes resemble the tight junctions which are considered to act as low-resistance surfaces which permit ionic or electrical communication between cells, as a barrier to the passage of substances through the intercellular spaces between the cells and as a sole contact holding cells together in the cells of different tissues. The occurrence of such junctions between corpus cardiacum neurosecretory cells may be of a considerable importance in their function.

Comparative Studies in Crustacean Neurosecretory Hyperglycemic Hormones

L. H. KLEINHOLZ and R. KELLER

Biology Department, Reed College, Oregon (USA)

Studies with hyperglycemic hormone (HGH) indicate molecular differences in HGH from *Cancer magister* (Crab), *Pandalus jordani* (Prawn) and *Orconectes limosus* (Crayfish), the three species examined in detail. The evidence comes from (1) interspecific differences in response to injected extract; (2) differences in anion exchange chromatography under standard conditions; (3) differences in electrophoretic mobility on gel acrylamide.

After control injections, blood glucose levels are 11 mg-% in Uca and 20 mg-% in Procambarus. Crude eyestalk extract was injected into Uca and Procambarus in doses containing 80 µg and 375 µg respectively of protein. In Uca, increases of 800—1200% were produced by HGH from Uca and Cancer; extract from Pandalus and three genera of crayfish had no hyperglycemic effect. With Procambarus as test animal, HGH from the three genera of crayfish increased glucose levels more than 500%, while that from Uca (about 50%), from Cancer (about 20%) and from Pandalus (about 100%) gave much lower or not significant increases. HGH activity is eluted from columns of DEAE cellulose in fractions Number 60—90 (Pandalus), 100—160 (Cancer), and 150—200+ (Orconectes). Disc electrophoresis shows HGH activity associated with bands whose R_f's differ for the three species.

Peptidergic Regulation of the Dogfish Pituitary

Sir FRANCIS KNOWLES, LUTZ VOLLRATH, and PATRICK MEURLING

King's College, London (Great Britain), and Department of Zoology, Lund (Sweden)

The dogfish pituitary is a suitable subject for an investigation of hypothalamic control because its four lobes (rostral, median, neuro-intermediate and ventral) have largely independent blood supplies. In this investigation attention has been focussed on the median lobe which receives a blood supply which has drained a restricted area, the posterior median eminence. There is evidence that the median lobe contains a gonadotropic substance (Firth and Vollrath, 1973) and that hypothalamic extracts are capable of stimulating this part of the pituitary, as indicated by Deery (this volume, p. 299).

Electron microscopic studies of the posterior median eminence have shown that the portal vessels are bordered by neurosecretory fibre terminals with microvesicles containing also electron-dense vesicles of the A-Type, i.e. spherical, regular uniformly dense and c. 2000 Å in diameter. Light microscopic studies showed that this area contained Gomori+ ve material.

The close proximity of fibres of the peptidergic type to portal vessels supplying part of the dogfish adenohypophysis provide an interesting comparison to studies on amphibians (Dierickx, this volume, p. 170), and together with the experimental observations indicate that pituitary releasing factors, contained in peptidergic neurosecretory nerves are present in primitive vertebrates.

Firth, J. A., Vollrath, L.: J. Endocr. 58, 347—348 (1973).

Extracellular Spaces of the Adenohypophysis in Normal and Castrated Rats

J. Krsulovic

Department of Physiology, Faculty of Mathematics and Natural Sciences, University of Chile, Valparaiso (Chile)

Essentially similar adenohypophysial cells limiting extracellular spaces sealed by junctional complexes have been described by Farquhar (1957), Rodriguez (1969), Kurosumi (1968), Lagios (1973) and were termed follicular, marginal, stellate, non-granulate, etc. Their nature and functional role still remain unknown due to the absence of significant morphological reactions under experimentally induced endocrine changes. Dingemans and Feltkamp (1972) have considered them to be involved in the digestion of waste material from other cells. The cells seem to form an actual hypophysial canalicular system, which appears hypertrophied in castrated rats (Krsulovic, 1973). In the present work the ultrastructural changes observed after castration are analyzed in more detail in order to obtain new histological and physiological data about the cells and the system that they form.

Cells limiting special extracellular compartments sealed by junctional complexes seem to form a network of canaliculi throughout the whole adenohypophysis. This specialized class of apparently non-endocrine epithelial cell presents common and specific characteristics according to the topographic region. They border virtual or real cavities (most of them not visible by light microscopy) in the pars tuberalis, pars distalis, pars intermedia and the hypophysial cleft.

The hypophysial canalicular system presents its largest diameter in the upper and central part of the gland. At this level the cells show abundant microvilli, ovoid or piriform nucleus, and an undeveloped perikaryon, which shows a tendency to form processes which determine the frequently irregular shape of these elements. Other essentially similar elements, the hypophysial cleft boundary cells, are provided with clusters of cilia (9—2 morphology) and associated ciliary rootlets. All these cells are attached apically by specialized tight junctions. These junctions are characterized by a closer approximation of the cell membrane and resemble the zonula occludens (and also the zonula adhaerens and desmosomes). In the pars distalis the cellular network forms folds and interdigitations. The Golgi complex, a poorly developed rough endoplasmic reticulum, lysosomes, abundant mitochondria and free ribosomes are usually found within the cytoplasm of all these cells. The typical secretory granules of the glandular epithelia are not present, but near the Golgi complex small granular vesicles (smooth or bristle coated) may be observed occasionally.

Castrated animals sacrificed one week after the operation show hypertrophy of the limiting cells in the pars distalis, increase of folds and interdigitations. Within the lumen a colloid content or non-homogeneous electron dense material may be observed.

In animals sacrificed after one month of castration folds and interdigitations appear significantly increased forming an actual "labyrinth".

After one year of castration the canalicular system increases in amplitude and duct diameter and the limiting cells send long and slender processes among a large part of the glandular cells of pars distalis. The canalicular system, significantly modified after castration, may represent a pathway of humoral communication for the neural control of the adenohypophysis.

Dingemans, K. P., Feltkamp, C. A.: Z. Zellforsch. **124**, 387—405 (1972).
Farquhar, M. G.: Anat. Rec. **127**, 291 (1957).
Harris, G. W.: Neural control of the pituitary gland. London: Edward Arnold 1955.
Kalimo, H.: Z. Zellforsch. **122**, 283—300 (1971).
Knowles, F., Bern, H. A.: Nature (Lond.) **210**, 271—272 (1966).
Krsulovic, J.: XI. Congreso Latinoamericano de Ciencias Fisiologicas. Resumenes de comunicaciones libres No. 30. Mendoza/Argentina 1973.
Kurosumi, K.: Arch. histol. jap. **26**, 329—362 (1968).
Lagios, M. D.: Gen. comp. Endocr. **20**, 362—376 (1973).
Reynolds, E. S.: J. Cell Biol. **17**, 208—215 (1963).
Rodriguez, E.: Z. Zellforsch. **104**, 1—13 (1970).
Vila-Porcil, E.: Z. Zellforsch. **129**, 338—369 (1972).

Microfluorimetric Quantitation of Catecholamines in Rat Median Eminence

A. Löfström, G. Jonsson, and K. Fuxe

Department of Histology, Karolinska Institutet, Stockholm (Sweden)

A microfluorimetric method was applied to study three CA terminal systems in rat median eminence, using a Leitz microfluorimeter with epi-illumination. Fluorescence was measured in the subependymal layer (SEL), the medial (MPZ) and lateral palisade zone (LPZ) in a rostral, central and caudal region, employing a circular measuring diaphragm of 13.5 μ in diameter. Changes in amine turnover were estimated after tyrosine hydroxylase inhibition (H 44/68). A differential evaluation of NA and DA was attempted after dopamine-β-hydroxylase inhibition (FLA-63) using the caudate nucleus as a control area. Specific fluorescence was calculated and the data submitted to a computerized statistical analysis.

Tyrosine hydroxylase inhibition induced an exponential decline of fluorescence with a calculated T 1/2 of 2—$3^{1}/_{2}$ h in MPZ and more than 4 h in SEL. Dopamine-β-hydroxylase inhibition caused a marked fluorescence disappearance in SEL, and to a lesser extent, in the other systems. The studies *inter alia* indicated a preferential activation of NA after adrenalectomy and DA during pregnancy.

Andén, N.-E., Corrodi, H., Fuxe, K.: In: Hooper (Ed.): Metabolism of amines in the brain, pp. 38—47. London: MacMillan 1969.
Corrodi, H., Fuxe, K., Hamberger, B., Ljungdahl, Å.: Europ. J. Pharmacol. **12**, 145—155 (1970).
Falck, B., Hillarp, N.-Å., Thieme, G., Torp, A.: J. Histochem. Cytochem. **10**, 348—354 (1962).
The definitive paper will appear in J. Histochem. Cytochem.

Phospholipid Activity as an Indicator of Hormone Secretion by the Supraoesophageal Ganglion of *Nereis Virens*

J. Marsden

Department of Biology, McGill University, Quebec (Canada)

The uptake of ^{32}P from orthophosphate has been measured in the phospholipids of the supraoesophageal ganglion of *N. virens* in very young, sexually undifferentiated and in older, maturing or mature worms. *In vivo* injections at 3, 6, 18, 24, and 48 h before dissection of the "brain" and extraction of the lipids show a more extensive incorporation of tracer into phosphatidyl inositol than into any other phospholipid. At one week after injection phosphatidyl choline carries 6—8 × more isotope than does phosphatidyl inositol. Since measured phosphatidyl choline : phosphatidyl inositol ratios in the "brain" vary from 1.4—1.7 it appears that the slowly labelled phosphatidyl choline turns over more completely than does the rapidly phosphatidyl inositol. The incorporation of ^{32}P into all "brain" phospholipids is more active in young, growing animals than it is in mature individuals. In addition the ratio of activity in phosphatidic acid plus phosphatidyl inositol to that in phosphatidyl choline in sexually undifferentiated animals is about 10 × that in mature animals. It is suggested that the differentially high activity in the phosphatidic acid—phosphatidyl inositol pathway in ganglia of mature worms is a manifestation of the well-known relationship of this phenomenon to secretory activity and reflects the production of juvenile hormone at this stage of life. Localization of this activity among the nuclei of the "brain" by radioautography is now underway.

On the Nature of Hypothalamo-Neurohypophysial Neurosecretory Granules: Inferences from Their Appearance after Different Fixation Procedures

J. F. MORRIS

Department of Anatomy, The Medical School, Bristol (Great Britain)

Experiments using an aldehyde mixture (glutaraldehyde, formaldehyde and acrolein) at pH's 5.0—8.0 have revealed that the appearance of neurosecretory granules (NSG) is very dependent on the fixation procedures used. The reaction of the NSG-core constituents to the fixative solutions *in vitro* has also been studied.

In the neural lobe, NSG cores are electron-dense after fixation at acidic pH but progressively lose electron-density at pH's 7.0—8.0 with rupture of the granule membrane. Most core constituents are precipitated by the fixative at acidic pH but dissolve at pH's 7.0 and 8.0. This suggests that the core may be present in a "solid" state *in vivo*.

The hormone content of NSG's may affect their electron-density, oxytocin containing granules appearing less dense, since oxytocin and its neurophysin dissolve in fixative much more than do vasopressin and its neurophysin.

The maturity of NSG's can be inferred from their reaction to fixation in different parts of the hypothalamo-neurohypophysial system. Immature granules are less prone to lose electron density at pH's 7.0—8.0.

Fine connexions between NSG's and neurotubules and between adjacent NSG's are seen in aldehyde-fixed unosmicated material. The possible significance of such connexions is being investigated.

Cannata,M.A., Morris,J.F.: J. Endocr. **57**, 531—538 (1973).
Morris,J.F., Cannata,M.A.: J. Endocr. **57**, 517—529 (1973).

Neurosecretory Control of Reproduction in the Bivalve, *Katelysia Opima*

R. NAGABHUSHANAM

Department of Zoology, Marathwada University (India)

The role of neurosecretion in the reproductive cycle in the marine clam, *Katelysia opima*, was investigated. The histological picture of the different ganglia showed the presence of two types of neurosecretory cells when stained with Gomori's chrome-haematoxylin-phloxin: (1) Gomori-positive cells with blue-black neurosecretory material and (2) phloxinophilic cells with red neurosecretory material. Histochemical tests indicate that the neurosecretory material from the central ganglia contains lipoprotein. The intense staining of the secretory substance with Baker's acid hematin before pyridine extraction but not after, suggests the presence of phospholipid. This substance may be incorporated in the membrane bounding the secretory granules. The PAS-positive reaction suggests that the secretory material might be a glyco-protein. Monthly observations of the changes in the reproductive system and neurosecretory cells throughout the year revealed a parallelism between the neurosecretion and reproductive cycles. The general effect caused by extirpation of cerebral ganglia in the clams showed that the ablation of cerebral ganglia hastened the spawning reaction.

(Supported by grant ONR contract (NOOO 14-70-C-0172 from Office of Naval Research, Washington, USA.)

Neuroendocrine Control of ACTH Secretion in the Pars Intermedia

D. V. NAIK

Department of Anatomy, Faculty of Medicine, University of Sherbrooke, Sherbrooke, Quebec (Canada)

Naik (1970, 1972a) has proved the existence of a stimulatory influence exerted by the neuro-hypophysis on the glandular cells in the pars intermedia (PI). Besides showing the presence of true ACTH cells similar to those found in the pars distalis (PD), in the PI, pars tuberalis (PT) and the rostral zone (RZ), he has recently demonstrated immuno-electron microscopic localization of both MSH and ACTH in the same glandular cell of PI in rats and mice. He has also demonstrated that the glandular and ACTH cells in PI of rats and mice are innervated by 3 types of nerve fibers: 1) Peptidergic neurosecretory, 2) Adrenergic or Aminergic, 3) Cholinergic. Some of these nerve fibers have synaptic contact with PI glandular and ACTH cells (Naik, 1972b). To investigate whether these neural contacts or the hypothalamic releasing factors influence these PI cells, tiny isolated PI tissues were auto-transplanted in the evacuated pituitary capsule of totally hypophysectomized rats by the recent method of Naik and Sheriff. Five to six weeks after transplantation, the PI cells organized into many groups, showing mainly 2 types of cell growth: 1) cell growth away from the reorganizing neural lobe, consisting mostly of PI glandular cells and 2) cell growth very close to, or in contact with, the reorganizing neural lobe, consisting mostly of ACTH cells as identified by electron microscopy. These ACTH cells are innervated by many nerve fibers. The experiments suggest that the development of ACTH cells from PI glandular cells is influenced and controlled by neurosecretory, CRF and aminergic fibers and/or releasing factors from the hypothalamus. As suggested earlier (Naik, 1972a), the releasing factors could be either vasopressin and/or a type of CRF.

(Supported by MRC Canada, grant No. MA-5160).
Naik, D. V.: Z. Zellforsch. 107, 317—342 (1970).
Naik, D. V.: Z. Zellforsch. 125, 460—479 (1972a).
Naik, D. V.: Z. Zellforsch. 133, 415—435 (1972b).

Hypothalamic Lesions in *Xenopus Laevis* Tadpoles: Their Effect on Metamorphosis and on the Pars Nervosa of the Pituitary Gland

C. D. NOTENBOOM

Zoologisch Lab., Utrecht (The Netherlands)

During investigations with *Xenopus laevis* tadpoles the preoptic nucleus was divided into a rostro-dorsal, ventral and caudo-dorsal region. Osmotic stimulation of the tadpoles resulted in a disappearance of the neurosecretory material from, and a higher metabolic activity of, the cells of the caudo-dorsal region. This may indicate the cells of this region to be involved in osmoregulatory processes, probably by synthesizing posterior lobe hormones. In order to obtain additional information lesions were made in the hypothalamic region by means of an electrocoagulation technique, developed by Mrs. Dodd (Bangor, Great Britain). Lesioned animals which showed a retardation of metamorphosis (as compared to control animals) appeared to have a lesion in the rostro-dorsal region. In animals which demonstrated a regression or even disappearance of the pars nervosa, the caudo-dorsal region appeared to be obliterated. These observations indicate that in the preoptic nucleus there are at least two functionally different regions: the rostro-dorsal region being important in the regulation of thyroid activity, the caudo-dorsal region being related to the pars nervosa.

Dopaminergic Control of Prolactin Secretion in Eels

MADELEINE OLIVEREAU

Lab. Physiol. Inst. Océanographique, Paris (France)

In pituitaries autotransplanted 2 months earlier, prolactin cells appear stimulated (Olivereau and Lemoine, 1971), a result suggesting the presence of a hypothalamic prolactin inhibiting factor (PIF); however plasma sodium and N-acetyl-neuraminic acid (NANA) skin content, under prolactin control in freshwater eels, are often subnormal (Olivereau and Lemoine, 1971); this partial maintenance may be due to the lack of a prolactin releasing factor (PRF) and/or to the reduced size of the graft. In order to test whether catecholamines were involved in prolactin secretion, intact eels were injected with reserpin, but no typical and constant effect was noted in prolactin cells of male eels (Olivereau and Lemoine, 1973a). Two intracisternal injections of 6-OH-dopamine induced a marked development of the endoplasmic reticulum (ER) and a rapid degranulation in most cases. Conversely, L-dopa injections promoted a granule retention, a significant nuclear atrophy, the nucleus migrating to the cell periphery where the ER was no longer discernible (Olivereau and Lemoine, 1973b). CB 154 (2-Br-α-ergocryptine Sandoz) injections induced an evident granular storage and an increased cytoplasmic erythrosinophilia; plasma sodium level and NANA skin content were reduced after L-dopa or CB 154 administration (Olivereau and Lemoine, 1973a) corroborating the hypothesis of an inhibition of prolactin release. These data suggest that dopamine acts as a PIF on prolactin release and perhaps its synthesis, but a simultaneous regulation by a PRF remains possible.

Olivereau, M., Lemoine, A. M.: Z. vergl. Physiol. **73**, 44—52 (1971).
Olivereau, M., Lemoine, A. M.: C. R. Acad. Sci. (Paris) **276** D, 1325—1327 (1973a).
Olivereau, M., Lemoine, A. M.: C. R. Acad. Sci. (Paris) **276** D, 1883—1886 (1973b).

Ependymal Origin of Arginine Vasotocin

S. PAVEL

Department of Endocrinology, University School of Medicine, Bucharest (Rumania)

Pavel (Endocrinology, 89: 613, 1971) first advanced the hypothesis that pineal arginine vasotocin (AVT) is elaborated by secretory specialized ependymal cells. This hypothesis has been recently directly confirmed by the in vitro biosynthesis of an AVT-like peptide in ependymal cells from pineal glands of human fetuses (Pavel et al., Science, 181, 1252—1253, 1973). Using the same methods as for the pineal (Pavel et al., 1973), the present study demonstrates that ependymal neurohypophysial cells from human fetuses aged 4—5 months are also able to synthesize an AVT-like peptide when cultured in vitro (i.e., to release into their culture media the specific activities of AVT during 45 days of incubation). Although the non-incubated neurohypophyses of the same age contain pharmacological activities suggesting the presence of both arginine vasopressin and oxytocin, the neurohypophysial ependymal cells cultured in vitro release into their media only an AVT-like peptide. This strongly supports the suggestion that, whereas arginine vasopressin and oxytocin are synthesized in the hypothalamic neurosecretory nuclei, AVT, on the contrary, is synthesized in the ependymal neurohypophysial cells. Consequently, the fetal neurohypophysis appears not only as a storage site for neurohypophysial hormones but also as an endocrine structure that elaborates AVT by ependymosecretion.

Studies of Neurohypophysial Peptides during Foetal Life

A. M. PERKS and E. VIZSOLYI

Department of Zoology, University of British Columbia (Canada)

Early work on the neurohypophysial peptides has shown that the vasopressor/oxytocic ratios in the pars nervosa are unusually high in foetal life, and that foetal oxytocin appeared to be notably soluble in damp acetone. The studies carried out here were intended to find out whether these characteristics reflected the presence of new principles in the gland. Experiments on glands from foetal sheep and furseals showed that lyophilised glands gave high V/O ratios; this indicated that the ratios were not artifacts due to unusual solubility in acetone. Histological evidence suggested that the ratios reflected an earlier onset of vasopressin production by the supraoptic nucleus. Glands from foetal seals at mid-term were extracted and purified on G-15 Sephadex, CM-Sephadex, phosphocellulose and IRC-50 exchange resin. Arginine vasotocin (AVT), arginine vasopressin (AVP) and oxytocin were separated and identified by their pharmacology and amino acid analysis. The possible function of AVT was investigated. AVT acted on the isolated amniotic membrane of the guinea-pig to slow or reverse a materno-foetal flow of fluid. This effect was linearly related to the log of the dose administered. It is possible that foetal AVT (or AVP) passes in the foetal urine to the amniotic cavity, where it acts on the amnion to maintain amniotic volume. Foetal neurohypophysial peptides may form one method of control of foetal uterine fluids.

Perks, A. M., Vizsolyi, E.: In: Comline, K. S., Cross, K. W., Dawes, G. S., Nathanielsz, P. W. (Eds.): Foetal and neonatal physiology, pp. 430—438. Cambridge: University Press 1973.
Vizsolyi, E., Perks, A. M.: Nature (Lond.) **223**, 1169—1171 (1969).
Vizsolyi, E., Perks, A. M.: Canad. J. Zool. In press (1973).

The Effect of Testosterone Treatment on the Ultrastructure of the Nucleus Infundibularis Ventralis of the Green Frog (*Rana Esculenta*)

J. PEUTE and P. G. W. J. VAN OORDT

Zoological Laboratory, State University of Utrecht (The Netherlands)

Up till now in the hypothalamus of Amphibia two peptidergic neurosecretory nuclei have been described: the Gomori-positive nucleus praeopticus and the Gomori-negative nucleus infundibularis ventralis (NIV). The NIV is located in the lateral lobes of the caudal hypothalamus (Peute and Meij, 1973). Ultrastructurally its cells are characterized by a well-developed rough endoplasmic reticulum and Golgi apparatus, and in particular by the presence of neurosecretory granules. On the basis of the average diameter of these granules at least two cell types can be distinguished: Y cells (granules $\pm$ 1400 Å) and Z cells (granules $\pm$ 1800 Å). The localization in the caudal hypothalamus suggests that this nucleus is involved in the production of gonadotrophin releasing factor. Implantation of testosterone in the dorsal lymph sac of *Rana esculenta* induced an excessive dilatation of the rough endoplasmic reticulum in certain Y cells. Moreover, the swollen cisternae were filled with a dense, flocculent material, indicating the storage of peptidergic material. This observation may be interpreted in terms of a negative feed-back mechanism, exerted by testosterone on the Y cells of the NIV.

Peute, J., Meij, J. C. A.: Z. Zellforsch. **144**, 191—217 (1973).

Ultrastructural Cytochemical Observations on the Hypothalamo-Neurohypophysial System of the Rat

D. PICARD, M. MICHEL-BECHET, and F. TASSO

Faculté de Médecine de Marseille (France)

In normal rats, as well as during dehydration with or without subsequent rehydration, NSO cells have a cyclic secretory activity; therefore, individual cells in these various conditions were considered with regard to their Golgi complexes. The Golgi complex consists of three layers: (a) one layer composed of large cisternae directly related to E. R. and transfer vesicles, and demonstrated by prolonged osmication; in this layer accumulation of dense material takes place, leading to formation of neurosecretory granules; (b) an intermediate layer of flattened cisternae with a positive reaction for TPPase; (c) a third layer, made of polymorphous components, is a particularly conspicuous GERL complex with positive APase reaction; there, lysosomes of different shapes are formed, some of which happen to be dense bodies of the same size and appearance as N. S. granules, so that a reaction for APase is not a character of immature granules. Golgi complexes of N. S. neurons thus appear as functionally bipolar; the concept of a formation and a maturation face is inadequate in this particular case. The Thiery technique (periodic acid-thiosemicarbazide-silver proteinate) reveals too small amounts of glycoproteins in the Golgi apparatus and related structures for a dynamic experimental approach of secretory material synthesis; though it provides evidence of glycoproteins localized at the periphery of the dense core of N. S. granules, which might be interesting to compare with recent data on granule fractionation.

Novikoff,P., Novikoff,A.B., Quintana,N., Hauw,J.J.: J. Cell Biol. **50**, 859—886 (1971).
Picard,D., Michel-Bechet,M., Athouel,A.M., Rua,S.: Exp. Brain Res. **14**, 331—353 (1972).
Tasso,F.: J. Microsc. (In press).

Uptake and Transport of Horseradish Peroxidase (HRP) in the Hypothalamo-Neurohypophysial System of Rats

CH. PILGRIM, H.-J. WAGNER, and J. BRANDL

Fachbereich Biologie, Universität Regensburg (Federal Republic of Germany)

10—70 min after intraventricular injection, pinocytotic uptake of HRP is observed in nerve cells of the SON. The tracer can, however, not be detected in the pars nervosa.

12 h after injection, numerous dense bodies of the perikarya are filled with HRP. In the pars nervosa, a few HRP containing structures are seen in axons and axon endings. The tracer is present in tubular profiles of 300—600 Å width or, occasionally, in small round dense bodies. Pituicytes are still free of reaction product.

Animals injected three times on successive days: All perikaryal dense bodies are heavily loaded with the tracer. The pars nervosa now contains a number of axon endings which are filled with reactive tubules and dense bodies of variable size. In addition, dense bodies with a positive reaction for HRP can be observed in pituicytes. Lipid inclusions of variable size and free of reaction product are found attached to the HRP-positive matrix of dense bodies.

It is suggested that, after incorporation into lysosomes of the perikarya, HRP is transported down the axons and released at the terminals. It is then taken up and digested by lysosomes of pituicytes. Lipid inclusions are thought to represent residues of lysosomal activity.

Krsulovic,J., Brückner,G.: Z. Zellforsch. **99**, 210—220 (1969).
Whitaker,S., LaBella,F.S.: Z. Zellforsch. **125**, 1—15 (1972).
Whitaker,S., LaBella,F.S., Sanwal,M.: Z. Zellforsch. **111**, 493—504 (1970).

Binding Protein from Neurosecretory Granules with High Affinity for Vasopressin ("Native" Neurophysin?)

V. PLIŠKA, M. MEYER-GRASS, and D. SUNDE

Institut für Molekularbiologie und Biophysik, Eidg. Technische Hochschule, Zürich (Switzerland)

The association constants (K_a) for binding of oxytocin and the vasopressins to neurophysins have generally been reported to be of the order of 10^4 l/mol. We have recently found a minor population of binding sites in bovine neurophysin II with a high affinity ($K_a \sim 10^7$) for lysine vasopressin (LVP) (Pliška and Sachs, in press). The neurophysin in neurosecretory granules may differ (Mylroie and Koenig, 1971) from the material isolated in the usual way, by acid extraction of acetone-dried neurohypophyses. Since modification during isolation might also affect the binding properties, we have studied the binding of LVP to the protein obtained from lysed neurosecretory granules, isolated from homogenates of fresh bovine neurohypophyses by gradient centrifugation. The proteins in the $27\,500 \times g$ supernatant were separated from peptides on Sephadex G-25 with tris-HCl buffer, pH 7.8 (rather than the customary acetic acid). The eluates containing the protein ($300\,\mu g/ml$) were directly used to measure binding of tritiated LVP by equilibrium dialysis in a rotating-cell apparatus (Weder et al., 1971). The results were analysed as a nonlinear regression fit to the Hill equation. At least two "high affinity" populations of binding sites were found, with $K_a \sim 7 \times 10^5$ and 5×10^6 l/mol. The capacity of the fraction with higher affinity was sufficient to bind up to 40% of the hormones originally present in the granules, the total capacity of both fractions to bind 100%. We suggest that "native" neurophysin has a higher K_a than the material usually isolated. A physiological binding role of neurophysin has generally been discounted because of the apparently low K_a; this conclusion may now have to be revised.

This work was supported by Swiss National Science Foundation Grant No. 3.424.70.

Mylroie, R., Koenig, H.: J. Histochem. Cytochem. **19**, 738—746 (1971).

Pliška, V., Sachs, H.: Europ. J. Biochem. (In press).

Weder, H. G., Schildknecht, J., Kesselring, P.: American Laboratory **1971**, (10) 15—20.

Evidence for the Periventricular Localization of the Hypothalamic Osmoreceptors

E. M. RODRIGUEZ, Z. BAIGORRIA, A. RODRIGUEZ, and D. CIOCCA

Instituto de Histologia y Embriologia, Facultad de Ciencas Medicas U.N.C., Mendoza (Argentina)

Based on morphological and some experimental evidence we postulated, at the Kiel symposium, that the hypothalamic osmoreceptors are localized in the wall of the third brain ventricle. A long series of experiments carried out during these years supports this possibility. By applying some stimuli to the water-loaded alcohol-anaesthetized rat used for the assay of antidiuretic hormone (ADH) it has been possible to determine the exact moment at which the endogenous ADH of the experimental animal is released after a given stimulus. The antidiuretic response of the experimental animal, the increased urinary sodium concentration during the antidiuretic phase, the determination of the plasma AD activity of blood samples obtained during the antidiuretic period, and the inhibition of this AD activity after treatment with sodium thioglycollate were used as indications of ADH release. Eighty-four experiments have led to the following conclusions:

1. Perfusion of hypertonic saline in the jugular vein is followed by ADH release with a time-delay of 20 min.

2. Subperfusion of hypertonic saline in the third brain ventricle produces an immediate release of ADH.

3. Intraventricular infusion of isotonic saline is ineffective to promote ADH release.

4. Vascular perfusion of isotonic saline does produce a mild release of ADH.

5. Several stimuli, some of which are known to reach the hypothalamus by nervous afferents (hemorrhage, anesthetics, steroceptive stimuli) trigger the release of ADH with a time delay between 2 and 5 min.

The fact that the hypothalamic osmoreceptors are more rapidly stimulated by the CSF hyperosmolality than by the plasma hyperosmolality suggests that the osmosensitive elements are localized in some region of the ventricular walls or, alternatively, that they are localized in a region where the brain-CSF barrier is not present.

Regulation of Neurosecretory Activity in the Freshwater Snail, *Lymnaea Stagnalis* (L.)

E. W. ROUBOS and H. H. BOER

Department of Biology, Free University, Amsterdam-Buitenveldert (The Netherlands)

The neurosecretory Dark Green Cells (DGC) in the pleural and parietal ganglia of the freshwater snail, *Lymnaea stagnalis*, are involved in osmoregulation. They become activated when the snail is exposed to demineralized water, while placing in a 0.08% NaCl solution leads to inactivation (Wendelaar Bonga, 1971). To investigate whether these changes in DGC neurosecretory activity are under nervous control, isolated pleural and parietal ganglia were transplanted into acceptor snails. Using quantitative electron microscopy (synthesis and release rates of neurosecretory material were determined on the basis of several ultrastructural parameters) it was found that the transplanted DGC reacted in a quite similar way to variations in osmolarity of the environment as the DGC in the acceptor's own nervous system. Therefore it is concluded that these reactions are not evoked via afferent nervous pathways to the pleural and parietal ganglia (Roubos, 1973).

Techniques have been developed for the isolation and the *in vitro* cultivation of neurosecretory cells. This has been done to answer the following questions. 1. Do hormones play a role in the regulatory mechanism of the DGC? 2. Are the DGC osmoreceptors? 3. Do other neurons in the pleural or parietal ganglia have an osmoreceptor function?

Roubos, E. W.: Z. Zellforsch. In press (1973).
Wendelaar Bonga, S. E.: Neth. J. Zool. **21**, 127—158 (1971).

Central Adrenergic Neurons and Puberty in Rats

K. B. RUF and M. J. HOLMES

MRC Group in Developmental Neurobiology, Department of Neurosciences, McMaster University, Hamilton (Canada)

The process of puberty was studied in female rats following functional impairment of central adrenergic neurons produced by a single intraventricular injection of 6-hydroxydropamine

(6-OHDA; Malmfors and Thoenen, 1971) on day 23 of life. 6-OHDA dissolved in artificial CSF (yielding quinones and other oxidation products; Malmfors and Thoenen, 1971) produced a significant postponement of vaginal opening, first ovulation and onset of vaginal cyclicity without interference with body growth. 6-OHDA dissolved in dilute HCl (unoxidized form; Malmfors and Thoenen, 1971) caused, in addition, some retardation of body growth, as did repeated injections of 6-OHDA in newborn rats (Ruf and Holmes, 1973). Uni- or bilateral irritative electrolytic lesions placed in the vicinity of the medial forebrain bundle reliably produced precocious vaginal opening and ovulation within 4—5 days. The effect of such lesions was duplicated by local injections of $FeCl_3$ (Everett and Radford, 1961), but counteracted by local deposition of colchicine or s.c. injections of reserpine. The results are compatible with our hypothesis (Ruf, 1973) that the maturation of central adrenergic pathways is a component of the pubertal process and that lesions advance puberty through local stimulation rather than removal of brain tissue.

Everett, J. M., Radford, H. M.: Proc. Soc. exp. Biol. (N. Y.) **108**, 604—609 (1961).
Malmfors, T., Thoenen, H. (Eds.): 6-Hydroxydopamine and Catecholamine Neurons. Amsterdam, London: North-Holland Publ. 1971.
Ruf, K. B.: Z. Neurol. **204**, 95—105 (1973).
Ruf, K. B., Holmes, M. J.: Submitted to J. Endocr. (1973).

Calcium and Stimulus-Secretion Coupling in the Neurohypophysis

J. T. RUSSELL and N. A. THORN

Institute of Medical Physiology C, University of Copenhagen (Denmark)

5 halved rat neurohypophyses were stimulated for 10 min in a medium containing 56 mM potassium or by application of a field current (20 Hz, 2 msec, 40 mA). Both stimulations resulted in a 5—8 fold increase in the release of vasopressin which was inhibited (in a dose related way) by $LaCl_3$ (4×10^{-4}, 4×10^{-3} M/l), Prenylamine (2×10^{-5}, 1×10^{-4} M/l) and D600 (a verapamil derivative) (4×10^{-6}, 1×10^{-5}, 2×10^{-5} M/l). Increasing the Ca^{2+} concentration in the medium to 14 mM abolished the inhibitory effect or D600. D600 also inhibited vasopressin release caused by introducing Ca^{2+} into a Ca^{2+} free medium during continued electrical stimulation.

Using the same stimuli, uptake of Ca^{2+} by bovine neurohypophysial slices (20—40 mg wet wt) was calculated from the kinetic analysis of the $^{45}Ca^{2+}$ washout curve. It was found that while 56 mM K stimulation increased entry of Ca^{2+} into the cells, no significantly increased uptake was observed with electrical stimulation, although hormone release was of a comparable magnitude. Similar results were obtained using the lanthanum method (Mayer et al., 1972) for quantitation of presumably intracellular Ca^{2+} uptake.

It is concluded that an inward movement of Ca^{2+} across the stimulated nerve membrane is essential for release. It may be so small that it is not detected by the sensitive methods currently available. Evidence is also presented for a possible intracellular mechanism whereby the axoplasmic free Ca^{2+} concentration may be augmented during release.

Mayer, C. J., van Bremen, C., Casteels, R.: Pflügers Arch. ges. Physiol. **337**, 333—350 (1972).

Identification and Ultrastructural Characterization of Seven Types of Protocerebral Neurosecretory Cells in the Colorado Beetle

H. Schooneveld

Laboratory of Entomology, Agricultural University, Wageningen (The Netherlands)

The cerebral neurosecretory system of the Colorado beetle, *Leptinotarsa decemlineata* SAY, shows the most complex architecture and the widest variety in types of neurosecretory cells (NSC) hitherto found in insects (Schooneveld, 1970). On the basis of light microscopical analyses of paraldehyde fuchsin-stained sections seven different types of neurosecretory cells could be distinguished. The medial group of NSC comprises 3 types of Gomori-positive NSC (the so-called A-, A_1-, and C-NSC) and 2 -negative NSC (B- and E-NSC). Lateral groups comprise the -negative D- and L-NSC. A-, A_1-, B-, C-, and L-NSC carry their secretion to the neurohaemal organs, the corpora cardiaca, where at least two additional kinds of secretions are produced.

Electron microscopical studies revealed that each type of NSC can be characterized and differentiated from the other types by the nature of the elementary particles produced therein, e.g. elementary granules (EG), dense-core vesicles (DCV), or vesicles (EV) with varying electron transparency and size. No relation exists between the nature of these particles and the corresponding Gomori-stainability. For instance, A-NSC contain EG of approx. 1250 Å, A_1-NSC: EG of 2100 Å, C-NSC: EV of 1700 Å, B-NSC: DCV of 1300 Å, and L-NSC: EG of 1300, resp. 1700 Å.

The aim of recently initiated work is to relate hormonal activities extracted from corpora cardiaca with exactly known places of synthesis.

More extensive paper submitted for publication in Z. Zellforsch.
Schooneveld, H.: Neth. J. Zool. **20**, 151—237 (1970).

Scanning Electron Microscopy of the Ventricular Lining of the Hypothalamus of Some Birds

P. J. Sharp

Poultry Research Centre, Edinburgh (Great Britain)

The surface topography of the ventricular lining of the hypothalamus has been investigated in quail and fowl using the scanning electron microscope. The ventricular walls were generally densely ciliated except in the regions of the ventro-lateral hypothalamus and the median eminence. Here the ventricular lining has a glandular appearance and is associated with different forms of tanycyte processes (Sharp, P. J.: Z. Zellforsch. **127**, 552—569, 1972). In the fowl, cilia were rare in this area but persisted in isolated tufts in the quail. The glandular ependyma of the ventrolateral hypothalamus was characterized by various types of cytoplasmic protrusions. In the fowl, these included microvilli, blunt villiform processes, small blebs of various sizes, and large blebs covered with irregular bulges. In the quail, irregular non-ciliated ridges covered in cytoplasmic leaflets were observed. The ventricular lining of median eminence in both species also showed signs of cytoplasmic activity although large cytoplasmic protrusions were absent. These observations support the suggestion (Sharp, P. J.: Z. Zellforsch. **127**, 552—569, 1972) that the glandular ependyma of the avian basal hypothalamus may be involved in the transport of material between the cerebrospinal fluid and the hypophysial portal vasculature.

Effect of Rat Pineal Gland on the Hypothalamo-Hypophyseo-Gonadal Axis

A. R. SMITH and J. ARIËNS KAPPERS

Netherlands Central Institute for Brain Research, Amsterdam (The Netherlands)

Serotonin and yellow autofluorescent cells were observed both in the pineal and in the arcuate and part of the ventromedial nucleus of the hypothalamus. They were quantified using fluorescence histochemistry. Microelectrophoresis and special staining methods revealed the autofluorescent substance to be a protein containing relatively much tryptophan. The possible relation between the pineal and the hypothalamic nuclei mentioned has been studied under the following experimental conditions: (1) pCPA administration, (2) castration, (3) pinealectomy, and (4) pinealectomy followed by substitution using rat and sheep pineal extract.

pCPA administration causes a decrease in number of serotonin containing cells and an increase in that of autofluorescent cells, both in the pineal and in the hypothalamic nuclei. Castration is, however, followed by an increase in number of autofluorescent pinealocytes, but a decrease of autofluorescent neurones in the nuclei, the number of serotonin containing cells increasing in the pineal, but decreasing in the nuclei. After pinealectomy an increase in number of autofluorescent and a decrease of serotonin containing neurones occur in the hypothalamic nuclei, while the normal contents are restored by substitution using either rat or sheep pineal extract.

The investigation brings histological evidence of an influence, exerted by the pineal on nuclei forming part of the hypothalamic hypophysiotropic area. On the ground of the presented and literature data the hypothesis is put forward that serotonin inhibits the production of hypothalamic gonadotropic regulating factors.

Hypothalamic Monoaminergic Neurosecretion and the Regulation of Pars Intermedia Activity in *Xenopus Laevis* Tadpoles

M. TERLOU and P. G. W. J. VAN OORDT

Zoological Laboratory, Utrecht (The Netherlands)

Monoaminergic centres in the caudal hypothalamus are involved in the regulation of pars intermedia activity in *Xenopus laevis* tadpoles. This is based upon the following data:

1. With the Falck-Hillarp method in the caudal hypothalamus two paired fluorescent nuclei were demonstrated. From these nuclei a tract originates, running towards the median eminence and the pars intermedia. In the latter the aminergic fibres intermingle between the glandular cells.

2. The histochemical localization of the enzyme monoamine oxidase, which catalyzes the breakdown of monoamines, confirms the localization of fluorescence-histochemically demonstrated monoamines.

3. The development of monoaminergic neurons in the hypothalamus coincides with the acquisition of the ability of the tadpole to regulate MSH secretion by the pars intermedia cells.

To identify the monoamine involved, spectrofluorometrical studies were carried out. The excitation and emission spectra of models, consisting of formaldehyde-induced fluorophores of known monoamines were compared with those of fluorophores in the above-mentioned nuclei. It appeared that the nuclei contain catecholamines. Experiments to differentiate between dopamine and noradrenalin are in progress.

Terlou, M., Ploemacher, R. E.: Z. Zellforsch. **137**, 521—540 (1973).
Terlou, M., Stroband, H. W. J.: Z. Zellforsch. **140**, 261—275 (1973).
Terlou, M., van Straaten, H. W. M.: Z. Zellforsch. In press (1973).

Ultrastructural Studies on the Caudal Neurosecretory System, Spinal CSF Contacting Neurons and Filum Terminale

B. VIGH

2nd Department of Anatomy, Semmelweis University Medical School, Budapest (Hungary)

In previous studies we demonstrated cerebrospinal fluid (CSF)-contacting neurons around the central canal of the medulla oblongata and spinal cord of different vertebrates. Each neuron sends a dendritic process into the CSF to form an ending provided with numerous stereocilia and one kinocilium. As the ultrastructure of the spinal CSF-contacting terminals resembles that of known mechanoreceptors we suppose the CSF-contacting neurons to be receptor cells. Furthermore, we found CSF-contacting neurons in the region of the urophysis caudalis of fishes.

In our present work, we describe mainly bipolar CSF-contacting nerve cells in the filum terminale of *Cyprinus carpio*. Their cytoplasm contains granulated vesicles besides of elements regularly present in nerve cells. Numerous axons containing granulated and synaptic vesicles build up synapses on these CSF-contacting neurons. The CSF-contacting nerve cells are dissimilar to Dahlgren cells present in the upper part of the filum. Furthermore, we found axon terminals forming neurohormonal synaptic semidesmosomes on the basal lamina of the outer surface of the filum terminale. In addition to synaptic vesicles these terminals contain the same type of granulated vesicles that is present in the CSF-contacting neurons. This finding suggests that the axon endings may belong to the CSF-contacting neurons. As in our opinion synaptic semidesmosomes are the most characteristic structure of neurosecretory or "hormonsecretory" neurons we regard the CSF-contacting nerve cells and the neurohormonal axon terminals of the filum terminale to represent a second spinal neurosecretory system in addition to the urophysis caudalis.

Vigh,B., Vigh-Teichmann,I.: Acta biol. Acad. Sci. hung. **22**, 227—243 (1971).
Vigh,B., Vigh-Teichmann,I.: Int. Rev. Cytol. **35**, 189—251 (1973).
Vigh,B., Vigh-Teichmann,I., Aros,B.: Z. Zellforsch. **122**, 301—309 (1971).

Fiber Connections of Hypothalamic CSF Contacting Neurosecretory Cells

I. VIGH-TEICHMANN

2nd Department of Anatomy, Semmelweis University Medical School, Budapest (Hungary)

In previous studies we demonstrated in a wide range of species cerebrospinal fluid (CSF)-contacting neurons in the magnocellular preoptic and paraventricular neurosecretory nuclei as well as in the parvocellular infundibular nucleus. All these CSF-contacting neurosecretory cells are summarized by us under the term of "CSF-contacting neurosecretory system". These neurons form special dendritic terminals in the CSF. We suppose them to be receptory in function.

At present, we do not know whether all neurosecretory cells are CSF-contacting neurons or only a part of them. It is also unknown where the axons of the CSF-contacting neurons terminate. Therefore, in our present work we have studied the preoptic nucleus of fishes (*Anguilla vulgaris, Cyprinus carpio*) and the paraventricular nucleus of reptiles (*Emys orbicularis, Lacerta agilis, Lacerta viridis*) by light and electron microscopy. Most of the neurosecretory cells of the *preoptic nucleus* form CSF-contacting dendrite terminals. The axons of these CSF-contacting neurons enter the hypothalamo-neurohypophysial tract. In the *paraventricular nucleus* the pattern is more complicated as the nucleus consists of a hypendymal and a distal part. The hypendymal neurosecretory cells are all CSF-contacting neurons. In the distal part of the nucleus we could not demonstrate any CSF-contacting dendrites convincingly. The distal neurosecretory cells may bear cilia of type $9 \times 2 + 0$. We observed three kinds of axo-dendritic and axo-somatic synapses containing either large peptidergic (diameter about 1500 Å), or small (diameter about 600 Å), or medium-sized (diameter about 1000 Å) granulated vesicles presynaptically. These findings suggest synaptic connections between the CSF-contacting and the other neurosecretory neurons as well as afferents coming from outside the paraventricular nucleus. We propose that independently from their cholinergic, aminergic or peptidergic nature only those neurons should be called "neurosecretory" or "hormonsecretory" whose axons terminate as synaptic semidesmosomes on the basal lamina of blood-vessels or brain surface.

Vigh, B., Vigh-Teichmann, I.: Int. Rev. Cytol. **35**, 189—251 (1973).
Vigh-Teichmann, I., Vigh, B.: In: Ependyma and neurohormonal regulalion. Symposium in Smolenice, Sept. 20—22, 1972. Endocrinologica exp. (Prague) 1973.
Vigh-Teichmann, I., Vigh, B., Aros, B.: Z. Zellforsch. **144**, 139—152 (1973).

Subcellular Distribution of Hormones and Enzymes in the Neural Lobe of the Bovine Pituitary Gland

H. VILHARDT, R. V. BAKER, and D. B. HOPE
Department of Pharmacology, South Parks Road, Oxford OX1 3QT (Great Britain)

In the present investigation the distribution of subcellular components in fractions of homogenates of the neural lobe of bovine pituitary glands has been studied by means of ultracentrifugation. The findings are discussed in relation to previous studies in this field. Special interest is focussed on the distribution and behaviour of ATP hydrolysing activity. The ATPase activity is grouped into three categories:
1) a $Mg^{++} + Na^+ + K^+$-ATPase, 2) a Mg^{++}-ATPase, and 3) a Ca^{++}-ATPase, which are all membrane bound. Triton X-100 solubilized the Mg^{++}- and the Ca^{++}-ATPase activity. Polyacrylamide gel electrophoresis of such preparations followed by incubation of the gels with ATP and lead ions confirmed the presence of two enzymes: one of which was activated solely by Ca^{++} and another activated by either Mg^{++} or Ca^{++}.
  Ultracentrifugation of subcellular fractions on continuous and discontinuous sucrose density gradients for various lengths of time showed that the distribution of ATPases was different from that of vasopressin. These findings indicate that the ATPase activity found in preparations of neurosecretory granules is a consequence of a contamination of the preparations with other subcellular elements and that the granules themselves are free from ATP hydrolysing activity.

Influence of the Pineal Complex on the Hypothalamo-Hypophysial System of *Rana Esculenta* under Light/Darkness Conditions

H. VULLINGS
Zoologisch Lab., Utrecht (The Netherlands)

In *Rana esculenta* the activity of the hypothalamo-hypophysial system has been investigated in intact and blinded animals, after removal of the frontal organ and after elimination of the whole pineal complex.

In agreement with the findings in *Rana temporaria*, a difference in secretory activity of the preoptic nucleus can be found between light- and darkness-treated intact animals. After blinding this difference disappears. Even a reversal in rate of incorporation of ^{35}S-cysteine takes place. A difference between the two other groups (without frontal organ and without pineal complex) can hardly be demonstrated. Compared with the intact animals the latter two groups show a marked increase in incorporation of ^{35}S-cysteine in the preoptic nucleus. It appears that an absence of the frontal organ has the same effect on the preoptic nucleus as the elimination of the whole pineal complex.

The enhanced synthesis of labelled material in the preoptic nucleus results in an increased transport along the hypothalamo-hypophysial tract, mainly to the outer zone of the median eminence and not to the posterior lobe.

Rapid Transport of Horseradish Peroxidase (HRP) from CSF to Pars Distalis in Rats

H.-J. WAGNER and CH. PILGRIM

Fachbereich Biologie, Universität Regensburg (Federal Republic of Germany)

Median eminence and pituitary of rats were examined 10, 30, 70 min, 12 and 24 h after injection of HRP into the lateral ventricle.

As early as 10 min after injection, the tracer has penetrated the extracellular space of the median eminence. At the same time, the pars distalis is intensely stained whereas the pars nervosa is free of reaction product.

This finding suggested a rapid transport of the tracer, the mechanism of which was examined in the electron microscope. Endothelial cells of median eminence blood vessels show rows of HRP filled pinocytotic vesicles budding from the basement membrane. Furthermore, numerous free vesicles and vesicles fusing with the luminal plasmalemma are observed. This is interpreted as a transport mechanism by which HRP may reach the blood stream of the portal vessels. The tracer is then seen to be diffusely distributed in the perivascular spaces of the pars distalis. From here it is absorbed to the plasma membrane of the hypophysial cells and, occasionally, taken up by pinocytosis.

Ependymal tanycytes do not seem to participate in this rapid transport although there is an uptake into lipofuscin-like structures after longer time intervals. Diffuse uptake into single tanycytes is considered to be due to cell damage.

Neurosecretery Innervation of the Reptilian Pars Intermedia: A Comparative Study

BRIAN WEATHERHEAD

Department of Anatomy, The Medical School, Birmingham (Great Britain)

In nearly all of the non-reptilian vertebrates studied to date there is evidence for the innervation of the pars intermedia by peptidergic and/or aminergic nerve fibres. However, in those reptiles in which the pars intermedia has been examined with the electron microscope i.e. the lacertilians *Klauberina* (Rodriguez and La Pointe, 1970), *Calotes* (Nayar and Pandalai, 1963) and the rhynchocephalian *Sphenodon* (Weatherhead, 1971), there seems to be no such neurosecretory innervation.

During a survey of the comparative cytology of the reptilian neuro-intermediate lobe the above findings have been confirmed in more species of lizards (*Anolis, Chamaeleo, Draco, Lacerta, Tarentola* and *Calotes*) and in some chelonians (*Clemmys, Emys* and *Pseudemys*).

However, it has proved possible to demonstrate the presence of neurosecretory fibres in the pars intermedia of some snakes viz. *Thamnophis* and *Eryx*, and in the single crocodilian representative examined, *Caiman*. The nerve fibres found in these species contain electron dense granules of c. 130—180 nm and are of the type presumed to be peptidergic and variously described as Type A or Type III. It was not possible to locate the source of the stainable neurosecretory material described by Bargmann, Knoop and Thiel (1957) in the pars intermedia of the snake *Natrix*.

This survey therefore reveals a hitherto unsuspected variability in the anatomical basis of the neuroendocrine relationships that exist between the hypothalamus and the pars intermedia in the major reptilian groups.

Bargmann,W., Knoop,A., Thiel,A.: Z. Zellforsch. **52**, 256—277 (1957).
Nayar,S., Pandalai,K.R.: Z. Zellforsch. **58**, 837—845 (1963).
Rodriguez,E.M., La Pointe,J.: Z. Zellforsch. **104**, 1—13 (1970).
Weatherhead,B.: Z. Zellforsch. **119**, 21—42 (1971).

Neuroendocrine Activity in the Organum Vasculosum of the Lamina Terminalis

ADOLF WEINDL and INGEBORG SCHINKO

Neurologische Klinik und Poliklinik der Universität München (Federal Republic of Germany)

The organum vasculosum of the lamina terminalis (OV) which is located between the optic chiasma and the anterior commissure belongs to the circumventricular organs of the vertebrate brain. Its specific function is still unknown. Like the median eminence and neurohypophysis, the richly vascularized OV differs from typical brain tissue structurally by a specialized angioarchitecture as well as by the ultrastructure of its vascular, neural, glial, and ependymal components (Weindl, 1973), functionally by the lack of a blood-brain barrier (Weindl, 1969). The OV of the golden hamster was studied by means of microvascular injections of microfil, as well as by light, transmission and scanning electron microscopy. The blood vessels form a well developed external and a less prominent internal plexus. The organ contains a large quantity of neurosecretory elements which like those of the median eminence are loaded with dense core vesicles with a mean diameter of $\sim$ 1000—1100 Å. At the light microscopic level staining with chrome-alum-hematoxylin is not seen. The axon terminals end at the peripheral basal lamina of the connective tissue space which surrounds the fenestrated capillary endothelium. In addition, a considerable quantity of neurosecretory axons is found above the specialized pleomorphic non-ciliated ependyma which covers the ventricular surface. Their content may be discharged into the ventricular fluid. By scanning electron microscopy, these neurosecretory processes can be identified as a part of a supraependymally located network of cells with branching processes.

Weindl,A.: In: Ganong,W.F., Martini,L. (Eds.): Frontiers in Neuroendocrinology. New York: Oxford University Press 1973.
Weindl,A.: Neurology (Minneap.) **19**, 295 (1969).

Functional Plasticity of the Neuro-Vascular Surface Area of the External Layer of the Median Eminence

W. WITTKOWSKI

Anatomisches Institut der Rheinischen Friedrich-Wilhelms Universität, Bonn (Federal Republic of Germany)

The vascular surface of the external layer of the median eminence is formed by nerve fibre endings and the endfeet of ependymal or glial cells. Penetration of nerve fibres into the peri-vascular space of the capillaries of the primary plexus as well as the occurrence of degenerating nervous material phagocytosed by connective tissue cells suggest that the storage and the release of hypothalamic hormones is associated with dynamic changes in the spatial distribution of neuronal and glial elements of the median eminence.

It is shown that the relative extent to which nerve fibres are bordering the perivascular space varies depending on functional conditions. In normal rats about 20% of the surface area is abutted on by neuro-vascular contacts. Bilateral adrenalectomy leads to an enlargement of the neuro-vascular contact area to 40% mean value, whereas after application of a crude extract of beef stalk median eminence tissue there is a decrease to about 15% mean value. These results suggest that the extent of the neuro-vascular contact area of the external layer changes in relation to the secretory activity of the median eminence.

Güldner, F. H.: Verh. d. Anat. Ges. 67, 279—283 (1973).
Wittkowski, W.: Z. Zellforsch. 139, 101—148 (1973).

Correlation of Degenerative Processes in the Hypothalamus after Neurotoxic Drug Administration with Serum Prolactin and LH and with the Corresponding Hypothalamic Hormones

W. WUTTKE, H. G. BAUMGARTEN, M. FENSKE, and L. LACHENMAYER

Max-Planck-Institut für Biophysikalische Chemie, Göttingen, und Abt. für Neuroanatomie, Hamburg (Federal Republic of Germany)

There is good evidence for a selectively destructive action of 6-OH-Dopamine (6-OHDA) on noradrenergic terminals in the hypothalamus. The tuberoinfundibular dopaminergic neurons are not influenced by this drug. Following intraventricular injection of 200 µg 6-OHDA into male rats a significant rise in serum prolactin and a decrease in serum LH was observed within 24 h. Serum prolactin levels remained elevated for 15 days and were lower than control levels at 37 and 71 days after 6-OHDA treatment whereas serum LH had increased. Hypothalamic PIF, as measured by bioassay, was not detectable and LRF content was significantly reduced 10 days after drug treatment. These results suggest that the reduced hypothalamic nor-adrenergic tonus after 6-OHDA administration is causally linked to the hormonal changes. They furthermore suggest a regeneration of noradrenergic terminals within approximately a month after drug treatment. This would explain the long term depressant effect on pituitary prolactin and the enhancing effect on pituitary LH release.

Intraventricular injection of 60 µg of the serotonin (5-HT) analogue 5.6-Dihydroxytrypt-amine (5,6-DHT) reduced hypothalamic 5-HT within 1 h to approximately 35% of control levels. The 5-HT levels remained low for 10 days and then progressively rose to control values within 60 days. Tryptophane hydroxylase activity was also reduced to approximately 40% of control levels within 1 h after 5,6-DHT treatment. The enzymatic activity recovered within

4 days, but decreased again 6 days after treatment. Serum prolactin levels in these animals had a triphasic pattern with high levels 1/2, 12 h—4 days and 12—23 days whereas serum LH displayed just the opposite pattern. Determination of hypothalamic factors 10 days after 5,6-DHT treatment evidenced a substance with prolactin releasing activity and a reduced LRF content. On the basis of these bioassay data for hypothalamic factors however it cannot be concluded as to whether or not the substance is indeed the prolactin releasing factor. An attempt to correlate serum hormone levels with hypothalamic 5-HT or tryptophane hydroxylase does not lead to conclusive results because relatively little is known about the action of 5,6-DHT on serotoninergic neurons.

List of Participants

ABRAHAM, A., Institute of Zoology, University of Szeged, Tancsics u. 2, Szeged, Hungary.

ADIYODI, K. G., Department of Zoology, Calicut University, Kerala 673635, South India.

ARIENS KAPPERS, J., Netherlands Central Institute for Brain Research, Ijdik 28, Amsterdam Ø, Netherlands.

AROS, B.*, 2nd Department of Anatomy, Medical University, Budapest IX, Tuzolto-u 58, Hungary.

BAKER, R. V., Department of Pharmacology, South Parks Road, Oxford OX1 3QX, U.K.

BARA, D., Institutum Anatomiae Pathologicae, Kossuth Lajos Sugarat 40, Postafiok 401, Szeged, Hungary.

BARGMANN, W., Anatomisches Institut der Universität Kiel, D-2300 Kiel, Neue Universität, Eingang F1/F3, Germany.

BARRY, J., Faculté de Médecine, Laboratoire d'Histologie, Place de Verdun, 59 Lille, France.

BAUDRY, N., Laboratoire de Zoologie, 7 Quai St. Bernard, Paris 5, France.

BAUMGARTEN, H. G., Anatomisches Institut der Universität, D-2000 Hamburg 20, Martinistraße 52, Germany.

BEIER, S., Schering AG, D-1000 Berlin 65, Müllerstraße 170—172, Germany.

BJÖRKLUND, A., Department of Histology, University of Lund, Biskopsgatan 5, S-223 62 Lund, Sweden.

BLISS, D. E., Department of Living Invertebrates, The American Museum of Natural History, Central Park West at 79th Street, New York, New York 10024, USA.

BOCK, R., Anatomisches Institut, Rheinische Friedrich-Wilhelms Universität, D-5300 Bonn, Nußallee 10, Germany.

BOER, H. H., Department of Biology, Free University, Amsterdam, Netherlands.

BOUNHIOL, J. J., Faculté des Siences, Biologie Animale B., Université de Bordeaux 1, 351 Cours de la Libération, Talence (Gironde), France.

BRUCE, I., Department of Biology, The University of Calgary, Calgary, Canada.

BUDTZ, P. E., Zoophysiological Lab. A., Universitetsparken 13, Copenhagen Ø, Denmark.

BURLET, A., U.E.R. Sciences Médicales A., Laboratoire d'Histologie, 31 Rue Lionnois, Nancy, France.

BURLET, C., U.E.R. Sciences Médicales A., Laboratoire d'Histologie, 31 Rue Lionnois, Nancy, France.

CALAS, A., Laboratoire de Physiologie Animale, Université de Montpelier, Place Eugene Bataillon, France.

CHEVINS, P., Department of Biology, University of Keele, Keele, Staffs. ST5 5BG, U.K.

CHRIST, J., Max-Planck-Institut für Hirnforschung, Neurobiologie-Abteilung, D-6000 Frankfurt a. M., Niederrad, Deutschordenstraße 46, Germany.

CORDINGLEY, J. L., Department of Anatomy, King's College, Strand, London WC2R 2LS, U.K.

CROSS, B. A., Department of Anatomy, University of Bristol, Bristol BS8 1TD, U.K. Present address: ARC Institute of Animal Physiology, Babraham, Cambridge, U.K.

DA LAGE, C., Faculté de Médecine, Necker-Enfants Malades, Laboratoire d'Histologie, 156 Rue de Vaugirard, 75730 Paris, France.

DAVEY, K. G., Macdonald Campus of McGill University, Macdonald College, Quebec, Canada.

DAVIES, D. T., Department of Zoology, University College of North Wales, Bangor, Caernarvonshire, U.K.

DEERY, D., Department of Anatomy, King's College, Strand, London WC2R 2LS, U.K.

DELLMAN, H. D., Department of Veterinary Anatomy, 103 Conaway Hall, University of Missouri, Columbia 65201, USA.

---

* Did not attend the Symposium.

DE MEY, J., Department of Embryology and Histology, State University, Godshuizenlaan 4, Gent, Belgium.

DIERICKX, K., Department of Embryology and Histology, State University, Godshuizenlaan 4, Gent, Belgium.

DODD, J. M., Department of Zoology, University College of North Wales, Bangor, Caernarvonshire, U.K.

DORN, A., Institut für Allgemeine Zoologie der Universität Mainz, D-6500 Mainz, Saarstraße 21, Germany.

DOUGLAS, W. W., Department of Pharmacology, Sterling Hall of Medicine, Yale University School of Medicine, 333 Cedar Street, New Haven, Connecticut 06510, USA.

DREIFUSS, J. J., Département de Physiologie de l'Université, École de Médecine, 1211 Genève 4, Switzerland.

DYBALL, R. E. J., Department of Anatomy, The Medical School, University Walk, Bristol BS8 1TD, U.K.

DYER, R. G., Department of Anatomy, The Medical School, University Walk, Bristol BS8 1TD, U.K.

FALCK, B., Institute of Anatomy and Histology, Department of Histology, Biskopsgatan 5, Lund, Sweden.

FASOLO, A., Universita di Torino, Instituti di Anatomia, Via Giolitti 34, Torino, Italy.

FIELD, P., Department of Human Anatomy, University of Oxford, South Parks Road, Oxford OX1 3QX, U.K.

FIRTH, J. A., Department of Anatomy, King's College, Strand, London WC2R 2LS, U.K.

FLAMENT-DURAND, J., Department of Neuropathology, Université Libre de Bruxelles, Brussels, Belgium.

FLEISCHHAUER, K., Anatomisches Institut der Rheinischen Friedrich-Wilhelms Universität, D-5300 Bonn, Nußallee 10, Germany.

FOLLENIUS, E., Laboratoire de Cytologie Animale, Institut de Zoologie, 12 Rue de l'Université, 67 Strasbourg, France.

FOWLER, D. J., WMU Kalamazoo, Michigan, USA.

FRANZONI, M. F., Universita di Torino, Istituto di Anatomia, Via Giolitti 34, Torino, Italy.

FUXE, K., Department of Histology, Karolinska Institutet, Stockholm 60, Sweden.

GELDIAY, S., Ege Universitesi, Fen Fakultesi, Genel Zooloji Kursusu, Bornova-Izmire, Turkey.

GOOS, H. J. T., Zoologisch Lab., Janskerkhof 3, Utrecht, Netherlands.

GOOSSENS, N., Department of Embryology and Histology, State University, Godshuizenlaan 4, B-9000 Gent, Belgium.

GRAINGER, F., Department of Experimental Pathology, Charing Cross Hospital Medical School, London, W.6., U.K.

GÜLDNER, F. H., Max-Planck-Institut, D-3400 Göttingen-Nikolausberg, Am Faßberg, Germany.

HAASE, E., Institut für Haustierkunde, D-2300 Kiel, Neue Universität, Olshausenstraße 40—60, Germany.

HARRIS, M., Department of Physiology, Medical School, University of Birmingham, Edgbaston B15 2TJ, U.K.

HARTWIG, H. G., Anatomisches Institut der Justus-Liebig-Universität, D-6300 Gießen, Friedrichstraße 24, Germany.

HELLER, H., Department of Anatomy, The Medical School, University Walk, Bristol BS8 1TD, U.K.

HOPE, D. B., University Department of Pharmacology, South Parks Road, Oxford OX1 3QT, U.K.

HOWE, A., Department of Physiology, Chelsea College, Manresa Road, London, S.W.3, U.K.

HYYPPÄ, M. T., Department of Neurology, University of Turku, SF-20520 Turku 52, Finland.

JITARIU, P. J., Biological Centre Rechesch, Jasi, Romania.

JONES, C. W., Department of Anatomy, The Medical School, University Walk, Bristol BS8 1TD, U.K.

JONES, M. T., Sherrington School of Physiology, St. Thomas's Hospital Medical School, London, S.E. 1.

JUBERTHIE, C., Laboratoire Souterrain, Centre National de la Recherche Scientifique, 09410 Moulis, France.

KANTARJIAN, A., Department of Anatomy, King's College, Strand, London WC2R 2LS, U.K.

KAUL, S., Department of Anatomy, King's College, Strand, London WC2R 2LS, U.K.

KELLER, R., Freie Universität Berlin, D-1000 Berlin 41, Grunewaldstraße 34, Germany.

KLEFBOHM, B., Department of Zoology, University of Lund, S-223 62 Lund, Sweden.

KLEINHOLZ, L., Biology Department, Reed College, Portland, Oregon 97202, USA.

KNOWLES, F.G.W., Department of Anatomy, King's College, Strand, London WC2R 2LS, U.K.

KRATZSCH, E., Klinikum Steglitz, D-1000 Berlin 45, Hindenburgdamm 30, Germany.

KREIKENBAUM, K., Univ. Frauenklinik, Abt. Endokrinologie, D-3400 Göttingen, Humboldtallee 3, Germany.

KRSULOVIC, J.*, University of Chile, Laboratory of Electron Microscopy, Casilla 130 V, Valparaiso, Chile.

LARSSON, L., Department of Zoology, University of Lund, S-223 63 Lund, Sweden.

LEDERIS, K., Division of Pharmacology and Therapeutics, The University of Calgary, Calgary 44, Alberta, Canada.

LEONARD, B. E., Pharmacology Department, Organon International B.V., Oss, Netherlands.

LICHTENSTEIGER, W., Pharmakologisches Institut der Universität Zürich, CH-8006 Zürich, Gloriastraße 32, Switzerland.

LINCOLN, D.W., Department of Anatomy, The Medical School, University Walk, Bristol BS8 1TD, U.K.

LÖFSTRÖM, A., Department of Histology, Karolinska Institutet, Stockholm, Sweden.

MARTINET, J., Laboratoire de Physiologie de la Lactation, CNR2 78 Jouy-en-Josas, France.

MARTINI, L., Department of Endocrinology, University of Milan, Milan, Italy.

MARSDEN, J., Department of Biology, McGill University, P.O. Box 6070 Montreal 101, Quebec, Canada.

MASON, C. A., Department of Zoology, University of California, Berkeley, California 94720, USA.

MCKENNA, O., Department of Physiology, New York University Medical Center, 550 First Avenue, New York, N.Y. 10016, USA.

MCKEOWN, B. A., Department of Zoology, University of Guelph, Guelph, Ontario, Canada.

MEURLING, P., Zoological Institute, University of Lund, S-223 63 Lund, Sweden.

MEYER, M., Eidg. Technische Hochschule, Zürich-Honggerberg Institut für Molekularbiologie und Biophysik, CH-8049 Zürich, Switzerland.

MÖLLER, M., Copenhagen University, Medicinsk Anatomisk Inst., Universitetsparken 1, 2100 Copenhagen Ø, Denmark.

MÖLLGAARD, K., Copenhagen University, Medicinsk Anatomisk Inst., Universitetsparken 1, 2100 Copenhagen Ø, Denmark.

MORRIS, J.F., Department of Anatomy, The Medical School, University Walk, Bristol BSQ ITD, U.K.

MÜLLER, E. E., Universita degli Studi, Facolta di Medicina, 20129 Milano, Via Vancitelli 32, Italy.

MURRAY, J.R., Faculty of Pharmacy, University of Manitoba, Winnipeg, Canada.

NAGABHUSHANAM, R.*, Department of Zoology, University Campus, Marathwada University, Aurangabad, Marathtra, India.

NAIK, D.V., Département d'Anatomie, Faculté de Médecine, Université de Sherbrooke, Sherbrooke, Quebec, Canada.

NOBIN, A., Department of Histology, University of Lund, Biskopsgatan 5, S-223 62 Lund, Sweden.

NORDMANN, J., Département de Physiologie de l'Université, CH-1211 Genève 4, Switzerland.

NORSTRÖM, A., Institute of Neurobiology, Medicinaregatan 5, 400 33 Gotenborg, Sweden.

NOTENBOOM, C.D., Zoologisch Lab., Janskerkhof 3, Utrecht, Netherlands.

ÖZTAN, N., Department of Zoology, University of Istanbul, Vezneviler, Turkey.

OKSCHE, A., Anatomisches Institut der Justus-Liebig-Universität, D-6300 Gießen, Friedrichstraße 24, Germany.

OLIVEREAU, M., Institut Océanographique, 195 Rue Saint-Jacques Ve, Paris, France.

PATERSON, A., Department of Anatomy, King's College, Strand, London WC2R 2LS, U.K.

PERKS, A. M., Department of Zoology, University of British Columbia, Vancouver 8, Canada.

PETER, R.E., Department of Zoology, University of Alberta, Edmonton 7, Canada.

PEUTE,J., Afd. E.M. Subf. Biologie, Lange Nieuwstraat 106, Utrecht, Netherlands.

PICARD,D., Faculté de Médecine, 13385 Marseille Cedex 4, Boulevard Jean Moulin, Marseille, France.

PICKERING,B.T., Department of Anatomy, The Medical School, University Walk, Bristol BS8 1TD U.K.

PILGRIM,C., Fachbereich Biologie, Universität Regensburg, D-8400 Regensburg, Universitäts-straße 31, Germany.

PICKFORD,M., King Sterndale, Near Buxton, Derbyshire, U.K.

PLIŠKA,V., Eidg. Technische Hochschule, Zürich-Honggerberg, Institut für Molekularbiologie und Biophysik, CH-8049 Zürich, Switzerland.

PRASADA RAO,P.D., c/o Prof. A. Oksche, Anatomisches Institut, D-6300 Gießen, Friedrich-straße 24, Germany.

PROVANSAL,A., Laboratoire de Zoologie, Université Paris VI, 7 Quai Saint Bernard, Paris 5, France.

RAABE,M., Equipe de Neuroendocrinologie, C.N.R.S. No. 24, Laboratoire de Physiologie des Insectes, 9 Quai Saint-Bernard, Paris 5e, France.

RAISMAN,G., Department of Human Anatomy, University of Oxford, South Parks Road, Oxford OX1 3QX, U.K.

RICHARDS,S.G., F. Hoffmann-La Roche & Co., CH-4002 Basle, Switzerland.

RODRIGUEZ,E., Instituto de Histologia y Embryologia, U.N.C., Casilla de Correo 56, Mendoza, Argentina.

ROUBOS,E.W., Department of Biology, Free University, Amsterdam, Netherlands.

ROSENBERG,L.L., Department of Physiology and Anatomy, University of California, Berkeley, California 94720, USA.

RUF,K.B., Department of Neurosciences, McMaster University, Hamilton 16, Ontario, Canada.

RUSSELL,J.T., Institute of Medical Physiology C., University of Copenhagen, 71 Radmands-gade, 2200 Copenhagen N., Denmark.

SCHINKO,I., Institut für Histologie, Universität München, D-8000 München, Pettenkofer-straße 11, Germany.

SCHARRER,B., Department of Anatomy, Albert Einstein College of Medicine, 1300 Morris Park Avenue, Bronx, N.Y. 10461, USA.

SCHOONEVELD,H., Laboratory of Entomology, Agricultural University, Binnehaven 7, Wageningen, Netherlands.

SCOTT,D.E., Department of Anatomy, University of Rochester, School of Medicine and Dentistry, 260 Crittenden Boulevard, Rochester, New York 14620, USA.

SHARP,P.J., Poultry Research Centre, King's Building, West Mains Road, Edinburgh EH9 3JS, U.K.

SLOPER,J.C., Department of Experimental Pathology, Charing Cross Hospital Medical School, London, W.6., U.K.

SMITH,A.J., The Netherlands Central Institute for Brain Research, Ijdik 28, Amsterdam Ø, Netherlands.

STENEVI,U., Department of Histology, Biskopsgatan 5, S-223 62 Lund, Sweden.

STERBA,G., Sektion Biowissenschaften der KMU, Talstraße 33, Leipzig 701, DDR.

STOECKEL,M.E., Laboratoire de Physiologie Générale, Institut de Physiologie et de Chimie Biologique, 67000 Strasbourg, Rue René Descartes, France.

STUTINSKY,F., Laboratoire de Physiologie Générale, Institut de Physiologie et de Chimie Biologique, 67000 Strasbourg, Rue René Descartes, France.

SWANN,R.W., Department of Anatomy, The Medical School, University Walk, Bristol BS8 1TD, U.K.

TERLOU,M., Zoological Lab., Janskerkhof 3, Utrecht, Netherlands.

THORN,N.A., Universitets Medicinks-Fysiologiske Institut C., Radmandsgade 71, 2200 Copen-hagen N. Denmark.

THORNLEY,A.L., Department of Zoology, Katholieke Universiteit, Nijmegen, Netherlands.

THORNTON,V., Department of Anatomy, King's College, Strand, London WC2R 2LS, U.K.

TIXIER-VIDAL,A., Collège de France, Laboratoire de Biologie Moléculare, 11 Place Marcelin-Berthelot, Paris Ve, France.

VAN HERP, F., Department of Zoology, Katholieke Universiteit, Nijmegen, Netherlands.

VAN OORDT, P. G. W. J., Zoologisch Lab., Janskerkhof 3, Utrecht, Netherlands.

VIGH, B., 2nd Department of Anatomy, Medical University, Budapest IX, Tuzolto-U 58, Hungary.

VIGH-TEICHMANN, I., 2nd Department of Anatomy, Medical University, Budapest IX, Tuzolto-U 58, Hungary.

VILHARDT, H., Department of Pharmacology, South Parks Road, Oxford OX1 3QT, U.K.

VINCENT, J. D., Laboratoire de Neurophysiologie, Faculté de Médicine, (Annexe 2), 24 Rue Paul Broca, 33 Bordeaux, France.

VOGEL, I., Inst. f. Histolog. d. Univ. München, D-8000 München, Pettenkoferstraße 11, Germany.

VOGT, M., Agricultural Research Council, Institute of Animal Physiology, Babraham, Cambridge, U.K.

VOLLRATH, L., Department of Anatomy, King's College, Strand, London WC2R 2LS, U.K. Present address: Anatomisches Institut der Universität, D-6500 Mainz, Saarstraße 19/21, Germany.

VULLINGS, H. G. B., Zoologisch Lab., Janskerkhof 3, Utrecht, Netherlands.

WAGNER, H. J., Fachbereich Biologie, Universität Regensburg, D-8400 Regensburg, Universitätstraße 31, Germany.

WAKERLEY, J. B., Department of Anatomy, The Medical School, University Walk, Bristol BS8 1TD, U.K.

WARBURG, M. R., Department of Biology, Technion—Israel Institute of Technology, Haifa, Israel.

WATKINS, W. B., Postgraduate School of Obstetrics and Gynaecology, University of Auckland, National Women's Hospital, Claude Road, Auckland 3, New Zealand.

WEATHERHEAD, B., Department of Anatomy, The Medical School, University of Birmingham, Birmingham 15.

WEINDL, A., Neurologische Klinik und Poliklinik der Universität München, D-8000 München 80, Mohlstraße 28, Germany.

WEITZMAN, M., Albert Einstein College of Medicine, 1300 Morris Park Avenue, Bronx, New York 10461, USA.

WITTKOWSKI, W., Anatomisches Institut der Rheinischen Friedrich-Wilhelms Universität, D-5300 Bonn, Nußallee 10, Germany.

WUTTKE, W., Max-Planck-Institut, D-3400 Göttingen-Nikolausberg, Am Faßberg, Germany.

Organiser:

KNOWLES, Professor Sir Francis, F.R.S., Department of Anatomy, King's College, Strand, London WC2R 2LS, U.K.

Subject Index

S.L. Palay, V. Chan-Palay

Cerebellar Cortex

Cytology and Organization
267 figures incl. 203 plates
X, 348 pages. 1974

ISBN 3-540-06228-9 Cloth DM 156,—;
ISBN 0-387-06228-9 Cloth US $60.10

This atlas with its splendid light and
electron micrographs illustrates the
modern approach to the morphology
of the cerebellar cortex, its cytology
and organization, particularly that of
the synapses. Wherever possible structure is related to function. Much of
the work is based on the author's own
research.

**Contemporary Research Methods
in Neuroanatomy**

Editors: W.J.H. Nauta, S.O.E. Ebbesson
Proceedings of an International
Conference, held at the Laboratory of
Perinatal Physiology, San Juan, Puerto
Rico, in January 1969, under the
auspices of the National Institute of
Neurological Diseases and Stroke and
the University of Puerto Rico
190 figures. VIII, 386 pages. 1970

ISBN 3-540-04785-9 Cloth DM 110,—
ISBN 0-387-04785-9 Cloth US $34.30

This is the only available comprehensive book on neuroanatomical methodology. Each chapter contains a historical
sketch, a detailed description of the
method, abilities and limitations of the
technique, sources of misinterpretation,
and a bibliography.

J.M. van Buren, R.C. Borke

**Variations and Connections of the
Human Thalamus**

Part 1: The Nuclei and Cerebral
Connections of the Human Thalamus.

Part 2: Variations of the Human
Diencephalon. In two parts, not sold
separately.
98 figures, 187 plates
XXI, 587 pages. 1972

ISBN 3-540-05543-6 Cloth DM 670,—
ISBN 0-387-05543-6 Cloth US $196.60

Distribution rights for Japan:
Igaku Shoin Ltd., Tokyo

The first part reevaluates the morphology and cerebral connections of the
human thalamus using a wide variety of
exclusively human material. Part 2
provides a three-plane variation atlas
of the brain with a special study of the
thalamus for the stereotaxic surgeon.

C. Pilgrim

**Morphologische und
funktionelle Untersuchungen
zur Neurosekretbildung**

Enzymhistochemische, autoradiographische und elektronenmikroskopische
Beobachtungen an Ratten unter osmotischer Belastung. 29 Abb. 79 Seiten.
1969 (Ergebnisse der Anatomie und
Entwicklungsgeschichte. Band 41,
Heft 4).

ISBN 3-540-04461-2 DM 34,—
ISBN 0-387-04461-2 US $10.60

Zusammenfassende Darstellung der
zellulären Vorgänge bei der Neurosekret-
entstehung mit besonderer Berücksichtigung des Lysosomenproblems.

Preisänderungen vorbehalten

Prices are subject to change
without notice

**Springer-Verlag
Berlin
Heidelberg
New York**

Acta Neuropathologica

Organ of the Research Group for Neuropathology, of the Research Group for Comparative Neuropathology, and of the Research Group for Neurooncology of the World Federation of Neurology. Editorial Board: W. Blackwood, L. von Bogaert, E. Frauchiger, P.F. Girard, W. Haymaker, I. Klatzo, W. Krücke, F. Lüthy, G. Peters, F. Seitelberger (Managing Editor), H. Shiraki, K. J. Zülch

1975, Vols. 31-33 (4 issues each): DM 564,—; US $230.20 plus postage and handling

Experimental Brain Research/ Experimentelle Hirnforschung/ Expérimentation Cérébrale

Editorial Board: O. Creutzfeldt, D.R. Curtis, P. Dell, J.C. Eccles, R. Jung, D.M. MacKay, D. Ploog, J. Szentagothai, V.P. Whittaker, V.J. Wilson

1975, Vols. 273-277 (5 issues each): DM 474,—; US $193.40 plus postage and handling

Histochemistry

Editorial Board: M. Chèvremont, P.B. Diezel, P. van Dujn, F. Duspiva, O. Eränkö, P. Gedigk, W. Gössner, W. Graumann, W.A. Jensen, Z. Lojda, F. Moog, H. Padykula, A.G.E. Pearse, W. Sandritter, T.H. Schiebler (Managing Editor), A.M. Seligman, G. Siebert, M. Wolman

1975, Vols. 43-46 (4 issues each): DM 656,—; US $267.70 plus postage and handling

Journal of Neural Transmission

Formerly "Journal of Neuro-Visceral Relations". Journal of the International Society for Neurovegetative Research. Founded Foundet in 1950 as "Acta Neurovegetativa" by Carmen Coronini and Alexander Sturm. Editorial Board: J.Ariëns Kappers, W. Birkmayer, A. Carlsson, O.-J. Grüsser, W.J.H. Nauta, R.J. Wurtman

Springer-Verlag Wien 1975, Vol. 36 (4 issues): DM 156,—; US $63.70 plus postage and handling

Prices are subject to change without notice

Springer-Verlag
Berlin Heidelberg New York